Piaget before Piaget

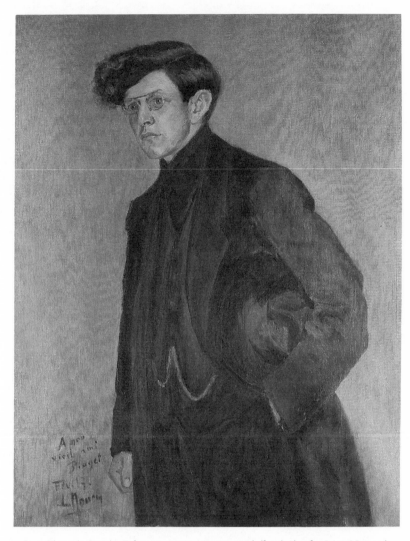

Jean Piaget in Leysin, February 1917, age twenty (oil painting by Léon Nancey)

PIAGET
BEFORE
PIAGET

Fernando Vidal

Harvard University Press
Cambridge, Massachusetts
London, England
1994

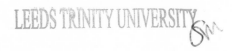
This book is printed on acid-free paper, and its binding materials
have been chosen for strength and durability.

Library of Congress Cataloging-in-Publication Data

Vidal, Fernando.
  Piaget before Piaget / Fernando Vidal.
    p. cm.
  Includes bibliographical references and index.
  ISBN 0–674–66716–6 (alk. paper)
  1. Piaget, Jean, 1896– —Childhood and youth. 2. Psychologists—
  Switzerland—Biography. I. Title.
BF109.P5V53 1994
155.4′13′092—dc20
[B]
93–43068
    CIP

To Brigitte

Acknowledgments

Several institutions and many individuals helped to smooth my path in researching and writing this book. A grant from the Fonds National Suisse de la Recherche Scientifique enabled me to begin my research with the freedom to do a lot of exploratory investigation. The University of Geneva supported related projects with the Jean-Louis Claparède Prize and the Théodore Flournoy Scholarship. A leave of absence from the University of New Hampshire in 1992–93, a grant from the Central University Research Fund, two Summer Faculty Fellowships, a Liberal Arts Faculty Research Support Grant, a Center for the Humanities Program and Projects Grant, and a Humanities Program Library Stipend allowed me to finish writing. A small grant from the Fondation Jean Piaget pour Recherches Psychologiques et Epistémologiques supported the final stages of the editorial process. The oversize manuscript became this book thanks to the skill and acumen of my editor, Ann Hawthorne. I also thank Clark University Press for permission to quote from Jean Piaget, "Autobiography," in Edwin G. Boring, Heinz Werner, Robert M. Yerkes, and Herbert S. Langfeld, eds., *A History of Psychology in Autobiography*, vol. 4 (Worcester, Mass., 1952); and Cambridge University Press for permission to use material included in Fernando Vidal, "Jean Piaget and the Liberal Protestant Tradition," in Mitchell G. Ash and William R. Woodward, eds., *Psychology in Twentieth-Century Thought and Society* (New York, 1987).

Professor Ruth Turner and other members of the Mollusk Department at Harvard's Museum of Comparative Zoology provided invaluable help on malacological taxonomy. I am also grateful to Professor Bärbel Inhelder for the opportunity to spend a summer at the Archives Jean Piaget in Geneva, and to Olivier Rod, the Archives' former librarian, for ensuring a supportive working environment. With their invitation to write a chapter for their *Psychology in*

Twentieth-Century Thought and Society, Mitchell Ash and William Woodward gave me a timely incentive to move ahead with my research.

Gaston Rod guided my very first steps in Neuchâtel. Dr. Paul Ducommun gave me liberal access to the papers of the Club of the Friends of Nature before they were deposited at the local Musée d'Art et d'Histoire. Maurice de Tribolet, the state archivist, patiently fulfilled all my requests and taught me much about Neuchâtel's social and mental universe. Also invariably helpful were Maryse Schmidt-Surdez, at the Bibliothèque Publique et Universitaire; Jean-Pierre Jelmini, at the Musée d'Art et d'Histoire; and Jean-Marc Barrelet, at the Archives Cantonales.

Among the many people who answered my questions over the years, I wish especially to mention the late Mme. Marthe Burger, Jean Piaget's sister, who kindly shared her memories; Mme. Jenny Humbert-Droz, widow of the socialist leader Jules Humbert-Droz, who did likewise; and the historian Marc Perrenoud, who directed me to archival material in La Chaux-de-Fonds.

Several mentors played roles larger and more varied than can be adequately described here: Antonio Battro, Howard Gruber, Daniel Hameline, Jerome Kagan, the late Jacques Roger, Jacques Vonèche, and Sheldon White. I am also thankful for the help and advice of Christiane Gilliéron, Mireille Cifali, Wolfgang Edelstein, and Françoise Perot.

A final word of gratitude is reserved to Jacqueline, Lucienne, and Laurent Piaget for their encouraging trust and for permission to use the portrait of their father as a young man; and to Hélène and Albert Leupin, whose generous hospitality helped greatly to make this book possible.

Contents

Preface xi

Introduction: Biography and Autobiography 1

1 Neuchâtel, an Orderly Little Town 10

2 Mollusk Taxonomy 23

3 Natural History 34

4 The Friends of Nature 44

5 Piaget Discovers Bergson 51

6 Natural History and Creative Evolution 57

7 At the Threshold of Biology 72

8 The Protestant Context 92

9 The Problem of Religion 113

10 From Catechism to Philosophy 123

11 *The Mission of the Idea* 132

12 The Making of a New Identity 162

13 *Recherche* 182

14 The Theory of Equilibrium: From Personal Crisis
   to Universal Salvation 195

Epilogue 219

Notes 235

Bibliography 243

Index 269

Preface

In a text titled "La vie est un conte" (Life Is a Tale), Paul Valéry wondered if anybody had ever wanted to write a biography trying to know, at each moment, as little about the next as the biography's subject did at the corresponding moment of his or her life—trying, in sum, to restore chance at every instant instead of constructing an inevitable teleological sequence. He rightly implied that the task is impossible. Because biographers know the end of the story, they can hardly avoid transforming lives into destinies, and destinies into lessons for those who read about them. The writing of history, however implicit its critical function, necessarily entails unceasing cognizance of the present and evaluation of the past. Thus, although in this book I avoid retrospective predictions and write independently of psychological controversy, I hope to contribute to the continuing debate over the Piagetian oeuvre and its legacies. The young Piaget was engaged in a moral crusade, and while his youthful worldview and life program should not be the sole basis for judging his later work, it is not legitimate to ignore them entirely.

In the following pages I aim at reconstructing Piaget's early development and the biographical and contextual roots of his psychological and philosophical system. I wish I could make him as intensely alive to the reader as he became to me. The young Piaget was zealously committed to his intellectual and moral choices, and passionately desirous of making a contribution to humanity. He took himself seriously; he was absorbed more with his own self than with anything or anyone else. In his thinking and style are traces of the pompousness that often accompanies immoderate ambition, self-confidence, and self-centeredness. The young Piaget fully embodied what he would later describe as the adolescent's egocentrism, which manifests itself in a messianic desire to reform the world.

The self-proclaimed reformer tends to find it necessary to control himself and others. Piaget was no exception. Rarely are we able to see him unguarded. But when we do, he is obliging, lively, and good-humored. In 1913 J. Duplain, a graphologist, detected the following traits: "Remarkably vivid, bright, and very active intelligence . . . Clear mind; quest for original views, with a more or less secret desire to stand out! Very gifted at repartee. Good intellectual equilibrium, combining intuition and logical sense . . . Pride, with consciousness of your own merits. Kindness, always very controlled by intelligence . . . Great distinction, sustained by an unusual reserve. Sure taste and loathing of vulgarity. Irony, mask of a marked sensibility. In sum: temperament of a very understanding intellectual, very critical, very loyal in the domain of ideas and feelings. Perhaps a bit of that noble candor that makes one take principles and ideas seriously."

Although these characteristics persisted into adulthood and are occasionally discernible in the surviving documentation, they are not the ones Piaget chose in constructing his adolescent persona.

A portrait made of Piaget in February 1917, at age twenty, shows a serious, even grave young man (see the frontispiece). The pince-nez does not lessen the intensity of his light blue eyes, but the fixed gaze is turned inward. The face is framed by a dark mass of romantically rebellious hair and austere, dark clothing; its compositional weight is only mildly balanced by the right fist, clenched as if to denote a certain inner tension, and the unobtrusive watch chain barely attenuates the picture's dominant verticality. Nothing reveals his social situation: the viewer is made to focus on the visage, and the character is made to concentrate upon his own thoughts. We are not drawn into the painting, nor are we able to communicate with a subject that makes no gesture toward us other than to let himself be portrayed in the act of introspection. But such was the young Piaget's characteristic stance.

In his autobiographical novel, *Recherche*, finished about the time the portrait was done, Piaget described his hero's life as "purely intellectual. His friendships, his emotions, and even the little love he allowed himself, everything revolved about his philosophy"; he lived "through his brain alone. His emotions, his sympathies, his religion, his morality, everything had crystallized into ideas, and this tremendous abstracter had never known life itself." Though undoubtedly sincere, this self-portrait was tailored to the message Piaget wished to communicate to his contemporaries; it is also consistent with the traces he left for posterity. Years of research reveal little of Jean Piaget's life outside his ideas. But this fact alone makes it clear that those ideas remained the very substance of his life.

Introduction: Biography and Autobiography

Jean Piaget (1896–1980) is unanimously recognized as one of the most influential figures in modern psychology and education, and certainly as the most important one in the field of child development. Whether celebrated or criticized, "the classroom's Freud" (*Hommage,* 63) seems indeed second only to the founder of psychoanalysis. By the time of his death, the grandfatherly silhouette of the "Einstein of psychology" (ibid., 109)—a humble sage, beret on the head and pipe in the mouth, immersed in the lonely creative disorder of his study or surrounded by admiring collaborators and world-renowned scientists, exploring nature, interviewing children, or pedaling along the streets of Geneva—had blended with the ever-appealing image of the precocious genius who published his first scientific paper at age eleven and chose, as an adolescent, the single intellectual project he would pursue for the rest of his long life.

Piaget's project was to elaborate a "biological" explanation of knowledge. Postulating that knowledge is a form of adaptation continuous with, and functionally equivalent to, organic adaptation, he wished to trace through the psychological development of children the basic notions and operations that make scientific knowledge possible.[1] It cannot be denied that elaborating such a "genetic" (that is, developmental) epistemology became his dominant project, nor that its pursuit led to major insights into the growth of the human intellect. Nevertheless, the historical record contradicts in fundamental ways the most widespread version of the origins of Piaget's vocation and oeuvre. This book seeks to correct the commonplace but inaccurate view of Piaget's early development.

The first misconception concerns Piaget's allegedly biological training.

Piaget claimed that he started his scientific career as a "biologist," and that he was formed by empirical issues about organic adaptation, evolution, and the relations between genotype and phenotype. I do not wish to deny the existence of vital links between his early scientific activity and his later thought, nor provide definitive answers to ever-debatable questions of continuity and discontinuity. Those links, however, must be redefined. The young Piaget worked on the classification of mollusks; the processes that make us call an organism a *living* organism were foreign to his early science, which is better characterized as natural history than as biology; his "biological" perspective originated less in scientific biology than in a metaphysics of life which he related in peculiar ways to questions of zoological classification.

The second biographical misconception about the origins of Piaget's thinking concerns his epistemological calling. In 1912 Piaget first encountered perhaps the most famous (for some, infamous) philosophical work of the early twentieth century, Henri Bergson's 1907 *Creative Evolution*. Bergson asserted that the theory of knowledge and the theory of life were inseparable. This idea indeed became the foundation of Piaget's thought. Yet, contrary to current belief, his discovery of Bergson did not immediately give rise to his vocation as an epistemologist. Only gradually did epistemology become his central concern, and probably did not establish itself as such until the 1920s. By 1914 Piaget had incorporated key notions of Bergson's metaphysics both into the practice and theory of classification, and into a conception of religion and faith. In the years 1914–1918 it was issues related to faith, and particularly to the renewal of Christianity and postwar society, that seemed most pressing to Piaget; and it was to those issues, about which he said nothing when recalling his youth, that his intense philosophical speculations were subordinated.

This book tells the story of the young Piaget—an individual who, by the age of twenty-two, had published scores of articles in malacological taxonomy, a prose poem identifying the mission of young people as bringing about the new birth of Christianity, and an autobiographical novel proposing a grand theory that resolved its hero's personal difficulties and set allegedly scientific foundations for reconstructing society. Our story stops in 1918, a year which serves as a threshold in Piaget's life: he finishes his doctoral dissertation on the classification of mollusks—and never again deals with the subject; he publishes his autobiographical and philosophical novel, *Recherche*—and henceforth leaves behind metaphysical speculation; he breaks away from the French-speaking Swiss milieu where he grew up—but rediscovers it after crucial sojourns in Zurich and Paris. Only then begins the career of Jean Piaget as we know it.[2]

Some Ideas about Contextual Biography

In the spirit of Max Weber's (1905, 115) remark that "methodology can only bring us reflective understanding of the means which have *demonstrated* their value in practice by raising them to the level of explicit consciousness," I offer here the considerations that shaped my approach in the following pages.

Like Thomas Hankins (1979, 2, 8), I support the notions of integrating science into the rest of the "human endeavor" and of bringing together "the different aspects of the subject's life as much as possible into a single coherent picture." But in the case of a figure such as the young Piaget, whose scientific work was not always his top priority, and whose "intellectual" concerns were often inseparable from "personal" issues related to self and identity, it is necessary also to provide "nonscientific" (and nonphilosophical) documentation. In this respect I find myself in agreement with Susan Sheets-Pyenson's (1990) idea that scientific biography should be allowed the same opportunities as literary biography, and with Thomas Söderqvist's (forthcoming) statements about the importance of an individual's "existential projects."

My approach to biography has also been inspired by Howard Gruber's (1974, 1980a, 1980b) study of Darwin and subsequent theorizing on "scientific creativity." Although Gruber's vocabulary of the "network of enterprise" is absent from this book, it underlies much of its form and contents. A "network of enterprise" is the collection of an individual's activities; each enterprise is composed of projects and tasks that evolve and interact; the image of the network thus provides a heuristic for depicting the individual both synchronically and diachronically. Moreover, it implies that the person is a "system" (which does not mean that he or she is always coherent and self-consistent), whose intellectual development or scientific oeuvre belongs in the context of an entire life. The detailed study of an evolving enterprise demands reconstructing what F. L. Holmes (1981, 1986) calls the "fine structure" of scientific creativity—the slow emergence of an idea, the complex path that leads to a discovery or an insight.

In Piaget's case, it can be shown that his well-known "epistemological enterprise" was preceded and then accompanied by a "moral enterprise." The goal of this enterprise was the establishment of a foundation for the reconstruction of the individual and society after World War I. Its evolution can be traced through Piaget's *The Mission of the Idea* (1915), his desire to "base morality on science" (thus formulated in 1917), and the theory of equilibrium set forth in *Recherche* (1918). Only in the 1920s does it become structured as a series of empirical and theoretical projects (for example, to study children's moral judgment and to respond to Durkheim's sociology). During that decade, the main feature of Piaget's network is the coordination of the moral and the epistemological enterprises—until the former is brought to a halt with *The Moral Judgment of the Child* (1932).

However one conceptualizes it, the individual's development always occurs in a context. Since, like Robert M. Young (1988) and L. Pearce Williams (1991), I believe that biography and social constructionism are not incompatible, the account presented here is expressly not the story of an isolated individual mind. Neither, in my view, is a context a collection of distant figures and "isms." By 1918 the young Piaget had actively participated in an amateur naturalists' club, in a Christian students' association, and in a young socialists' group. Each of these microcontexts provided norms and models that nourished his evolving identity, and from which he could demarcate himself. Thus I attempt to reconstruct Piaget's immediate environments and his place within them, examining not only dominant ideas but also codes of behavior, modes of expression, sensibilities, social practices and representations—that is, what the French call *mentalités*.

My attachment to context determines my attitude toward the place of psychology in biography. It is possible, even easy, to apply to Piaget's life story schemes borrowed from psychological theories. They all fit, but none captures the particulars of the case. For example, Piaget's discovery of the conflict between religion and science can be interpreted in terms of cognitive dissonance, the Oedipus complex, or Piagetian or Eriksonian stages. Yet it can also be shown that undergoing that conflict was a social norm for young Christian intellectuals, and that Piaget's personal experience is best understood in relation to this norm. In the terms of the Russian "semioticians" of cultural history (Nakhimovsky, 1985), the fact that Piaget experienced a religious crisis demonstrates that he had acquired the language of his culture; an ideal representation of the young Christian, communicated in print and speech, was thus transformed into actual behavior within a real life story. As illustrated by a recent study (Schepeler, 1993), the very limited amount of independent documentation concerning Piaget's personal life dooms psychobiographers, especially those of psychoanalytic orientation, to reach conclusions that are applicable to most creative individuals or that do not go beyond what Piaget himself said in his autobiographical narratives.

Psychological frameworks can certainly be of use to the biographer: Michael Sokal (1990) sensibly uses concepts from life-span developmental psychology, and I think of Piaget's story partly as a process of socialization. The tendency of psychobiography to disappear as a separate genre and become absorbed into biographical literature (Shore, 1980) seems to me utterly reasonable. But the attempt to validate a theory through its extended application to an individual case is antithetical to what I try to do. With the Genevan critic Jean Starobinski (1966, 81), I believe that for the historian, an affective experience exists only after it attains linguistic status. The inner life of an individual of the past can be apprehended only through culturally determined intermediates that give it a communicable form. Hence my systematic attention to Piaget's own "voice"—to his style, the details of his language, and his own self-directed attention.

All this looks, and is, eclectic; but a biography is the story of a person, and the more one wishes to focus the story on the person, the more difficult it is to impose a rigid methodology.

The Problem of Autobiography

Piaget's autobiographical writings have commanded unquestioned factual and interpretative authority in narratives of his development. They are, however, documents to be critically examined. More fundamentally than a documentary source, an autobiography is a self-interpretation, even an act of self-creation.[3] Autobiographers speak from the standpoint of their own present. Omissions and distortions in their stories do not necessarily result from intentional mystification, but from their desire to give a sense and a coherence to their lives and, often, to commend their experience to others. The existential meaning of an autobiography lies beyond the test of empirical accuracy; the narrative, however, must be put to the test and placed in the perspective of its author's purpose if we are to use it as a source of information.

Thus, an autobiography can be read in at least three different ways: literally, to obtain factual information; critically, to check this information and to expose distortions and omissions; and interpretatively, to discover its principles and account for its biases. Piaget's autobiographical statements have been read from the literal standpoint; we must now understand them otherwise.

Jean Piaget's best-known autobiographical text was written in 1950 and published in English in 1952. The French version was subsequently updated in 1966 and again in 1976. In 1959 he published "An Outline of Intellectual Autobiography," and the first chapter of his 1965 *Insights and Illusions of Philosophy* is an autobiographical narrative. In addition, his conversations of the early 1970s with Richard I. Evans and Jean-Claude Bringuier contain many remarks of biographical interest. Most biographical narratives about Piaget, however, are explicitly based on the 1950/1952 text.[4]

The 1952 autobiography appeared in the fourth volume of *A History of Psychology in Autobiography*. The basic purpose of this multivolume work begun in 1930 was educational. One of the contributors to the first volume alluded to the complexity of fulfilling the editors' invitation "to write one's own 'intellectual history,' accompanied as it is by the suggestion that this may be helpful to younger men with their lives still to make" (Spearman, 1930, 299). In 1952 the editors pointed out that although every autobiography can "go far toward instructing the reader as to how human motive moves to make science progress," nobody "can hope to deal adequately with the springs of his motivations" (Boring et al., 1952, vi).

Piaget was aware that writing with a pedagogical purpose would generate distortions. After noting that the 1952 autobiography "tried to bring out the motivations and phases of the contributions I might have made to our discipline," he added, "An autobiography is never objective, and it is naturally the role of the reader to rectify it in the sense of impersonal truth"; rather, its chief value lies in furnishing "some indications about what an author wished to do, and about the ways in which he understands himself" (1976a, 23–24). Clearly, then, Piaget recognized autobiography as a self-interpretation; he also knew that it could serve an apologetic function.Similarly, in the "Outline" of 1959 Piaget sought to justify his increasing use of abstract formal models (1959a, 8–9). And in the opening autobiographical chapter of *Insights,* he tells of the "disenchantment" that made him break with philosophers, and thus legitimizes an intellectual position on the basis of a personal life story.

Piaget's self-presentation is typical of the traditional scientific autobiography (Shortland, 1988). Conforming to the norms of the scientific style, it effaces the self, pursues objectivity rather than sincerity, and relates a career rather than a life. Such features are announced in what Philippe Lejeune (1971) calls the "autobiographical pact," a statement of intention whereby the author delimits the topic, clarifies his motives, sets conditions, and anticipates criticism. Piaget presents his 1952 autobiographical pact in three paragraphs:

> An autobiography has scientific interest only if it succeeds in furnishing the elements of an explanation of the author's work. In order to achieve that goal, I shall therefore limit myself essentially to the scientific aspect of my life.
>
> Many persons doubtless are convinced that such a retrospective interpretation presents no objective value, and that it is to be suspected of partiality even more than an introspective report. I myself had originally subscribed to this view. But, on re-reading some old documents dating from my years of adolescence, I was struck by two apparently contradictory facts which, when put together, offer some guaranty of objectivity. The first is that I had completely forgotten the contents of these rather crude, juvenile productions; the second is that, in spite of the immaturity they anticipated in a striking manner what I have been trying to do for about thirty years.

There is therefore probably some truth in the statement by Bergson that a philosophic mind is generally dominated by a single personal idea which he strives to express in many ways in the course of his life, without ever succeeding fully. Even if this autobiography should not convey to the readers a perfectly clear notion of what that single idea is, it will at least have helped the author to understand it better himself. (1952, 237)

Each paragraph has a different function. The first one demarcates the text's contents. "Scientific interest" points to the educational aims of the history of psychology in autobiography. At the same time, it intimates that some events will be omitted, and that others will be recounted only from the angle of their "scientific" significance. It therefore comes as no surprise that in this text Piaget minimizes the consequences of his discovery of Bergson's philosophy and omits any mention of his 1915 poem *The Mission of the Idea*, his aspiration to base morality on science, his youthful moral, social, and political concerns, or his 1920s writings on religious matters.

The second paragraph seeks to establish the autobiography's objectivity by recounting a personal psychological experience: Piaget rereads some long-forgotten youthful works and is struck by the extent to which they anticipate his later ideas. These early pieces thus help to define a lifelong project, and demonstrate its precocity and continuity. Pointing out, as Piaget does, that they are of little intrinsic value in fact reinforces their function as warrants of objectivity.

The theme of continuity reappears in the third paragraph, this time to emphasize the unidirectional character of Piaget's development. Later in the text Piaget claims to have been dominated by "one idea developed under various aspects," the idea "that intellectual operations proceed in terms of structures-of-the-whole. These structures denote the kinds of equilibrium toward which evolution in its entirety is striving; at once organic, psychological and social, their roots reach down as far as biological morphogenesis itself" (1952, 256). By reducing his youthful interests to "one idea," Piaget bestows coherence on his life story. It would be of course absurd to diminish the magnitude of his ambition to produce a psychological and biological epistemology. But it is also important to realize that such an ambition was initially inseparable from a larger set of purposes of which no traces are left in the autobiography.

All of Piaget's autobiographical statements are consistent with his theories, research, and projects as they stood in 1950, as well as with his own theory of developmental progress. At the time, Piaget was involved with projects that could genuinely have seemed remote from those that had most occupied his youth. In the 1940s he had concentrated on three areas: the empirical study of logico-mathematical operations (manifested in his work on the child's conception of geometry, representation of space, and notions of time, movement, and speed), the theoretical systematization of operational logic, and the major synthesis of 1950, *Introduction to Genetic Epistemology*.

In his autobiography, Piaget focused on those elements of his life that apparently anticipated the main features he attributed to his mature thinking: the scientific approach, the logical and biological perspective, and the epistemological target. In so delimiting his account, Piaget treated himself as a subject of his own psychological theory. His intellectual development from 1912 to 1918 appears as a progress toward objectivity, experimental and empirical reasoning, and in general toward scientific knowledge, away from the egocentrism typical of the speculations and dreams of adolescence.

Most presentations of and commentaries on Piaget's work open with a biographical sketch based chiefly on the 1952 autobiography. Such sketches tend to intensify the originals' biases. For example, Piaget writes: "Having seen a partly albino sparrow in a public park, I sent a one-page article to a natural history journal of Neuchâtel. It published my lines, and I was 'launched'!" (1952, 238). The "article" was a short note of about one hundred words, published in 1907 in the modest, handcrafted magazine of a local Neuchâtel amateur naturalists' club. Although Piaget does not provide this context, the quotation marks around "launched" give the story a touch of irony that nobody seems to have taken into account. By universal consensus, the article on the albino sparrow was Piaget's first scientific publication, and an obvious foreshadowing of his genius. Also in his autobiography, Piaget recalls that discovering Bergson made him feel an "intellectual shock" that inspired him to look for a "biological explanation of knowledge," as well as an "emotional shock" and "an evening of profound revelation" during which he identified God with life (1952, 240). This account is often abbreviated, with the shock and revelation omitted entirely, and the young Piaget portrayed as having been immediately devoted to epistemology.

By including the legendary "Albino Sparrow" and other youthful works in their annotated anthology *The Essential Piaget* (1977), Howard Gruber and Jacques Vonèche have done much to promote an increasing awareness of Piaget's own development (see especially Chapman, 1988; Kesselring, 1988; Balestra, 1980, is among the first to recognize Bergson's role). But a biographer who relies on Piaget's autobiography or on a partial (in both senses) compilation of documents cannot hope to present an authentic account of that development (see in particular Ducret 1984; Vander Goot 1985; Elkind 1986a, 1986b; and the extensive review of these publications in Vidal 1988).

As for my own contribution, I certainly do not believe that any biography can be definitive: each biographer's background, motives, emphasis, techniques, and sources are bound to differ and lead to different results. But I do hope that the following chapters will counteract Piaget's autobiographical suppressions in ways that enlarge our understanding both of the youth he was and of the person he became.

1

Neuchâtel, an Orderly Little Town

Jean Piaget is usually identified with Geneva, and rightly so in terms of his adult life. He arrived there in 1921 to work at the Rousseau Institute, and except for the years 1925–1929, when he taught at the University of Neuchâtel (but maintained links with the Institute), his whole career and international renown are based on work carried out in Genevan institutions. But the young Piaget was not in any sense Genevan. He was born and brought up in Neuchâtel, and although the two cities are only about sixty miles apart, they are different worlds, and were even more so at the turn of the century. Piaget evolved in specific Neuchâtel subcultures. Even the larger Christian and socialist groups in which he participated maintained special links to his native canton.

The Birthplace

Neuchâtel, where Piaget was born on 9 August 1896, is the capital of the canton of Neuchâtel, in the western part of Switzerland, on the border with France.[1] It is situated near the northeast corner of the lake of Neuchâtel. In 1900 the population numbered 134,014 persons, for the most part French-speaking and Protestant. The canton is located entirely in the Jura, a mountain range extending between the Rhine and Rhone and forming the border between France and Switzerland. Its territory is made up of three regions, known as "The Vineyard" (along the lake, and including the city of Neuchâtel), "The Valleys" (Val de Ruz and Val de Travers), and "The Mountains" (upland valleys including the industrial cities of Le Locle and La Chaux-de-Fonds). Another traditional way of dividing the canton is between the *Haut* (especially the

Mountains), and the *Bas* (especially the city of Neuchâtel), representing a social divide. While these are only oversimplified clichés, they are a constitutive
part of the local mentality.

By the mid-eighteenth century, inhabitants of the Mountain tended to be
peasants and shepherds from spring to fall, and home-based workers for the
growing watchmaking industry during the very rough winters. Their diligence
and ingenuity aroused the admiration of many travelers, and they were sometimes idealized as models of harmony between nature and industry, manual
labor and cultivation of the intellect. Thus, in his 1758 *Letter to d'Alembert,*
Rousseau described the *montagnons* as members of an autonomous, half-pas-
toral, half-industrial idyllic community. Later on, the Mountains, and particularly the industrial cities in the second half of the nineteenth century, became
centers of political activism and played a significant role in the histories of an-
archism, communism, socialism, and the social Christian movement (see, for
example, Perrenoud, 1988).

The *Bas,* in contrast, represented conservatism, tradition, aristocracy, the
defense of traditional privileges, and the artificiality of city life. By the time
Piaget was born, it also embodied the stiffness and conformity of a prosperous
and self-confident middle class active in a striking number of philanthropic,
religious, social, and cultural associations (see Guillaume, 1881). Rousseau,
again, thought the inhabitants of Neuchâtel pretentious, pompous, and
amoral. André Gide (*Journal,* 1 May 1927), who actually liked the city, found
its streets so clean that he feared to throw his cigarette on the ground; watching
people leave church on Sunday, he commented that all their thoughts "have
been bleached and ironed by the sermon they just heard, and tidily put away in
their head as in a chest for clean linen." In a depiction of the local "castes" at
an evening concert, the Neuchâtel writer William Ritter (1891, 16–17) asserted: "In Neuchâtel, everyone is a boarding-house owner, the town being
characterized by Protestant honesty, pedagogical pedantry, Prussian haughti-
ness, Dutch cleanliness, catacomb-like tranquillity, and pastoral stupidity."
Ritter also left kinder recollections, however, close in tone to those of Guy de
Pourtalès, Blaise Cendrars, and Henry de Montherlant recalling the studious
atmosphere of the town, full of students and pensions for foreign girls, as well
as the unassuming, calm, monotonous, somewhat sad but charming ambience
of the lake.

The stereotype of the *Bas* patrician and bourgeois has been linked with the
outstanding continuity in social and political organization that characterized
Neuchâtel from the early eighteenth to the mid-nineteenth century. When
Piaget was born in 1896, Neuchâtel had been a republic for merely half a cen-

tury; in the 1940s, Denis de Rougemont (1948, 13), one of Neuchâtel's best-known writers, still noticed vestiges of aristocratic traditions "in the oldest democracy of the world."

In 1504, as a result of alliances, the principality of Neuchâtel passed to the house of Orléans-Longueville, a bastard line of the royal house of France. In 1707 the Longueville house became extinct, and a great struggle arose for the succession. The local parliament elected Frederick I of Prussia prince of Neuchâtel. In practice, however, Neuchâtel was autonomous. From 1806 to 1814 it was held by Marshall Louis Alexandre Berthier, to whom it was given by Napoleon. In 1814 it returned to Prussia and at the same time joined the Swiss Confederation—a double anomaly, since Neuchâtel was neither a republic nor a sovereign state. In 1848 a peaceful revolution brought about the republican form of government; and only a year after a failed royalist attempt to regain power in 1856, the king of Prussia renounced his rights over Neuchâtel.

In 1896 Switzerland itself had been a federal state for merely half a century. With the 1848 Constitution, and under the leadership of the dominant Radical Party, the cantons lost their character as sovereign states and were obliged to adapt their constitutions and political regimens to the federal one. The second half of the nineteenth century saw the formation of a Swiss national consciousness. Such major developments as legal, political, and monetary unification, industrialization, and the construction of railroads and tunnels were accompanied by the emergence of the traditional rural village as a national symbol (one such village, reconstructed beside an artificial mountain, was the centerpiece of the Swiss National Exhibition in Geneva in 1896).

But national unity was (and in some respects remains) a fragile idea. During the late nineteenth century, numerous Swiss-French worried about the increasing dominance of Germany and German-speaking Switzerland; a Swiss-French Union was founded in Neuchâtel in 1908 to defend and preserve the local French and "Latin" culture against Germanic infiltration. This was part of a more general rivalry between France and Germany (Digeon, 1959; Paul, 1972), but in Switzerland it touched the country's political essence.

During World War I the "gulf" (*fossé, Graben,* as it was called) between the French-speaking and German-speaking parts of Switzerland deepened (Du Bois, 1980, 1983). The Swiss-French openly and passionately sided with the Allies and accused the federal government and the army chiefs of preferring Germany and German military methods. This feeling was intensified by several "scandals"; the biggest one involved the virtual acquittal of two colonels who had communicated documents from the army staff to the military attachés of Germany and Austria-Hungary. Starting in 1916 a latent antimilitarism, combined with a worsening economic situation and the growing influence of pacifism and socialism, led to social action (workers' demonstrations, calls for revolution, civil disobedience, and refusal to join the army), to which civil and military authorities sometimes reacted violently. The culmination of this process was the general strike of November 1918, which led to the army occupation of several cities, including Zurich, where Piaget was at the time (on the strike, see, for example, Vuilleumier, 1977).

At the same time, the cultural atmosphere of French-speaking Switzerland during the war was outstandingly rich: literary and political magazines sprouted up; through meetings and publications, the entire region led political and aesthetic debates that had become impossible in the belligerent countries, and it seemed for a while to concentrate in itself the responsibility of preparing a better world.

It is in this general context of turmoil and anxiety, but also of hope and cultural effervescence, and in close relation to many of its movements and participants, that the personality and projects of the young Piaget evolved.

The Family

Jean Piaget was the only son of Arthur and Rebecca Piaget; he had two younger sisters, Madeleine (1899–1976) and Marthe (1903–1985). In his autobiography he speaks of his parents' role in his development. His father, the historian Arthur Piaget, "a man of painstaking and critical mind, who dislike[d] hastily improvised generalizations," taught him "the value of systematic work, even in small matters" (1952, 237). Piaget (1977, 7) says that he got his "love of facts" from his father, and that Arthur advised his son not to study history, because "it isn't a true science."

Arthur Piaget (1865–1952) was born in Yverdon, a town close to Neuchâtel but in the canton of Vaud, where his father, a royalist, went into exile after the failed royalist rebellion of 1856. He was trained in medieval literature, and by the early 1890s had become a well-known Romanist. In 1895 he left Paris, where he had lived since 1889, for Neuchâtel, where he was appointed to the chair of Romance languages and literatures at the university. In his inaugural lesson, Arthur Piaget (1896) demonstrated that the *Canons' Chronicle,* the most revered document of Neuchâtel's history, was not a medieval original but an eighteenth-century forgery. His demonstration displeased conservatives; years later, it still gave rise to passionate debates (Ph. Godet, 1902; Perrochet, 1914). The government, however, appointed him state archivist in 1897; this appointment was the beginning of his ground-breaking research in local history and of a complete renewal of Neuchâtel historiography. Arthur Piaget's exposure of the *Chronicle* was not the only iconoclastic gesture of his career:

his critique of the genealogies established by a reputed local historian, his lectures on the 1848 revolution, and his sketch of the history of the university inevitably made some people unhappy for sentimental or political reasons. His incisive and ironical style often extended to his personal relationships: at least, Piaget (1952, 238) recalls that after his father's "ironic remarks" on a book on birds he composed at about age ten, he "had to recognize [it], regretfully, as a mere compilation" (a graphologist later perceived in the young Piaget's handwriting traces of inherited causticity; Duplain, ms. 1913). In sum, although Arthur Piaget was a highly respected and widely known figure of Neuchâtel, conservative circles long considered him a troublemaker.[2] Certainly he did not represent the proverbial qualities of the *Bas*.

Nor is Piaget's mother remembered for self-effacement and conformity to tradition. Those who knew her agree that she was an eccentric woman; one person I interviewed described her as being "as impossible as her handwriting." According to Piaget, Rebecca-Suzanne Jackson (1872–1942) was "very intelligent, energetic, and fundamentally a very kind person" but had a "rather neurotic temperament" that made "family life somewhat troublesome" (1952, 237–238). Piaget's sister, Marthe Burger, confirmed this recollection to me in 1981, asserting that Rebecca Piaget was an authoritarian woman who made their childhood unhappy. One of the "direct consequences of this situation," Piaget writes, "was that I started to forgo playing for serious work very early; this I obviously did as much to imitate my father as to take refuge in both a private and a non-fictitious world. Indeed, I have always detested any departure from reality, an attitude which I relate to the second influential factor of my early life, viz., my mother's poor mental health" (ibid., 238). The same factor, he adds, made him interested in psychoanalysis and pathological psychology. In the 1920s he went so far as to try to psychoanalyze his mother (see Vidal, 1986a). In a 1927 letter, Piaget (ms. 1927) characterized Rebecca Piaget's troubles not as "a simple neurosis" but as a "case of alienation"— more precisely, as a paranoia, or *folie raisonnante,* in which the patient is lucid and reasons quite well, but on the basis of false premises (in his mother's case, ideas of persecution).

The background to this diagnosis, which lacks further documentation, calls for a word of caution. In the same letter Piaget mentions that his mother had recently spent three months at Dr. Bersot's clinic. Henri Bersot (1896–1955), director of the Bellevue clinic at Le Landeron (canton of Neuchâtel) and a member of the national Swiss committee for mental hygiene, was the author of several general-information publications on "nervous diseases," including a brochure titled *The Nervous Woman.* Bersot (1932) considered that the features characteristic of the female "temperament" (such as intuition, delicacy, sentimentality, and curiosity) made women more susceptible than men to neurosis and psychosis. In 1929, he reported, his clinic admitted "for psychoses, ideas of persecution, etc., 698 men and 1089 women" (ibid., 5). From the perspective of Bersot's brochure, any mild state of female "nervousness" could rapidly degenerate into a full-blown psychiatric case; the line between such a state and mania, melancholy, or paranoia was extremely thin, and easy to cross in the course of diagnosis.

Like Bersot's ideas, the easy crossing of diagnostic lines was commonplace in the area of "nervousness." Launched in French as *nervosisme* in the 1860s, it encompassed from the start a variety of afflictions; it later fused with neurasthenia but remained popular in French as a name for the most widespread malady of the *fin-de-siècle* middle class. Paranoia, a psychosis, was a less popular and more narrowly psychiatric notion than nervousness; it was reported as being rare among hospitalized patients, and its nosographic boundaries were the object of specialized debate. Paranoid states, however, were sometimes considered as forms or consequences of nervousness.[3]

Medical matters aside, Rebecca Piaget certainly had strong convictions and was outspoken about them. She was French, and during World War I it was clear that she sided with the Allies. Early in the war she was involved in an episode typical of a time when the wildest rumors spread unimpeded. In October 1914 she published in a local newspaper her impressions of a visit to refugee camps on the French side of Lake Geneva (R. Piaget, 1914a). She called the Germans "the invader" and "those barbarians" and mentioned having heard many horrible stories, including one about German Red Cross nurses poisoning soldiers from the Allied armies. In a later letter to the newspaper (R. Piaget, 1914b) she explained that, having received letters filled with complaints and insults, she decided to check the story. So she went to Paris, where some German nurses were indeed imprisoned, accused of stealing and waiting to be tried. Samuel Cornut, her son's godfather, helped her through several judiciary administrations. At the end of her investigation she concluded that the nurses were innocent of the crime attributed to them by the rumor; in her second letter to the newspaper she observed that it was necessary to be wary not only of exaggerations but also of fabrications. The story did not end there: in February 1915 the president of the German Red Cross brought legal action against her for libel. After a series of trials and appeals, it was recognized that Rebecca Piaget was guilty of reporting a slandering rumor, but that she could not be formally condemned for slander because she had not defamed anybody in particular, not even an identifiable body of persons.[4]

Rebecca Piaget's political commitments may have influenced her son. In 1912 she became the first socialist woman elected to the local school commission (Liniger, 1980, 50), and during World War I she supported a socialist minister who was imprisoned as a conscientious objector. While there is evidence (see Chapter 9) that the young Piaget tried to liberate himself from the education given by his mother, it is also imaginable that Rebecca Piaget was not an altogether negative figure in the development of his identity.

The Educational Institutions

One of the most distinctive aspects of Piaget's youth was his membership, beyond school obligations, in the institutions that contributed to Neuchâtel's reputation as an educational center. According to the local writer and literary critic Philippe Godet (1901, 52), some of the ponderous buildings constructed between 1880 and 1900, such as the Museum of Fine Arts and the future university, bore witness to the city's "intellectual effort" toward "justifying better and better its renown as a *ville-école* [school town]." In the young Piaget's urban landscape, these buildings were the highly visible emblems of progress and modernity whose "blatant utilitarianism" Godet melancholically reproved.

Prominent among Neuchâtel's educational institutions were various private learned societies and amateur clubs aimed at fostering knowledge through mutual instruction and independent research. Individuals, ideas, information, and values circulated freely among all levels of the public and private systems. It is within such an institutional network—a small community where everybody knew everybody, and where learning was openly shared—that the young Piaget was initially educated.

In 1907 Piaget entered the Collège Latin, or "Latin School," originally established in the sixteenth century with the goal of educating future magistrates and pastors. Instruction there lasted five years, starting at the age of ten. After attending the Latin School from 1907 to 1912, Piaget pursued his studies in the gymnasium from October 1912 to July 1915. Until 1896 the gymnasium had been attached to the university-level structures as a sort of preparatory school. It was divided into a literary, "Latin" section, aimed at preparing for entrance at the university; a scientific section, with a similar goal but more focused on technical and scientific studies; and a shorter (two years instead of three) pedagogical section, intended to train kindergarten and primary school teachers. (On both schools, see *Histoire de l'instruction;* and Quartier-la-Tente, 1898; see also *Gymnase.*) The young Piaget was in the literary section. Most academics, including Paul Godet, Pierre Bovet, and Arnold Reymond, all important figures in his education, taught at the gymnasium before starting a career at the university or other higher levels of the educational system.

At the university, the academic year went from mid-October to mid-March (winter semester) and from mid-April to mid-July (summer semester). Piaget entered the university in the winter of 1915 and remained enrolled, except for the summer term of 1916, until July 1918, when he received his *licence* in natural sciences. From a letter (ms. 1918g), we know that his doctoral thesis was finished by November 1918. In all but two of his courses and for his dissertation he received the highest grade of six; in the two exceptions, a course in human anatomy and physiology, and another in botany, he received a five.[5]

The University of Neuchâtel was established in 1909. It was preceded by two "Academies." The first Academy (1840–1848), founded by the monarchical régime, was suppressed when the republic was established. Louis Agassiz (1807–1873), Neuchâtel's first professor of natural history (since 1832), was in the United States at the time and decided not to return. He soon received an appointment at Harvard College, started a brilliant career as a builder of scientific institutions, and was followed by his main Neuchâtel associates (Jones, 1931; Lurie, 1960, 1974). Until 1896 the second Academy (1866–1909) combined the cantonal gymnasium and a university level.[6]

Turn-of-the-century Neuchâtel academics unanimously considered that the first Academy had been the most brilliant moment of their country's intellectual history. Political and academic authorities used the example of Agassiz and his group to argue for increased support for the sciences. The émigrés illustrated an ideal of science that was still dear to the local savants, a science in which the study of nature through direct observation went hand in hand with the doctrine of progress, an educational mission, democratic ideals, and Christian values (see, for example, Tribolet, 1899). Accordingly, in the 1890s grand buildings were erected, the Academy was renamed University, high costs were borne to further the ideal of science as a source of material and spiritual progress in the individual and society, and science and its institutions were celebrated as embodiments of the highest human values (see, for example, the speeches included in *Le cinquantenaire*).

Learned Societies

The idea of science grandiloquently formulated in official speeches was more modestly and concretely expressed at other levels. Societies and clubs brought together enlightened amateurs, specimen collectors, lovers of nature, and established professionals. Founded largely with the goal of improving citizens' knowledge of their country, such societies especially flourished after 1815, during the post-Napoleonic restoration.

The Natural Sciences Society of Neuchâtel was created in 1832. Its founders (one of whom was Louis Agassiz) saw the formation of learned societies as characteristic of "civilized nations" and considered that everybody's help was needed to exploit and disseminate nature's hidden "treasures." For Agassiz, societies were essential "to spread . . . the taste and the love of study, and to exert . . . the beneficial influence that results from the propagation of healthy doctrines and from the facts of science applied to social development" (quotations in L. Favre, 1883, 8, 9–10).

The Society was the seat of serious debates (such as the one on the glacier theory in the 1830s), participated actively in the study of practical problems (such as irrigation and canalization), and set up the detailed exploration of the canton of Neuchâtel. Through its activities and publications, it became the soul of local scientific life; and through its members' participation in youth groups, it furthered the educational and moral missions deemed inherent to science. Piaget joined it in 1912.

The Jura Club and the Club of the Friends of Nature were the two young naturalists' groups in turn-of-the-century Neuchâtel. Although by the 1910s the latter was more popular, the two clubs shared basic values. Piaget belonged only to the Friends of Nature, but like many other Friends he published his first texts in the Jura Club's magazine, *Le rameau de sapin* (The Fir Branch). His natural history teacher, Paul Godet, was at the same time a member of the Jura Club, an assiduous contributor to *Le rameau,* and one of the Friends' first mentors.

The Jura Club was founded in 1865 at the initiative of the physician Louis Guillaume (1833–1924), a member of the local parliament and at different times a director of the Neuchâtel penitentiary and of the Federal Statistics Bureau, as well as a professor at the Academy (1878–1889). In 1864 he had also helped found the local Society of History and Archaeology and launch its journal, *Musée neuchâtelois* (Neuchâtel Museum). The Jura Club and the historical society had much in common.

The founders of the historical society believed that each citizen's interest in the history of his country was the basis of political life, and did not judge it imperative "to have in-depth historical and philological knowledge" in order to observe the things worthy of being recorded (see, for example, Junod, 1923). Because the Society's aim was to consolidate a regional and national conscience, all discussion of religious or political questions was by statute excluded from its meetings.

The Jura Club was the natural-historical counterpart of the historical society. Its founders, "professors and friends of youth," wished to acquaint young people aged nine to eighteen with the study of the natural sciences, with a focus on the fauna and flora of the Jura. Their goal was to occupy youth with "healthy, elevated things, necessary during the often dangerous moment of transition when, having finished school, the adolescent has not yet taken his place in society, and is lured by frivolous pleasures and material enjoyments" (L. Favre et al., 1874, 1; see also *Le Club Jurassien*). Even before the Club was established, Guillaume and others organized outings that combined an introduction to the natural sciences (observation and the collection of specimens) with the development of patriotism and character. For them, such excursions for young people were the equivalent of national feasts for the adults. While giving youth the opportunity to exert their "observational instinct and innate taste for collecting," they made them acquainted with local history and helped them acquire principles of discipline, esprit de corps, respect, comradeship, and hygiene (Guillaume, 1864, Introduction). For the renowned French *Dictionary of Pedagogy and Primary Education,* the Jura Club was "a model of intelligent pedagogy," capable of promoting work in common and self-esteem, as well as morality and personal responsibility (Buisson, 1882).

The significance of institutions such as the Jura Club thus rested on the belief that the natural sciences had educational and utilitarian value for the individual and society. A related ideology encouraged a health tourism that by the end of the nineteenth century became one of Switzerland's main export products. Cleanliness, healthy habits, spotless interiors, active contact with nature, mountain air if possible, were all supposed to be morally and physically invigorating (Heller, 1979). To the extent that the natural sciences were based on the direct observation of natural facts, and that nature could not corrupt, introducing young people to natural history served to inculcate rules of bodily and mental hygiene, patriotic feelings, and moral values. Thus, in a letter to the Friends of Nature the naturalist Paul Godet, Piaget's future mentor, wrote (ms. 1894): "The study of nature is an inexhaustible source of enjoyment, and nothing is more useful to the soul, and sometimes to the body, than to devote one's spare time to it. This study develops the spirit of analysis and observation; it helps clarify ideas, and furnishes an admirable means of fighting ennui, often a bad adviser, and always hard to bear."

Like the Jura Club, but with more independence vis-à-vis the adult world, the Club of the Friends of Nature channeled adolescent energy in healthy and morally acceptable directions. Reserved to and run by secondary-level students with no direct adult supervision, it constituted a unique setting for autonomous socializing and intellectual exchange. It furnished occasions for the emergence of durable friendships and for personal beginnings in science and philosophy.

In early twentieth-century Switzerland, the "friend of nature" was still a familiar character, who matched the well-known prototype depicted by the

Genevan educator, author, and pioneer cartoonist Rodolphe Toepffer (1799–1846). The "friend of nature" was "a fifteen-year-old philosopher" capable of spending entire days looking for specimens, classifying, and perfecting his collections. Toepffer (1858, 65–66), together with many other naturalists and pedagogues, was convinced that natural history was accessible to adolescents because it required practically no specialized background and suited their supposedly typical energy, curiosity, and individualism.

The history of the Club of the Friends of Nature embodies Toepffer's ideas on youth and natural history. The club was established in May 1893 by two fifteen-year-olds, Pierre Bovet and Carl-Albert Loosli, and was to be composed exclusively of secondary students aged fourteen or above who would "apply themselves to the natural sciences with the goal of instructing each other in the branches of botany, zoology, etc., etc." (P. Bovet, 1943, 1). The Friends set themselves apart from the highly visible student societies, generally literary and of German inspiration, that prospered at the time in Swiss secondary schools and universities. These societies were usually governed by strict rules, and their members wore a uniform. In contrast, the Friends of Nature focused on science, and wished to work freely and inconspicuously. The club "was scientific, and working was its goal"; its motto was "To live free, let us live in hiding" (Ducommun, 1943, 24).

From its inception, serious naturalists helped the Friends and were thanked with honorary membership. The first honorary members were an artisan who was a missionary in Africa, two lepidopterist ministers, and Paul Godet. Early on, Godet taught his protégés the principles of natural history and zoological taxonomy; the eminent François-Alphonse Forel, a relative of the Bovets, introduced them to limnology, the science of lakes, which he pioneered; Otto Fuhrmann, Piaget's future professor at the university and Godet's successor as director of the Neuchâtel Museum of Natural History, showed them how to set up an aquarium.

Direct observation was the essence of the Friends' scientific activity. Godet wanted "not young people who talk, but young people who act"; he warned that "a beginner who limits himself to browsing through natural history books and does not feel the need for an immediate contact with nature will never be anything other than a failed naturalist" (P. Godet, 1875, 6). Such was indeed the Friends' intellectual creed.

Apart from regular sessions, the Friends organized botanical, paleontological, or zoological excursions. During the sessions, papers were presented, generally containing observations on animals, plants, or natural phenomena; readings were periodically held. Occasionally some collaborative projects were published in a local journal. The range of topics discussed grew over the years, apparently in parallel with science education in the schools. The initial focus on observation and description gave way to studies dealing with classification, anatomy, and physiology and eventually made room for general theories, the physical sciences, and mathematics.

In terms of active membership, the years 1900–1915 seem to have been remarkably prosperous, largely owing to the attraction still exerted by the observation of nature and its connection to social values. Adults supported the club. At the beginning, Bovet's parents paid for the rent of a room, which a visitor described as "looking more like a laboratory, or at least a scholar's study, than a society's quarters" (quoted in P. Bovet, 1943, 11). These quarters facilitated a social life judged to be healthier than that of other student societies, which the gymnasium's governing board had banned in 1859. The prohibition emphasized that it was not aimed at "preventing students from gathering for the purposes of recreation and instruction," but only at ending "functions in cafés and bars, banquets, and other events that have more than once given rise to disorders harmful to the intellectual and moral development of young people" (quoted in Quartier-la-Tente, 1898, 289). In contrast to those societies, the Club of the Friends of Nature was a self-conscious model of acceptable and safe socializing, an ideal for those concerned with the education of youth and the maintenance of public morality.

Conclusion

The ceremony of 9 June 1910 during which Piaget was admitted to the Club of the Friends of Nature illustrates the cohesion of the social context in which he grew up. The honorary members who attended were Paul Godet, Pierre Bovet, and Eugène LeGrand Roy. At the time, Godet was director of the local Museum of Natural History; he belonged to an old family, was the son of a well-known botanist and former city librarian, and was the nephew of a distinguished theologian; his cousin Philippe (mentioned above) was a famous writer and literary critic. Pierre Bovet, also of an ancient local family and one of the club's founders, was at the time professor at the university, whose rector was Arthur Piaget; in 1912 he became the first director of the Jean-Jacques Rousseau Institute of Geneva and still held that position when Piaget arrived at the Institute in 1921. LeGrand Roy, though not closely involved in Piaget's education, taught astronomy at the university, where he would be succeeded by Gustave Juvet, also a Friend of Nature and one of Piaget's best friends.

The simultaneous presence of Godet, Bovet, and LeGrand Roy during this ceremony reflects the structure of social relations in turn-of-the-century Neuchâtel. The same people and the same values circulated through different institutional levels. This phenomenon extended beyond the institutions mentioned here. Pierre Bovet, for example, was in his youth secretary of the Swiss Christian Students' Association to which Piaget belonged, and a lifelong contributor to *L'Essor*, a social and religious journal which published some of the young Piaget's work, and whose editor was a friend of his family.

The intertwining of institutions, people, and ideas in Piaget's youth produced a social network in which he continued to function for years to come. It helped define a range of existential possibilities and to shape early choices that in turn set directions for his later development. This applied not only to his precocious scientific activity, but also to his passion for grand social and intellectual causes. Paradoxical as it may seem, the young Piaget's desire to provoke and shock were expressions of an individual who was integrated in his milieu and who, early on, became a respected and well-known figure in his "orderly little town."

2

Mollusk Taxonomy

In 1907 ten-year-old Jean Piaget asked Paul Godet, the director of Neuchâtel's Museum of Natural History, permission to work there after hours. Godet (ms. 1907) granted permission and adopted Piaget as an assistant, had him stick labels on specimens, taught him how to collect, and introduced him to the classification of land and freshwater mollusks. Piaget responded with enthusiasm:

> For four years I worked for this conscientious and learned naturalist, in exchange for which he would give me at the end of each session a certain number of rare species for my own collection and, in particular, provide me with an exact classification of the samples that I had collected. These weekly meetings in the director's private office stimulated me so much that I spent all my free time collecting mollusks . . . every Saturday afternoon I used to wait for my teacher a half hour ahead of time! (1952, 238)

This early initiation to malacology afforded Piaget "a glimpse of science and what it stands for, before undergoing the philosophical crisis of adolescence," and allegedly protected him "against the demon of philosophy" (ibid., 238, 239).

The relationship between Piaget and Godet was decisive in the youngster's intellectual development. The biological concerns that later animated Piaget's thought, however, do not derive directly from this first "glimpse of science." Godet was seventy when he met his favorite disciple, and he taught him an increasingly outmoded sort of natural history, one that had little affinity with the practical and theoretical problems of biology as the study of living beings.

Paul Godet

Paul Godet (1836–1911) was born in Neuchâtel into an old bourgeois royalist family (see E. Godet, 1911). His father, Charles-Henri Godet (1797–1879), had been a well-known botanist. For the elder Godet, to know nature was to fit it into the Linnaean system; knowledge was identical with the correct identification of specimens, and identification was based solely on external characteristics. By the 1870s botanists had begun research on hybridization, fertilization, and pollination in the hope of shedding light on the questions of heredity and variation in an evolutionary perspective. According to his son, the older Godet rejoiced in such progress but "remained a man of the past" (P. Godet, 1879, 166). Much the same may be said of Paul Godet at the time he became Piaget's teacher, for he never ceased to focus on description and classification, impervious to the populational thinking and the evolutionary questions that, during his lifetime, started to enter into natural history (Farber, 1982).

Godet's devotion to natural history was total. In sixty years of travel in the canton of Neuchâtel, he asked countless individuals to gather shells for him, and his enthusiasm at the discovery of a "rare or unknown shell" never diminished (Dautzenberg, 1912, 359–360). From 1908 to 1918 the young Piaget likewise devoted a significant part of every trip and holiday to collecting mollusks (see remarks in 1911c, 1; 1921a, 49).

Godet encouraged his young disciple to collect specimens because, as he emphasized (1874, 1875), collections were useful to science. Moreover, he thought that natural history was emotionally beneficial. Godet (1879, ms. 1894) was fond of telling how his father had been saved from nostalgia by an old botany book that led him to collect and classify plants. Piaget, in turn, claimed to have found in science a refuge from a distressing family situation (1952, 238).

For Godet, natural history was an essential part of the education of youth. He pursued both actively throughout his long career as a teacher in local schools, as a mentor of the Jura Club and the Friends of Nature, and as a frequent contributor to *Le rameau de sapin*. He was an effective teacher whose enthusiasm was infectious to many young people. Piaget was not his only disciple; as a youngster, Pierre Jeannet, a Friend of Nature who as a pastor became a prominent figure among local Protestant youth, also spent "long hours" at the museum "dusting and labeling" under Godet's supervision (M. Du Pasquier, 1920, 123).

Godet was also a charitable Christian. The moving letter he sent to Piaget during an illness is filled with a spirit of Christian resignation and confidence

(Godet, ms. 1909). More importantly, for Godet natural science and religiosity went hand in hand. Nature was a God-written book, and reading it was equivalent to revelation. Like Neuchâtel's scientific idol, Louis Agassiz, the young Godet had sought to study "the unity of plan in the system of organized beings" (1862 letter quoted in L. C. Jones, 1929, 71). At least in print, however, he never exhorted young people to see nature as God's book; he preferred to speak of natural history as the simplest and most pleasant means of "relating to the mysterious and charming Isis" (P. Godet, 1875, 6). But he certainly retained beliefs that were closer to natural theology than to Darwinian evolutionism.

Godet was strongly interested in the question of the origins of species. Darwinian evolutionism seemed to him to give rise to two fundamental questions: whether or not there were fixed characteristics, and what was the origin of the human species and its place in the order of living beings. Godet (1874, 45) contrasted the generality of the "hypothesis" of a common ancestor (and thus of a "man-animal") with the idea of distinct creations (and thus of a separate "human kingdom"). Since he identified the existence of species with that of fixed characteristics, he must have embraced the "human kingdom" concept. In observing that certain forms "believed to be species, are rather the products of adaptation" (P. Godet, 1907a, 109), he implied that varieties were not to be considered as nascent species. Such issues, however, never received prominence in his written work.

In sum, Godet was above all a taxonomist. For him, knowing nature meant describing, classifying, and naming specimens, and the natural sciences were an ideal means of encouraging the moral and spiritual formation of youth. Unadulterated by experimental manipulation, nature itself was the best possible teacher: as Agassiz had said, "No one can warp her to suit his own views. She brings us back to absolute truth as often as we wonder" (Cary Agassiz, 1885, 2:775). Science, as the observation of nature, was inherently educational; and the best education was scientific.

Piaget and Godet

On 9 June 1910, thirteen-year-old Jean Piaget was initiated as a Friend of Nature. Tradition demanded that he give a talk. He began by quoting Paul Godet, who, he explained, had demonstrated the existence of several mollusks unique to Lake Neuchâtel and its surroundings (1910a, 1); his subject was to be one of them, the *lacustris* variety of the *Limnaea stagnalis*.

After describing the external features of this "beautiful species," Piaget examined his chosen variety, taking as type a specimen given to him by Godet and expressing gratitude to his mentor. He then gave a detailed description of the type, which he compared with the *stagnalis* variety found in agitated waters. Finally, he cataloged the different *lacustris* forms on the basis of shell morphology and named them in accordance with Godet's nomenclature.

Traces of Godet's teachings are omnipresent in Piaget's malacological work between 1910 and 1915. Godet's methods and interests dictated form and content, and classifications often derived from his catalog of Neuchâtel's mollusks. At first Piaget relied entirely on his teacher. In his first note in *Le rameau de sapin* (1909), he recounted how he found a certain shell and took it to Godet, who established its geographic origin. Piaget often adopted as types specimens given to him by Godet (1910a; 1913a, 464), who also provided or revised his classifications (for example, 1911b, 31; 1911c, 2). From 1907 to 1911 Godet taught Piaget to observe and describe a specimen, compare it with others, and use catalogs and illustrations to identify and categorize.

Trust and affection between master and pupil developed around scientific questions. In turn, these questions were colored by the personal touches that characterized their transmission. Piaget did not hesitate to invoke Godet. An anecdote involving the master could encapsulate the problems raised by the variability of *Limnaea*: "having shown Godet the same specimens at a relatively short interval, he—who had been studying our mollusks for sixty years— identified them, first as *L. ampla* var. *obtusa,* and later as *L. ovata* var. *patula!*" (1911a, 312). While describing the habitat of a certain species, he recalled Godet's surprise at its location (1913a, 510).

In 1911 Piaget announced Godet's death to the Friends of Nature, recalled everything the club owed to its mentor, and asked the members to rise in sign of mourning (PV, 11 May 1911). Later he often made use of Godet as an intellectual warranty. While writing about a species that had apparently disappeared from the local fauna, he mentioned that it was at least "sufficiently rare to have escaped Mr. P. Godet's conscientious investigations" (1913b, 165). He called Godet his "dear and venerated master," and honored him by naming after him at least one variety and one species (1913c, 78; 1914b, 255). He felt free to criticize him, but always did so with deference. For example, he could find Godet's nomenclature "too cumbersome" and at the same time observe that his master had "pushed scientific prudence to the point of naming only two [new] species in his whole lifetime" (1912a, 104).

Piaget had access to Godet's collections before they were inherited by the Friends of Nature. In his publications, he presented himself as Godet's scientific successor. He reported having closely examined Godet's "beautiful collection of shells" and possessing a large number of his manuscript notes (1912a, 104–105; 1913a, 510), which he sometimes cited (1913a, 465). He knew Godet's own books well enough to mention marginalia (ibid., 510). He completed his master's catalog of mollusks (1912b) and took over other projects in which Godet had been involved before his final illness: classifying a collection of Colombian mollusks (1914b) and preparing a monograph on Jura mollusks to accompany an atlas that Godet had offered to the Swiss Natural Sciences Society (1914c).

Some of Piaget's projects were realizations of Godet's explicit wishes. A catalog of batrachians (Piaget and Juvet, 1913) was his idea and was partly based on previous work by him. Godet (1907a, 110) had pointed out the interest of studying mimicry; Piaget would quote him at length before developing his own observations on the topic (1911d). Having received criticism from Godet for discussing geographic distribution in a presentation on shell collections, and thus covering too much ground, he made distribution the subject of a separate paper (1910c, 1).

Piaget's first article in a professional journal opened with an anecdote that epitomized and publicized his relationship with Godet: "When, after having vainly attempted to classify certain ill-defined specimens of *Limnaea,* I would bring them to my revered master, the late Dr. Paul Godet, he would not miss the opportunity to repeat to me all the aversion he felt for these nasty animals that are the despair of malacologists because of their variability. Then he would light a cigar, saying that he needed strength, examine the shells that I was showing him, and give his opinion with extreme circumspection" (1911a, 311). The whole article is in fact Piaget's homage to Godet, its subject and method being exemplary of the problems, techniques, and scientific values transmitted from master to disciple.

Malacological Taxonomy

Godet's scientific projects related above all to the description and classification of regional mollusks. His approach, which was typical of turn-of-the-century malacological taxonomy, defined both the form and content of his disciple's research. Everything in Piaget's early work was subordinated to systematics. He was aware, for example, that the discovery of species in regions where they had never before been found (1911e, 1914e–g) might give rise to important theoretical questions. Yet his priority was always to compile the most complete catalogs possible (see remark in Piaget and Romy, 1912, 145).

Cataloging

The typical product of Godet's and Piaget's research activity was the taxonomic monograph (or "taxonomy" for short). A taxonomy usually comprises several sections. The longest one, a systematic "catalog," is based on the "determination" of specimens, that is, the attribution of a name taken from an existing classification.

If the specimen being classified is used to create a new species or variety, its "diagnosis," or description, must be given. Piaget gave concise diagnoses in Latin, followed by longer ones in French. Since Linnaeus' invention of the binominal system, "naming" a specimen has meant assigning to it a name composed of the name of the genus followed by that of the species. Naming must follow the rules of nomenclature, or system of names applied to taxonomic units (taxons). Nomenclature was still barely codified at the turn of the century, and systematists tended to multiply names corresponding to categories below the species: the subspecies, the variety, the subvariety, sometimes the "form." Catalogs also include a list of the works used for determining and naming; if necessary, a "synonymy," or inventory of names (together with dates and authors) previously attributed to the taxon; and brief descriptive notes on the specimen's origins and biogeography or on the reasons for choosing the proposed taxonomy. The methods used, the decisions made, and the difficulties encountered in systematics were often traceable to theories about the nature of taxonomic categories. (See Coutagne, 1895, for a particularly full exposition of freshwater mollusk systematics at the time.)

The Morphological Species Concept

Freshwater organisms tend to display great phenotypic variability. *Limnaea,* a genus of an extremely common gastropod on which the young Piaget worked, is no exception. These variations occur on both the shell and the body of the organism (see, for example, 1912d). For taxonomic purposes, however, shell variability was of greater importance.

Turn-of-the-century malacological taxonomy was dominated by the morphological species concept. The determination of species and lower categories was based on the exterior aspect of the shells rather than on functional, anatomical, or biological factors. The difference between species and varieties was established on the basis of the stability of a characteristic: the less it changed, the better criterion it provided for defining a species. Less stable features were used to define the variety and lower categories.

Because of the vast range of variation in conchological characteristics, the morphological species concept was a persistent source of dispute. Mollusk shells are sensitive to such factors as the force and volume of water currents, and therefore offer numerous environmentally induced individual variations. The range of variation is further increased by the fact that many mollusk species include several closely related subspecies. Not until the 1920s did zoologists begin to use anatomical considerations to address the taxonomic problems generated by the morphological species concept; and not until 1950 was the number of species for the genus *Limnaea* reduced from more than a thousand to about forty (Hubendick, 1951).

The following is a typical comment on the "disorder" generated in malacological systematics by the use of conchological characteristics: "Everybody knows about the reigning confusion . . . in the delimitation of species. Many species have never been graphically represented by their authors, and since anatomy furnishes no criteria to differentiate them, the systematist is guided exclusively by shell morphology. Under such conditions, determining specimens often means discerning subtle quantitative differences—estimating, for example, if the shell is 'oval, somewhat elongated' or 'oval, somewhat short,' or even 'quite elongated, a bit enlarged'" (Cardot, 1912, 197). There is no hint here that determination could be based on criteria other than shell morphology. Hence the paramount importance of form description. Yet because of great variability in the characteristics of mollusk shells, descriptions were approximative and full of adverbial nuances. Piaget's work demonstrates his early mastery of the conventional syntax of description (for example, 1913g, 166–167; 1914b, 254–255).

Illustration was the essential companion to verbal description. Most catalogs, however, include complaints about the lack of appropriate iconography. As one taxonomist remarked, "without very enlarged photographs or images . . . it is difficult to choose a name in the labyrinth of purely verbal descriptions that have been given" (Dollfus, 1911, 182). Godet was known as a skillful illustrator; his grandest project (never published and now lost) was a collection of 150 plates including more than 2,500 drawings depicting in anatomical and structural detail the mollusk species, varieties, and "forms" of the canton of Neuchâtel.

Nomenclature

One consequence of the importance attributed to form in the classification of extremely variable individuals was the use of categories such as "subvariety," "form," and "mutation." It seemed taxonomically relevant to establish categories that took into account even the most unstable morphological features. As Piaget explained, "each species, each type, each variety, subspecies, or subvariety offers . . . a certain number of more or less individual, accidental, or aberrant variations, designated by the general names of *forma* or *mutatio; forma* indicates a difference in form alone, and *mutatio*, only in color. Thus, for almost every mollusk, one can distinguish *f. major, minor, maxima, minima, depressa, elevata,* or *f. monstrosa, scelaris, contraria,* etc., etc., and *mut. alba, lutes, fasciata,* etc., and *mut. monstrosa, albina,* etc., etc." (1912a, 106). Such an approach to nomenclature inevitably generated such complex names as *"Clausilia Dubia* Drap. var. *Gallica* Brgt. *forma minor."*

Another consequence of the morphological species concept was that names were based on combinations and proportions of characteristics. The subtle art of naming was undoubtedly one of the first things Piaget learned from Godet; as early as 1910 he was capable of explaining it in detail. He did so in the first article of the many he would devote to *Limnaea.* Highly variable and endowed with a chaotic nomenclature, *Limnaea* was a challenging group to work with. Piaget (1910a) started by focusing on the *lacustris* variety of the *L. stagnalis,* particularly on its different "forms," that is, on the variety's variations.

Following Godet (1907a), Piaget distinguished *varietates ex colore* and *ex forma* and, among the latter, the *formae typica, major, minor, producta, abbreviata, conica,* and *ampliata.* All these distinctions were a matter of relative proportion and combination of characters. Thus, *forma major* is bigger than the type; *minor* is smaller. *Producta* is elongated, whereas *abbreviata* is more globular; it can also be found in combination with *ampliata,* which shares most dimensions with the type, except for a much larger aperture. *Forma conica* is "swollen toward the top, and thinner toward the bottom"; however, if the upper part is not very swollen, it may be named *attenuata.* In all cases, the choice of a name depended ultimately on details and fine degrees, the perception of which took an experienced eye, and a mastery of nomenclature and of the language of description.

Variability and Continuity

The existence of the species is a classical problem of natural history. During the eighteenth century, the idea of a perfectly continuous "chain of being," as well as the observation of gradations and transitions between species, often led to the conclusion that the species did not exist as a real object in nature (Lovejoy, 1936, chap. 8). To the extent that it seemed impossible to define natural and clear limits between groups of organisms, the species was judged not to be real, but only nominal.

With the advent of evolutionary theory, the problem of diachronic, phylogenetic continuity often combined with the older problem of synchronic, morphological continuity. The Darwinian species concept was nominalistic for both morphological and evolutionary reasons. Following traditional practice, Darwin (1859, 51–52) thought that varieties and species differed only in the degree to which they were "distinct and permanent." The main taxonomic consequence of the evolutionary perspective was that a "well-marked variety may be justly called an incipient species" (ibid., 52). Nominalism, therefore, also followed from the difficulty of deciding when a variety should be elevated to the rank of species.

An extreme example of how variability could lead to the proliferation of species is furnished by the French naturalist Jules-René Bourguignat (1829–1892), for whom any form characterized by three distinct signs of the shell should be ranked as a species (see especially Bourguignat, 1880–81). The consequence of his approach was that minor morphological features were considered as species traits; in his lifetime, Bourguignat defined 112 new genera and about 2,540 new species. He was an extreme "splitter." Most malacologists, however, tended to be "lumpers"; for them, the most challenging task was to reduce the number of species in a given genus by lumping together established species.

Godet was attracted to variable genera because, he said, "nowhere can one observe better the minute transitions between apparently very different forms" (P. Godet, 1872, 146–147). Variations in shell characteristics used to define a species frequently form a continuous gradation or series. It was a common practice to consider that two groups or individuals linked by such a series belonged to the same species (the method of continuous series).

Piaget's main early scientific project—to reduce the number of species by the method of continuous series—was inherited from Godet. As he declared in his first independent substantial article, variability was what interested him most, and he wondered "whether it would not be possible to reduce the number of species" (1911a, 311). His depiction of the situation is a model of the malacologist's predicament: "when you are confronted with a frightening number of more or less clear-cut variations, offering imperceptible transitions among them, and when you try to discriminate species characteristics, varieties, and accidental forms, you are shocked at the lack of stability of those characters, and at the ease with which certain intermediate individuals show unexpected similarities to two varieties that had at first seemed very different, and that you thought you could not confound" (ibid., 319). Piaget's solution was to lump hitherto accepted species into a single larger species, of which they became varieties. He was most sensitive to the difficulty of choosing suitable characteristics to define species. He claimed, however, that in practice the question was "easily resolved": a characteristic was unacceptable if it varied from individual to individual or if it was not hereditary; given the near-impossibility of testing for heritability, the method of continuous series was *the* way to deal with variability (1912a, 103–104). The species concept remained in all cases morphological and entirely dependent on the stability and constancy of the chosen characteristics.

The "Problem of the Species"

Darwin (1859, 484) thought that if systematists accepted varieties as incipient species, they would no longer "be incessantly haunted by the shadowy doubt whether this or that form be in essence a species"; they would only have to assess degrees of difference and constancy, and focus on the study of variation rather than routinely apply the method of continuous series.

According to Godet, Darwin's work showed that taxonomy had to be entirely rethought. "At the present time," he wrote in 1874, "no naturalist knows, at least in practice, what the species is": "The characteristics we used to call *specific,* or *of species,* and that we used to consider as invariable, are all subject to more or less extensive variation. Does this mean that there are not any [immutable ones]? Or even, could not characteristics that are variable in certain animal or vegetable genera be fixed in others? It is clear that it would be premature to declare in an absolute manner that there are no invariable characteristics to distinguish species" (P. Godet, 1874, 46). When Godet encouraged young people to make collections, he knew that the study of variation was the clue to answering his question, and that the counterproductive habit of creating new species resulted from not sufficiently comparing populations. Thus, Piaget's tireless collecting of specimens made him Godet's worthiest disciple.

Things were different when it came to evolution. When Piaget started thinking about it, not only did he have no doubts about its universal presence in the zoological realm, but he also saw it from a viewpoint inspired by Bergson's philosophy. In contrast, although Godet sensed the significance of evolutionary theory for taxonomy, he did not believe it invalidated the existence of unchangeable characteristics. "The most important thing," he affirmed, "is to distinguish those [characteristics] that are constant from those that are simple individual variations" (P. Godet, 1904, 27).

The "type" of the species—that is, the specimen adopted as the model by the species' discoverer—therefore acquired enormous importance. Instead of being the individual to which the name of the species was attached and of having a purely nomenclatorial significance, it was supposed to exhibit the species' defining fixed characteristics. For Godet (1907b, 288), one of the great riches of Neuchâtel's Museum of Natural History was that it possessed "invaluable types"; the interest of collections came from the fact that they made it possible to compare specimens and types, and thus to determine beyond doubt which morphological traits were really invariable. Thus, for Godet, morphological fixity was the ultimate criterion of the natural definition of a species.

Piaget would eventually adopt a diametrically opposite view. After 1912, inspired by Bergson's philosophy, he postulated that a natural definition of species had to embrace the fact of evolution by focusing not on invariable characteristics, but on a population's "tendency" to become a species. But in the years immediately following his studies with Paul Godet, natural history—gathering, determining, cataloging, naming, and writing—was the heart of an active and organized life, a pretext for socializing, and the occasion of moving toward broader intellectual horizons.

3

Natural History

In 1912 Piaget was portrayed as a "great mind" surrounded by a chaos of books, bottles, and dust, absorbed by his mollusk specimens, spending his nights "catching cerebral anemia, working like a madman to spread his works among the learned, scientific, and conchological journals of the globe" (PV, 25 January 1912). This portrait captures the intensity of the commitment that by then had turned Piaget into a professional naturalist.

Some of Piaget's presentations at the Club of the Friends of Nature were portions of articles (1911a, 1911b, 1914a, 1914i); what could be explained to the amateur audience of the Friends overlapped with what could appear in specialized journals. Moreover, in addition to joining the Friends of Nature in 1910, Piaget became an active member of the local Natural Sciences Society in 1912, the Swiss Zoological Society in 1913, and the Swiss Natural Sciences Society in 1914.[1]

Piaget also followed the standard practice of exchanging specimens or information with colleagues in Switzerland and abroad. A voluminous correspondence and many references in his articles demonstrate that he rapidly built a large network that included several well-known malacologists. Three Swiss naturalists became particularly important for his scientific socialization: Otto Fuhrmann, Emile Yung, and Maurice Bedot.

Otto Fuhrmann (1871–1945), from Basel, was professor at the University of Neuchâtel and Godet's successor as director of the local Museum of Natural History (Delachaux and Baer, 1944, 1945; Dubois, 1976, 58–61). He therefore knew Piaget from at least 1911; the two were collaborating at the latest by mid-1912.[2] Fuhrmann was also an honorary member of the Club of the Friends of Nature.

Fuhrmann's field of research was helminthology (the study of worms), but he also worked in comparative anatomy and hydrobiology. While studying the plankton of the lake of Neuchâtel, he gave specimens to Piaget for classification (1913b). He also asked Piaget to write the monograph that was to accompany Godet's iconographic atlas, and to examine the Colombian mollusks that Godet had planned to classify (1914b; on the monograph, Vidal, 1986b, 24–25).

Fuhrmann was one of Piaget's professors at the university from 1915 to 1918, as well as chairman of his dissertation committee. In 1912 he was president of the session during which Piaget was elected to the Neuchâtel Natural Sciences Society; together with another future teacher of Piaget at the university, he introduced him to the Swiss Zoological Society in 1913. Yet, after his scientific apprenticeship with Godet, Piaget did not become anybody else's disciple in the natural sciences. Fuhrmann did no more than help him occasionally on methodological details, send him specimens to classify, and put him in touch with other members of the profession.

Fuhrmann had been Emile Yung's assistant at the University of Geneva. Yung (1854–1918) was one of Switzerland's best-known scientists (Pictet, 1918, 1925). He was a remarkable popularizer, active in many local and foreign committees and societies, the author of widely used textbooks, and an amateur writer. Yung published on all sorts of subjects, from "cosmic dust" to anthropology, hallucinations, sleep, hypnotism, and the psychology of the snail. The work that made his reputation, however, dealt with limnology (the study of fresh waters), and in particular with the histology, anatomy, and physiology of decapods, cephalopods, and gastropods.

Yung proved to be an important figure in the young naturalist's development. Piaget (1912c, 1913d, 1913e) classified the specimens Yung collected in the deep waters of Lake Geneva, and the study of those specimens gave rise to the scientific problems on which he focused from 1912 to 1914. Yung's interests were directly related to the only work Piaget devoted to the biology of *Limnaea* (1914d). Finally, in the Swiss scientific context up to the 1930s, there is a significant continuity between the two naturalists. In an attempt to gain support for the Lamarckian hypothesis, Yung studied the effect of physical and chemical factors on inheritable anatomical modifications. Piaget's (1929a) research on the adaptation of *Limnaea* to lake environments differed from Yung's in that it employed naturalistic (rather than experimental) methods, and in that it attributed a causal role to time and to the organism's activity. Yet it also advanced a form of neo-Lamarckism.

Otto Fuhrmann's appointment at Neuchâtel had been recommended by Maurice Bedot (1859–1927), director of Geneva's Natural History Museum, professor at the university, and founder of the *Revue suisse de zoologie* (see Pictet, 1928; Revilliod, 1928). Like Yung, Bedot was interested in a vast variety of subjects: ethnology, anthropology, numismatics, music. His specialty, however, was the taxonomic, anatomical, and physiological study of coelenterates (a phylum of marine invertebrates). Moreover, he was an active organizer and administrator, earnestly devoted to the training and promotion of young zoologists.

In 1912 Piaget started corresponding with Bedot, working at the Geneva museum, and extensively borrowing books from its library. The beginning of their collaboration suggests the speed at which Piaget's career developed. Sometime in 1912 Piaget submitted a paper on alpine mollusks to Fuhrmann, who in turn sent it to Bedot; in a letter to Fuhrmann dated 4 May 1912, Bedot suggested changes, mentioned a position as assistant in malacology that might suit the paper's author, and suggested that the same author might replace Godet in preparing the section on mollusks for the general catalog of Swiss invertebrates, which he edited. Fuhrmann communicated Bedot's letter to Piaget, who, on 10 May 1912, accepted responsibility for the mollusk catalog and added: "The position of assistant in malacology you are so kind to mention would please me very much, but I cannot consider it before the end of my high school studies, that is, three years from now" (ms. 1912). In the meantime he corrected for Bedot's journal his article on alpine malacology (1913a) and started working on the catalog of Swiss mollusks (which he would not finish himself; Mermod, 1930).[3] Thus, at sixteen Piaget was being treated as a mature professional in the domain of malacological taxonomy.

Piaget's scientific precocity was accompanied by ambition and determination. In his first letter to Bedot he claimed that the lengthy and time-consuming catalogs he was being commissioned to do "can easily be carried out at the same time"; and he unhesitatingly said he would take up the position at the Geneva museum if it was still open after he finished high school: "I would quickly leave Neuchâtel for Geneva," he wrote, "where I plan to study medicine" (ms. 1912). In fact there is no external evidence to confirm such a project; but whether studying medicine was a genuine consideration or only a strategic claim, Piaget's letter embodies a remarkable self-confidence, enthusiasm, and integration in the professional world.

Piaget's relation to Godet, Fuhrmann, Yung, and Bedot also illustrates the advantages and inconveniences of a precocious scientific socialization. His public recognition, in the form of requests and publications, must have been a powerful stimulus to pursue scientific work. The work thus rewarded, however, was confined to malacological taxonomy. Whereas Fuhrmann, Yung, and Bedot were primarily laboratory scientists, Piaget always collaborated with them from outside the laboratory. He was thus prematurely driven, by a division of labor that required him to perform classificatory tasks, into the role of Godet's successor, and was given little opportunity to expand his professional horizon beyond systematics.

Adaptation and Evolution

The great variability of the mollusk shell largely determined the problems and methodology of malacological taxonomy. Piaget often accompanied the examination of variability with observations on the two factors supposed to account for it, adaptation and the influence of the environment. Since those factors were also thought to be at work in speciation and evolution, catalogs contained remarks on these topics. But such remarks were always made for purely taxonomic purposes. Piaget describes his earliest scientific activity thus: "I catalogued and studied adaptation," specifically the changes "in the shell of the *Limnaea* relative to the agitation of the water" (1977, 8). He did catalog—but adaptive change to water movement is the subject of a 1929 monograph, not of any of his early papers. When Piaget affirms that he was "formed" by the problem "of species and their indefinite adaptations as a function of the environment" (1959a, 9), he fails to mention that his goal in studying variation was classification, not a better understanding of adaptive or evolutionary mechanisms. He was not concerned with the processes of adaptation that might account for variability, but with variability itself as a topic of descriptive zoogeography, an obstacle to classification, or a means of reducing the number of species with a continuous series. In short, when Piaget identifies an essentially taxonomic problem as "that of the relations between genotypes and phenotypes" (ibid.), he describes his scientific activity anachronistically, making it look much more like biology than it really was.

Already at the very beginning of his career as naturalist, Piaget shared with Godet an interest in the phenomenon of acclimatization. This interest derived from the classifier's need to record the origins and distribution of the cataloged species. For example, in a 1910 note Piaget wondered whether two species Godet considered to have been "accidentally brought into Neuchâtel by vegetable merchants from the south of France" will acclimatize themselves to local conditions (1910b). Two years later he concluded that one of those species "may be presently considered as part of the Neuchâtel fauna, since it is definitively acclimatized" (1912b, 80). By 1913, an imported species that Piaget had discovered in 1909 was quite common in the Alps (1913a, 468–

469). From such local cases Piaget concluded that "the most recently immi-
grated species are almost always the most abundant," an observation that
turned out to be useful for the study of mollusks in other regions (1916a, 82).

The question of provenance and migration led Piaget to examine "origins,"
that is, to compare the cataloged organisms with the organisms of other regions. For example, from the European distribution of certain *Limnaea* species
of the Savoy area, he inferred that they were related to the mollusks of the
Danube basin (1913a, 179–180). Since Lake Neuchâtel had belonged to the
Danube basin (1911a, 314–315), those mollusks had a Danubian "origin."

Distribution was analyzed in terms of each species' "habitat region." Piaget
gathered mollusks at different altitudes (from lake shores to mountain
heights), and thus often devoted a portion of his catalogs to hypsometric distribution, as well as to other zoogeographical factors related to distribution
(such as geology and climate). In his dissertation (1921a), which is a malacology of the Valais, each determination is accompanied by information on geographic and hypsometric distribution, origins, habitat, and range of variation
of conchological characteristics.

Piaget's articles contain scattered remarks on the "adaptation" of organisms
to their environment. Most of them are statements of fact and tend to fore-
shadow the biometric approach he adopted in the 1920s. His early focus on
correlations between morphological variation and environmental change (for
example, between size and altitude) led him to speak of "laws" of adaptation.
Piaget's comments betray a Lamarckian position; they are not at all, however,
concerned with adaptive mechanisms, but remain squarely within the framework of systematics. Considerations of adaptation might even dictate taxonomic decisions, as when Piaget created a new variety because, although it was
not very distinct from other varieties, it lived isolated in a different milieu and
must therefore have followed "the laws of adaptation to the environment" by
acquiring new hereditary characteristics (1912c, 221). Since the environments
of the different varieties were markedly different, the organisms themselves
must be as markedly different as their habitats. He explained the presence of
Arctic mollusks in the Alps by the fact that during glaciation certain organisms
"adapted so well to the rigorous temperature, that the improvement of climate
make them flee, some toward high altitudes, others toward northern regions"
(1914h, 5). Certain species with very few varieties were for him "exceptions to
the law of variability," since their Alpine origin exempted them from adapting
to glacial conditions (1914i, 255; see 1916b, 49, for other "apparent exceptions
to the law of adaptation").

This "law" implied correlations that were empirical but not yet quantitative.
Very early, Piaget (1911e, 333) observed that "the size of certain mollusks di-

minishes greatly owing to altitude"; he later confirmed this observation in several regions (for example, 1913c). In the domain of Alpine malacology, he determined the existence of species peculiar to each climatic region (1913a). But only after his stay in Zurich in 1919 would Piaget (1920a) effectively use statistics to establish correlations.[4]

In his early taxonomic work, Piaget spoke of "evolution" in two different ways: by asserting that a particular organism has evolved, or by explaining evolution in terms of adaptation. He often affirmed, without justification, the existence of phyletic relations. His language remained vague. To say that species A "replaces" species B may mean that A "generates [*donne naissance à*]" B; thus, "the primitive type, obliged to change [*se transformer*] by certain causes, will necessarily disappear, and is replaced by [*laissant la place à*] the new variety" (1911a, 322–323). It is unclear whether or not *se transformer* has an evolutionary meaning. Even the sense of "to evolve" may be equivocal. When Piaget created the *subnaticina* variety of *Valvata piscinalis*, he described it as a *piscinalis* "evolved in the strongly flowing waters of the Areuse" (a Neuchâtel river), and compared it to the *V. naticina* of the Danube, which he characterized as a *piscinalis* "deeply transformed by its habitat" (1912b, 87). No distinction is made between speciation and adaptation.

The verb *donner* ("to give," here in the sense of "to give rise to," "originate") could also suggest evolution, as when Piaget wrote, "The *P[isidium] fossarinum* seems to have given the *P. candidum* in deep waters" (1913d, 621). Piaget offered no hint about what authorized him to conclude that one species descended from another. It is clear, however, that for him evolution resulted from direct adaptation. Thus, he noted that deep-water *Limnaea*, "forced to migrate [from shallow waters], necessarily had to adapt to their new conditions. They have shown such remarkable evolutionary flexibility that today those races support their exile very well" (1914d, 7). Another example of his Lamarckian outlook appears in his comments on the zoogeographical history of the marshy and alluvial Seeland region:

> [Terrestrial faunas] appeared and disappeared according to water fluctuations. Those animals did not have to change rapidly, because the surrounding areas offered them what they lacked in the Seeland. In contrast, water species had *to evolve* frequently and quite abruptly, because they were obliged *to adapt* to the new biological conditions, or else they would disappear.
>
> As everywhere else, this freshwater fauna was at first introduced by the rivers, and *adapted* only later to lacustrine life. [The "imperceptible transformation" of the region to a marshy state] favored . . . the *development* of certain marsh forms. The sudden increase in the water level of the lakes certainly

caused the largest changes. It is probably to this circumstance that must be attributed the *genesis* of a portion of the deep-water fauna . . . (1913g, 180; emphasis added)

Piaget assumed that direct adaptation takes place under the pressure of environmental changes. The correlation between morphological adaptation and environmental features thus explained geographic distribution and variability, and constituted a trace of the formation and evolution of species.

Biology

For Piaget, "biology" meant the "habits" that help determine an organism's adaptive reactions to the environment. The relation between environmental conditions and adaptation is circular, since habits themselves are adaptations. "Biology" retained this meaning throughout Piaget's early zoological writings.

The word *biology* usually appeared in comments accompanying classifications. The most elaborate example occurs in Piaget's revision of the classification of glacial mollusks of the Bern Natural History Museum. Each determination includes a section titled "Biol[ogy]," with observations such as: "Hygrophylic and sylvan species, lives under large humid stones, under moss and dead wood, on erratic blocs"; "the habits of this [morphologically] transitional form are intermediate between those of the two extreme types"; "Species with quite a supple biology, lives in the countryside and in woods, in humid as well as in dry places" (1914i, 216, 219, 233). To describe an organism's "biology" is to state its habitat, and thus, its "habits."

Piaget first used the word *biology* in a 1913 paper in which he declared that a certain littoral species may be found in deep water "because of its peculiar biology" (1913b, 163). He was alluding to the species' habits, since he added, "It is known that these [species] do not like to live too close to the shore." When describing the variability of a terrestrial frog, Piaget and Juvet noted that its gradually acquired habits "led it to very variable conditions of existence, and markedly different from its former, very uniform [aquatic] biology" (1913, 175). "As far as biology is concerned," they also noted, species living close to the lake "have a more aquatic inclination than those of other regions" (ibid., 185).

For Piaget, geographic distribution resulted from "physical and biological influences," consisting, respectively, of geology and climate, and "habits." The latter were "more vital" and acted in a "more delicate and detailed" manner than "purely physical" factors. Under the rubric "General Biology," for example, he wrote that "each species has its own habits; its presence or absence in a given region is determined by a very general physical setting, but it is the habits in question that regulate the detail of the habitat" (1914a, 104). Species able to live anywhere are described as having a "supple biology" (ibid., 109; see also the remark on those species' "very resistant biology," 1914i, 255, 263; and the same usage in 1916a and 1916b). "Biology," in sum, designated above all "habits," and "habits" indicated that which, apart from geological and climatic factors, determined the presence of an organism in an environment. Thus, the comparison of present-day specimens with shells found in alluvial strata could yield valuable information on "some facts resulting from each species' particular biology" (1913j, 45).

For Piaget, then, to study an organism's biology was essentially to study its habits. This he did from May to August 1913 while breeding deep-water *Limnaea* in an aquarium (1914d). Piaget's interest in such fauna and its biology is related to two elements in his scientific context.

One was that since 1912 (and at Piaget's initiative) he had classified the specimens collected by Emile Yung from his draggings in Lake Geneva.[5] Yung (as well as Fuhrmann, who gave Piaget deep-water specimens from Lake Neuchâtel) operated within an established Swiss tradition of lake studies. The existence of lacustrian deep-water fauna had been demonstrated at the end of the 1860s by the Vaudois naturalist François-Alphonse Forel (1841–1912). During the next twenty years Forel attracted numerous zoologists to the study of abyssal (deep-water) fauna and published abundantly on the topic, especially on Lake Geneva. In 1884 he published his major synthesis, *The Deep-Water Fauna of Swiss Lakes,* which became a classic and inspired further research for years to come.

In his study of *Limnaea* biology, Piaget followed the tradition inaugurated by Forel, and entered an exciting field of research of which Yung was a leading figure. At the same time, he followed the program that Yung advocated for biology as a whole. Yung (for example, 1917) deplored the excessive use of conchological characteristics in systematics; he exhorted the "young generation" to leave "those vast cemeteries, our museums," and to focus on the biological study of living organisms (Yung, 1904, 45). Piaget responded to the biologist's call, and on 18 November 1913 Yung presented to the Genevan National Institute his "Notes on the Biology of Deep-Water *Limnaea*" (1914d).

The second contextual element affecting Piaget's interest in deep-water faunas was the debate on the classification of deep-water *Limnaea* that occupied him from 1912 to 1914. The breeding of *Limnaea* enabled Piaget to confirm that abyssal organisms placed (or born) in a littoral (shallow-water) environment presented littoral morphology and habits. The research described in the "Note" aimed at elucidating the relations between abyssal and littoral *Limnaea*, in order to classify them correctly.

By the time Piaget bred *Limnaea*, he was already acquainted with the general biology of abyssal faunas. In February and March 1913 he talked to the Friends of Nature on "Animal Life in the Depths of Oceans and Our Lakes." His goal was to present "this abyssal fauna rendered so peculiar by its biological conditions" (1913i, 2): an environment that was dark, apparently poor in food, and characterized by a pressure that increased by one atmosphere every ten meters.

Piaget's presentation provided a global framework for the work he was carrying out on the materials furnished by Yung. His first article on those materials had already appeared (1912c), and "Animal Life" mentioned Yung's draggings (1913i, 18) and included biological observations. Abyssal *Limnaea* have a lung but are unable to reach the surface to breathe. Yet they adapt to their environment. How? "Nothing," Piaget answered, "could be simpler": "with an enviable good will, their lung is filled with water and keeps working as if nothing had happened. But if you take the animal out of deep water and place it in an aquarium, it will change its habits with admirable confidence, and will breathe as its shallow-water cousins do, even remaining for hours outside the water" even though it has always lived in deep waters (ibid., 20). Piaget here emphasizes vital functions, and does not even mention eventual modifications of the shell caused by the environmental change. What interests him in the quoted passage, as in the rest of his text, are the "biological conditions" (ibid., 19), or the adequacy of habits to the milieu.

The "Note on the Biology of Deep-Water *Limnaea*" shows the same orientation. "It seems interesting," Piaget wrote, "to study in an aquarium the biology of these animals . . . since they cannot be studied in nature. But we will only emphasize the points where their habits and instincts differ from those of littoral races" (1914d, 3). He thus observed that abyssal *Limnaea* are capable of pulmonate breathing, that they escape heat and sunlight, that they are not bothered by light alone, that their shell increases in size but remains typical of abyssal organisms, and that their mating periods are independent of seasons and temperature.

Piaget also reported that in an aquarium reproducing abyssal conditions, "the biology of *Limnaea Foreli* [abyssal] was entirely preserved in the new specimens [born in the aquarium] and resulted in the conservation of morphological characters" (1914d, 11). In contrast, abyssal specimens placed in littoral conditions acquired "littoral habits" and generated a shell similar to that of shallow-water *Limnaea*.

The "Note on the Biology of Deep-Water *Limnaea*" is Piaget's only laboratory research and does not mark the transformation of his scientific practice, which remained centered on morphology-based classification. The inspiration for the radical changes that take place in Piaget's projects and worldview starting in 1912 is biological—but only in the sense that it originates in a philosophy of evolution and aims at applying to all processes a certain metaphysics of life.

4

The Friends of Nature

Jean Piaget belonged to the Club of the Friends of Nature from June 1910 to September 1915, from ages fourteen to nineteen, during his last two years at the Collège Latin and throughout his time at the cantonal gymnasium. Although neither he nor any of his biographers ever mentions the Friends of Nature, the club was the center of his intellectual and social life, and remained a place he liked to return to in later life (Meystre, 1980). Piaget was deeply committed to it, and his presentations to the Friends furnish crucial elements for reconstructing his development during those years, especially his reorientation toward biological metaphysics.

In February 1910, when Piaget became a candidate for membership in the Club of the Friends of Nature, he was already called, with characteristic exaggeration, "professor of conchology" and author "of a famous dictionary" and of "many articles" (PV, 10 and 24 February 1910). In fact he had published only one malacological note, in *Le rameau de sapin* (1909); two others appeared in June, after his admission to the club. But his passion for mollusks was well known. At his "baptism" as a new Friend, it was declared that as a "[g]reat collector of shells, snails, etc., he will take the name of the snail; he is baptized 'Tardieu'" (PV, 28 September 1910). At the time, the Friends' nicknames were taken from the medieval *Roman de Renart*; Piaget's derived from Tardy the Snail.

According to the "official critique" of Piaget's first presentation at the club in June 1910, he demonstrated that the science of a pupil of the Latin school could be better than that of students in the scientific classes (Béguin, ms. 1910). Some months later, several Friends confessed that Piaget was ahead of them all: "We all agreed that, apart from a very knowledgeable conchologist, the club members are rather mediocre Friends of Nature" (PV, 13 July 1911). He was sometimes also said to be a bit pedantic. But to the charge that he used too many Latin terms, he replied that he could call shells only by their names (PV, 13 July 1911). Each year, during the club's first session, the secretary improvised some "philosophical discussions" about his peers; Piaget always survived brilliantly: "good associate secretary, perfect Toad Committee secretary, admirable conchologist; much more could still be said about him" (PV, 12 January 1911).

The Toad Committee had been established in the 1890s to study the batrachians of the canton of Neuchâtel. In 1912 it was formed again at the initiative of Gustave Juvet, another star of the club and Piaget's great friend. These two composed the new Committee and in 1914 published their researches jointly. Belonging to the committee was a proof of quality and motivation, to be recalled in relevant circumstances: "As usual, Piaget's work is well and very thoroughly done. I repeat, that is not surprising: he belongs to the Toad Committee" (PV, 27 January 1911). In every case, a piece by Piaget was "perfect in its content, perfect in its style, perfect in its length" (PV, 23 February 1911); his minutes of the club's sessions were equally "admirable." At a time when the Friends were accusing themselves of having abandoned the study of nature, one of Piaget's presentations elicited an enthusiastic comment: "His work is excellent! What can we say? It is by Piaget." His paper was found to be "splendid," but above all in accordance with "the Club's spirit: 1. it is personal; 2. it concerns the local fauna; 3. it is serious" (PV, 19 November 1914).

The Club of the Friends of Nature was the focus of an adolescent group's social life. This social life centered on intellectual preoccupations and scientific activity. The presentations made during the club's sessions were always discussed with a mixture of seriousness and mockery; the sessions themselves provided ample opportunity for songs, organizational matters (committees, outings, Christmas parties), and the reading and approval of the previous session's minutes. The minutes were almost invariably amusing, sharp, and, quite often, gently sarcastic. Even though the sessions tended to mock with exaggerated formality the rites of learned societies, they can hardly be described as purely academic. On the contrary, they allowed the Friends of Nature to socialize in an autonomous environment that operated entirely through their initiative and commitment.

Piaget contributed significantly to the club's social atmosphere. His minutes are among the funniest, and he often appeared as hilarious and uninhibited. But his essential contribution was intellectual. Since the club's inception in

1893, the Friends of Nature had presented papers outside the field of natural history and discussed philosophical, literary, or historical subjects related to the natural sciences or to science in general. But the years 1910–1915 seem to have been particularly rich in philosophical discussions, in large part because of frequent and passionate debates between Piaget and Juvet.

In 1912 the club was divided into sections. Piaget and Marcel Romy made up the malacology section; Juvet alone, the divisions of botany, and mathematics-physics-chemistry; Piaget and Juvet together formed the philosophy division (PV, 7 November 1912). A "literary section for the study of Nature in writers" was created two weeks later at Piaget's urging and despite Juvet's opposition (PV, 21 November 1912). In 1915, during a session in which both Piaget and Juvet lectured, one of the club's earliest members complained that the Friends' original ideal had not been "to philosophize," "not to do metaphysics . . . but to observe" (PV, 29 April 1915).

The status of science relative to other forms of knowledge was one of the Friends' favorite subjects. In 1913, for example, the "philosopher" Etienne Rossetti (who had been admitted to the club with a paper on "Nature in the Arts") compared scientism and pragmatism. He remarked that contemporary philosophy oscillated between those two "poles" or "tendencies," and perceived in their polemics "the anxieties and the hopes of the present moment." Rossetti's source turned out to be Abel Rey (1873–1940), the author of voluminous *Lessons of Psychology and Philosophy* widely used in French schools for preparation for the *baccalauréat*. Rossetti's "anxieties and hopes" came from Rey's popular *Modern Philosophy* (1908). Such borrowings were typical of the Friends, and document over and over their great reliance on French intellectual life.[1]

Rossetti (ms. 1913) stated that in spite of their fundamental differences, scientism and pragmatism shared the goal of "thinking science." Citing Henri Bergson and William James, he explained that, for pragmatism, science is just one particular orientation of instinct, of the "vital impulse creative of evolution," and that it is only "a technique adequate for certain needs." Pragmatism thus entailed the "failure of science as a real form of knowledge" and rehabilitated "ancient forms of human thought that scientific positivism had defeated since the eighteenth century." Everybody liked the paper, and Juvet and Piaget praised it (PV, 8 November 1913).

Rossetti's paper is interesting for three reasons. First, it dealt with debates that were at the forefront of contemporary French philosophy. In those years shortly before World War I, James and Bergson gave rise to more discussion than practically any other philosopher.

Second, Rossetti introduced one of the figures of French culture most intensely discussed among the Friends of Nature, the biologist Félix Le Dantec (1869–1917). Le Dantec was the author of a large number of books, many of them published in popular science collections. He was fanatically Lamarckian, atheist, monist, materialist, and determinist. He was widely read; and it is perhaps thanks to his peremptory and polemical style that he was so attractive to budding intellectuals. Rossetti placed him among the thinkers who helped "to chase the sterilizing specter of authority away from our thinking." Juvet was a committed disciple of Le Dantec, and Piaget spent much energy criticizing him.

Third, Rossetti's presentation highlighted the positive connotations of "scientism." Rey (1909, 478) had defined scientism as the point of view that applied "to the study of contemporary scientific thought the historical and critical methods." In spite of many individual differences, each Friend could subscribe to such a definition. None doubted that science was a valid source of knowledge: that was after all one of the club's conditions of existence.

Piaget's best friend among the Friends of Nature was Gustave Juvet (1896–1936), a future mathematician. In a tribute to Juvet, Piaget wrote that the years at the club were "happy years, when we united with passion the cults of the natural sciences . . . philosophical discussion, and friendship" (1937, 38).

Juvet was a Friend of Nature from 1912 to 1916. Very dynamic, he was with Piaget one of the club's driving forces. One of his favorite topics was the debate between Lamarckism and Darwinism, at the time very lively in France. He considered himself above all a champion of logical thinking, and often chastised the imprecision of biological language. He criticized teleological speech, claiming that it derived from man's belief in his absolute freedom, and that it was contrary to science's assumption of determinism (Juvet, ms. 1914). Biology, he maintained, must have its own language, if possible more precise than mathematics (Juvet, ms. 1915b).

Juvet's concern with determinism, teleology, and precision was largely derived from Félix Le Dantec. The mathematician Rolin Wavre (1896–1949), a longtime friend of both Juvet and Piaget, recalled that in 1913–1916 "only the title 'philosopher' seemed enviable to us; the particular sciences, no matter how enthusiastic we might be about some of them, seemed a superfluous game if they did not lead toward the synthesis we longed for of our rational, religious, and moral aspirations. Juvet, however, was more avid than the rest of us to gain positive knowledge. At the time, he did not look for it in higher mathematics, but largely in Le Dantec's chemical biologism" (Wavre 1937, 22–23; see also Reymond, 1937).

A widely read French handbook on evolutionary theories described the situation of early twentieth-century biology in the following way: "The natural selection of innate variations, or the heredity of acquired characteristics—such are the two possible solutions presently considered the essential problem of biology: to explain the general fact of adaptation . . . The heredity of acquired characteristics has thus become the crucial point, the most burning question of evolutionism" (Delage and Goldsmith, 1909, 186–187).

The opposition between Darwinism and Lamarckism was indeed a pivotal concern of French biology at the time, which leaned toward neo-Lamarckism. The very definition of the "most burning question of evolutionism" was typically French, and one of its authors, Yves Delage, was himself a prominent Lamarckian.

The neo-Lamarckian movement began in the United States in the 1860s and gained momentum in France in the late 1880s.[2] There was no formal neo-Lamarckian canon, but its adherents rejected the role of chance in the formation of species, minimized the evolutionary role of natural selection and Mendel's laws, believed in the heredity of acquired characteristics, sought the physicochemical mechanisms of variation, and focused on epigenesis.

All the Friends of Nature were firmly, if somewhat vaguely, Lamarckian. Juvet was its most articulate advocate. For him, as for Le Dantec, the hypothesis of evolution originated with Lamarck, and Darwin had not acknowledged his debt to the French naturalist. Juvet subscribed to the common Lamarckian criticism that natural selection could explain how adaptations were preserved but not how they originated. "Chance" was seen as an abomination. Juvet took one of his favorite assertions from Le Dantec: that natural selection is a "wonderful language," "very synthetic" and "very useful"—but also something obvious, worth keeping only because it can be applied "to the description of purely physical phenomena" (Juvet, ms. 1915a, 13v). Like Le Dantec, Juvet took an even more aggressive stance toward August Weismann (1834–1914) (compare Le Dantec, 1899a; and Juvet, ms. 1915a). The German cytologist's discovery of the separation between germ plasm and somatic plasm implied that the heredity of acquired characteristics was impossible—a conclusion totally unacceptable to the Lamarckians.

Juvet's Lamarckism was never contested. There are no traces, among the club's documents for 1910–1915, of a Darwinian Friend of Nature. Rossetti (ms. 1914) took for granted a certain "experimental evolutionism" that allegedly proved "that an environmental change gives rise to new and hereditary characters in individuals." Piaget never questioned Juvet's Lamarckism. But he disagreed with the materialist reductionism that his friend derived from Le Dantec.

Piaget participated in the club's sessions with readings of excerpts, original presentations, and occasional public lectures. In 1911 he read texts on mollusk embryology, the relationships between mollusks and other animals, zoological geography, and the octopus. By 1913 most of his presentations focused on philosophical aspects of science instead of on natural history per se and reveal the emergence of his Bergsonian worldview.

In 1913 a paper by Juvet on evolutionism (ms. 1913) excited everybody: Piaget, Rossetti, Romy, and Juvet alike were "seized by a furious burst of eloquence" (PV, 13 February 1913). At a certain point in the discussion Piaget compared "life to an arm plunging into a bucket of filings." This simile reveals the heart of the debate and evokes a famous dynamic image elaborated by Bergson in *Creative Evolution* to suggest how nature produced complex organic structures. Bergson asked the reader to imagine a hand going through compressed iron filings. He then speculated about the explanation an observer would give of the movement and arrangement of the filings if the hand and the arm were invisible. A mechanistic explanation would focus on the filings' composition and interactions; a teleological explanation would assume a plan presiding over the final arrangement. For Bergson (1907, 94), "the truth is that there has been merely one indivisible act, that of the hand passing through the filings," and such an act required a sui generis explanation, neither mechanistic nor teleological.

The purpose of the image was to elucidate the generation of organic form. According to Bergson (ibid., 95–96), "the relation of vision to the visual apparatus would be very nearly that of the hand to the iron filings that follow, canalize and limit its motion"; the analogy symbolized duration or life "inserting itself" into matter to create new forms—a process the philosopher called "creative evolution."

Clearly, by this time Piaget was using Bergson's ideas and vocabulary with facility. After this discussion on 13 February 1913, many sessions at the Club of the Friends of Nature focused on the friendly but fervent debate between Piaget and Juvet, the one supporting the philosophy of the *élan vital* and the other supporting mechanistic reductionism.

In May 1913, when Juvet read some passages from Le Dantec, Piaget was said to crave "to start all over again the legendary discussion of the fist in a box of filings" (PV, 8 May 1913). The debate was revived that October, when Piaget read "some fragments of Bergson's *Creative Evolution* against the mechanists, whom he disrespectfully call[ed] 'the new scholastics,' and against finalists"—fragments Juvet considered a "pure example of teleological style and scholastic idioms" (PV, 9 October 1913). In October 1914 Piaget read passages on "the genesis of thought from the biological point of view" by the French philosopher Alfred Fouillée (1838–1912). Fouillée (1890, 279) believed that mental states were "factors of evolution as much as purely mechanical factors." Once again, Juvet disagreed (PV, 22 October 1914).

At the celebration of the club's 400th session in 1915, Juvet read "The Neo-Darwinian Trend in Biology," and Piaget, "Biology and Philosophy." Juvet himself wrote the minutes of that "splendid, magnificent, idyllic, erotic, comical" session. Juvet found Piaget's presentation "a good paper, scientific, philosophical, etc., etc., but delivered with the help of grand words such as 'determinism,' 'bursting reality,' etc., etc." He was "very far from approving the personal conclusions of the lecturer, metaphysical and transcendental conclusions, based on Bergsonism and Piagetism, two philosophies that will perhaps lead the world for some time, but will finish in hell or in a junkyard" (PV, 29 April 1915).

The manuscript of "Biology and Philosophy" has not been found. It is clear, however, that Piaget's speech was yet another defense of Bergsonism—to the point of bearing the same title as a section of the first chapter of *Creative Evolution* where Bergson explains why neither mechanism nor teleology is an adequate approach to the study of life. This convergence illustrates Piaget's singular position among the Friends of Nature. He certainly believed in science as a form of knowledge; he was, after all, the only Friend who attained professional status within a scientific community. At the same time, however, he seems to have been the only strict partisan of a philosophy in which the other Friends tended to see, as Juvet would have put it, purely metaphysical and transcendental attitudes, and even the negation of science. Against the surrounding scientism and mechanism, Piaget affirmed himself as a Bergsonian. Like the other Friends, he proclaimed his rejection of Darwinism and other non-Lamarckian trends of modern biology. But the grounds for his rejection proceeded largely from Bergson's philosophy.

5

Piaget Discovers Bergson

The Vanity of Nomenclature," presented in September 1912, is Piaget's earliest extant synthesis of natural history and Bergsonian philosophy. That synthesis, which eventually extended to religious and social matters, must be traced to his first involvement with Bergson's thought. The circumstances in which he first encountered Bergson's ideas illuminate both Piaget's initial reaction and the path that he subsequently followed.

According to Piaget's autobiography, he first became acquainted with Bergson's thought after undergoing a course of religious instruction (in 1912) and reading the Protestant theologian Auguste Sabatier (see Chapter 9). Piaget's initial reaction to Bergson, as well as his first philosophical publication ("Bergson and Sabatier," 1914), suggests that such was indeed the sequence of events. His autobiographical novel, *Recherche* (1918a, 95), offers contradictory testimony. On the one hand, it implies that his introduction to philosophy took place about a year earlier: Sebastian, the protagonist, recalls that he was "aged fifteen" when philosophy "took hold of his being." In Piaget's life, this corresponds to 1911. But at this time Piaget was just starting to publish independently in the natural sciences, and he had not yet undertaken religious instruction. On the other hand, Sebastian also claims to have discovered philosophy "four years earlier" (ibid.). If we count backward from the time of the novel's composition, September 1916–January 1917, we arrive at 1912. Relying on these autobiographical hints, we can assume that Piaget discovered Bergson at the latest in July or August 1912.

In this, as in the rest of what concerns Piaget's discovery of Bergson, we are still largely indebted to the autobiography. Piaget recalls that one summer his godfather Samuel Cornut invited him to spend the holidays with him at Lake

Annecy (in French Savoy, close to Geneva). Piaget kept "a delightful memory of that visit: We walked and fished, I looked for mollusks and wrote a 'malacology of Lake Annecy,' which I published shortly afterward" (1952, 240).

According to Mme. Marthe Burger, Jean Piaget's sister, Piaget and his godfather were very close. They often went for walks together, and Cornut was one of the first persons with whom the youngster had long conversations. Piaget recalled that there was a purpose behind his godfather's invitation:

> He found me too specialized and wanted to teach me philosophy. Between the gatherings of mollusks he would teach me the "creative evolution" of Bergson. (It was only afterwards that he sent me that work as a souvenir.) It was the first time that I heard philosophy discussed by anyone not a theologian; the shock was terrific, I must admit.
>
> First of all, it was an emotional shock. I recall one evening of profound revelation. The identification of God with life itself was an idea that stirred me almost to ecstasy because it now enabled me to see in biology the explanation of all things and of the mind itself.
>
> In the second place, it was an intellectual shock. The problem of knowing (properly called the epistemological problem) suddenly appeared to me in an entirely new perspective and as an absorbing topic of study. It made me decide to consecrate my life to the biological explanation of knowledge. (1952, 240)

In another autobiographical text, Piaget (1959a, 9) remembers having been "seized by the demon of reflection, and focusing it almost immediately on the problem of knowledge." A third narrative adds another element to this "tremendous experience":

> in a moment of enthusiasm close to ecstatic joy, I was struck by the certainty that God is Life itself, under the form of the *élan vital,* of which my biological interests provided me at the same time with a small sector of study . . .
>
> On returning to school, my decision was made: I would devote my life to philosophy, whose central aim I saw as the reconciliation between science on the one hand, and religious values on the other. (1965, 5)

The religious overtones of his philosophical initiation are neither elaborated elsewhere in Piaget's autobiographical accounts nor considered essential by his commentators. Yet Piaget's initial reaction to Bergson clearly had an important religious dimension. The idea that dogmas evolved formed part of his religious background. But the particular mystical and enthusiastic quality of his response cannot be explained solely by that background. The figure of Cornut, whom Piaget (1959a, 9) described as "a *littérateur* enamored of general ideas," furnishes some important clues.

Samuel Cornut

Samuel Cornut (1861–1918) was born in the canton of Vaud, the son of a wine grower. He attended the classical gymnasium, did a thesis on Racine, and became a writer. In 1886 he settled in Paris, where he taught French literature; but he remained deeply attached to his native country, returning there for two months each year and frequently collaborating with local journals and magazines. His best friends were French-speaking Swiss artists and intellectuals, and his themes and style were familiar to a cultivated Swiss-French Protestant audience.

Cornut has been described as "impressionable, susceptible, prone to depression . . . very timid and incapable of managing in the world," but inclined to embark on generous crusades (Berchtold, 1963, 431); and as a melancholy, worried, enthusiastic and naive idealist living "in his dreams as in an ivory tower" (Brenner, 1929, 11). Arthur Piaget was his "intimate friend" (ibid., 14).

An essay titled "Peace!" (and dedicated to Arthur Piaget) provides a good example of the causes Cornut espoused. For him, most pacifists were hypocrites; and those who thought that peace would come from science were blind to the then-prevailing opposition between French and German science. "Laziness, egoism, cowardly discouragement lie hidden beneath the peace of thousands of families" (Cornut, 1910, 166): that was for him the "lie of peace," which he wished to combat by a revival of the will.

Cornut's emphasis on individual will was consistent with his religious attitude. He was a committed Protestant and a profoundly religious man, but his religion had neither church nor theology. His path was that of a "solitary consciousness . . . intimately linked to the living things of Creation" (Berchtold, 1963, 432).

Many of Cornut's writings are inspired by a vitalism that led him to celebrate what he called "joys without a cause"—without a cause because "they emerge spontaneously from life, from a life that perceives itself in its pure essence": "To live and to feel oneself live, that is the whole secret of happiness" (Cornut, 1910, 83). In the same spirit, he wrote a "Eulogy of Stupidity" in which he claimed that "to be intelligent is to forsake the great universal harmony" (ibid., 27). He believed that a future humanity would eliminate the limits "between matter and spirit, soul and body, man and animal, man and God. Everything is full of life, therefore, of soul; therefore, everything is full of joy" (ibid., 88). Such statements are unmistakably sympathetic to the philosophy of creative evolution and the *élan vital*.

Cornut's goal of expanding his godson's horizon was consistent with his belief that "at fifteen, we are as large as the world; our soul is vast; we are a poet, explorer, soldier, inventor, all at the same time" (ibid., 151). Youth was for him a "volcanic age" that "struggles in convulsions more resembling the painful becoming of a certain something that longs to be born, than to the action of somebody who is, knows, and wants" (Cornut, 1903, 153). Whereas in 1912 the prematurely professionalized Piaget was far from Cornut's ideal adolescent, by 1915 he had become a living image of his godfather's literary young man.

It is of course impossible to determine exactly how Cornut communicated Bergson to the young Piaget. Yet it is plausible that his teaching was consistent with the content of his writings: a mystical inclination, a vague mixture of pantheism and vitalism, a feverish and messianic tone, all concurring to exalt the feeling of communion with a creative nature. The version of Bergson that Piaget initially encountered might have been philosophically impoverished, but made especially exhilarating through mystical and pantheistic overtones. Nor was this solely a consequence of Cornut's temperament, for, as Bergson's critics never failed to stress, *Creative Evolution* lends itself easily to irrationalist or anti-intellectualist readings.

Henri Bergson

Henri Bergson (1859–1941) was the foremost French philosopher of his day.[1] In 1900 he became a professor at the Collège de France. His 1907 *Creative Evolution* generated much passionate debate among philosophers, made him familiar to a vast unspecialized audience, and marked the high point of his glory. In 1917 the French government charged him with the task of convincing the United States government to enter the war. In the interwar years he was involved in efforts to promote international peace through intellectual cooperation. Over the years Bergson, who was Jewish, came closer and closer to Catholic dogma in his views. Nevertheless, anticipating the development of anti-Semitism and wishing, as he wrote in his will, "to stay among those who shall be the persecuted of tomorrow," he chose not to convert (quoted in Béguin and Thévenaz, 1943, 11–12). At the end of his life, after the promulgation of racial laws by the Vichy government, he refused to be exempted by the régime and resigned all his honorary offices. According to some newspaper reports, a few weeks before his death on 4 January 1941 he left his sickbed and, aided by a servant, stood in line to be registered as a Jew.

In 1927 Bergson received the Nobel Prize for literature; on the whole, but particularly in *Creative Evolution,* his philosophy is inseparable from the non-technical, fluent, and elegantly imaged style in which it is couched. Calling Bergson "a magician," William James ecstatically compared his book's "after-taste" to that of *Madame Bovary* and spoke of its "flavor of persistent *euphony*" (in H. James, 1920, 2:290–291). For Julian Benda (1913, 34), on the contrary, this "pathetic philosophy" was merely a collection of gratuitous, unfounded, self-contradictory, and peremptory assertions. Most reactions to Bergson tended to be that extreme: his style and ideas either delighted or repulsed; they seemed to represent philosophy par excellence, or to be no philosophy at all.

Bergson's central concept is *durée,* duration. This term is intended as a con-trast to the notion of time used by the natural and physical sciences. On the one hand, the determinism of the sciences implies that every event unfolds preexisting conditions; on the other hand, scientific time is divisible, quantifiable—in short, a spatialized abstract construct. Duration, in contrast, is a continuous, irreversible, indivisible "flow." Time may be useful for under-standing matter; life, however, must be understood through duration.

For Bergson, life is a creative process that incessantly produces something new and unpredictable. It is thus endowed with the same essential features as *durée* in the form of a "vital impulse" *(élan vital).* Contrary to time, which we conceptualize on the basis of movement and represent by spatial images, dura-tion is possible only through memory; it is a process we know intuitively, from direct and immediate experience, not unlike William James's "stream of con-sciousness." As Bergson (1972, 1194) pointed out in a 1915 letter, "stream" and "duration" are in harmony, and differ mainly in their origins and explica-tive functions, the former psychological, and the latter epistemological or metaphysical.

The methodological parallel of Bergson's opposition between time and du-ration, matter and life, lies in the contrast between the analytical operations of the intellect, and "intuition," the nonconceptual operation whereby we grasp duration. Intuition, "the direct vision of mind by mind" (Bergson, 1934, 1273), is concerned mainly with "inner duration." Bergson identifies life with duration, and since the nature of the latter is psychological, "the evolution of the universe displays mind-like properties" (Kolakowski, 1985, 3). Matter is the proper domain of application of intelligence and science, life that of intu-ition and metaphysics. As long as each cognitive mode stays within its bounds, it is capable of knowing reality absolutely and in itself.

Bergson's partisans, and even some of his critics, considered his philosophy as a liberation from materialistic determinism, positivism, scientism, and such grand nineteenth-century systems as Auguste Comte's and Herbert Spencer's;

in France, it was also a welcome alternative to Kantian criticism and to the method-driven teaching that prevailed at the Sorbonne (Bergson was never a university professor). Bergson consistently thought in terms of a critique of existing philosophies: *Time and Free Will: An Essay on the Immediate Data of Consciousness* (1889) was written against associationist psychology, *Matter and Memory* (1896) against the materialist theory of mind, *Creative Evolution* (1907) against the "mechanistic" theory of evolution, and *The Two Sources of Morality and Religion* (1932) against the purely sociological interpretation of religion. Paul Valéry, who did not think highly of professional philosophy in general, noted that instead of renewing the problems (in his view, philosophy's most urgent need), Bergson responded in his own manner to the traditional questions: "He asked questions like a professor and answered—like a poet" (Valéry, 1930–31, 1:656).

Of Bergson's several books, only *Creative Evolution* made a direct major impression on the young Piaget—and a far less dissatisfying one than he later suggested. In *Recherche*, Sebastian looks back at the consequences of his discovery of philosophy. As he felt for the first time "the desire of the absolute," he contemplated "the illusions he had taken for the ultimate truth" and saw "the petty, hasty cadres" of his works in natural history collapse, dragged along by "the impulse of life, by the turns of an endless becoming" (1918a, 95). This vocabulary suggests the strength of the Bergsonian shock. And indeed, Piaget's first explorations outside the realm of malacological taxonomy were directly related to Bergson's philosophy and concerned, as *Recherche* also mentions (ibid., 96), the problem of the species. Starting at the latest in the summer of 1912, Piaget dealt with the ontological assumptions about taxonomic categories, the origin of adaptations, and the mechanisms of the formation and evolution of species. In all three cases, he elaborated a viewpoint in which Bergsonian philosophy and epistemology played a central role.

6

Natural History and Creative Evolution

In *Insights and Illusions of Philosophy,* Piaget underlines the significance of his adherence to the Bergsonian distinction between the vital and the mathematical: "Deeply interested in biology as I was, but understanding nothing of mathematics, physics, nor the logical reasoning they presuppose, I was fascinated by the dualism of the *élan vital* and of matter . . . or by that of the intuition of duration and of intelligence unable to understand life because its logical and mathematical structures are oriented in the direction of inert matter" (1965, 5). The most common image of his relation to Bergson comes from autobiographical recollections of his dissatisfaction with *Creative Evolution*'s unscientific character and of his decision to construct a biological theory of knowledge (1952, 240; 1959a, 9; 1959b, 44). More accurate, however, is his memory of having seen in his zoological interests "a small sector of study" of creative evolution (1965, 5).

Nominalism

Piaget's starting point was the problem of the species. As he asserted in "The Vanity of Nomenclature," a lecture he delivered in September 1912, if species are constantly evolving, if, "as Bergson says," it is "superficial to break up the flux of life" (1912a, 99), then the taxonomic notion of species is a useful and practical, but totally artificial, convention. To believe that such a concept corresponds to a stable reality of nature is nothing other than an expression of the nomenclator's vanity. In declaring the "immense importance of clearly establishing that the idea of species is a mere procedure" (ibid., 102), Piaget re-

mained a nominalist. But instead of basing nominalism on practical considerations of variation alone, as he and his colleagues had always done, he argued
for it with the help of Bergson's philosophy.

Variability and the existence of continuous series seemed to contradict the
idea that species have clearly defined natural boundaries. So did the fact that
species evolve. This evolutionary nominalism could take one of two forms.
The first one is based on the continuous variability of fossil specimens. Darwin
(1859, 485) had explained that "the only distinction between species and well-
marked varieties is, that the latter are known, or believed, to be connected at
the present day by intermediate gradations, whereas species were formerly
thus connected." Thus, for example, when Piaget could establish with fossil
specimens a continuous series between two modern species thought to be distinct, he chose to lump them together, just as he would if he had established
the series with modern specimens. The species were united because they were
presumed to be variations of a single ancestor. Yet the lumping together was
actually determined not by a demonstration of common descent, but by morphological continuity.

The second sort of evolutionary nominalism is much more radical and does
not require discovery of continuous series in the fossil record. It is based exclusively on the existence of evolution. "If the species is not immutable," Piaget
asked (1912a, 100), "where does it begin? How can it be delimited in the flux
of evolution?" Arbitrarily: "I believe that the specific unit [the species as cate-
gory] is a utopia. There is no more reality in a species than in the geographer's
meridians and parallels" (ibid., 99). In other words, no division of the continuous flow of evolution can possibly correspond to a reality that exists independently of the concept naming it.

In "The Vanity of Nomenclature" Piaget developed the arguments that,
some months later, enabled him to maintain that "if evolution is accepted,
then the notion of the species does not stand up" (1913f, 127). The question
Piaget asked in 1912 was whether taxonomic categories existed, or whether
they were "mere words" (1912a, 95). This question had immediate relevance
for his work. Its practical significance, Piaget explained, came from the fact
that certain "maniacs" were possessed by a "sick and pernicious passion" that
made them create new species indiscriminately, on the basis of the tiniest morphological difference. Perhaps, he ventured, such naturalists would be dis-
couraged if they knew that the species "is just a method" (ibid., 102–103).

Piaget also intuited a link between taxonomy and evolution. A classification
with many species, he said, gives the impression "that the species is totally unstable," and therefore implies the occurrence of rapid speciation. On the contrary, a classification that contains fewer species (and proportionally more va-

rieties) implies the existence "of a matter whose specific unity, relatively stable, is extremely variable but evolves in an infinitely slow yet uninterrupted manner" (ibid., 98). Piaget, however, was not sure whether evolutionary theory governed taxonomic systems, or the other way around. In the manuscript of "The Vanity," the whole passage where he deduces notions of evolution from classifications is marked with a long square bracket, accompanied by the remark "not clear." The confusion thus revealed accompanied Piaget's discovery of a new dimension to his own scientific activity. A conception of nature based on the language, methods, and problems of zoological classification was being replaced by a grander vision of evolution. Nominalism was their common denominator.

Just as Piaget wondered about the intellectual operation whereby specific characters are chosen—"weigh, establish, assess??" (ibid., 103)—he hesitated about the exact status of classification. "Definitions have been established that were excellent at the time they were made, but that . . . are not and can no longer be accurate" (ibid., 101). In the manuscript, "definitions" is underlined and accompanied by a question mark; "distinctions" is written just above it. The hesitation between the "definition" and "distinction" is not a matter of style: it signifies the difference between what is conventional and what is natural.

Similarly, when Piaget was about to explain why a morphological characteristic is "not practical in the method of nomenclature" (ibid., 103), he underlined the quoted words, placed two question marks on the adjacent margin, and finally changed the phrase into "not practical for the method that is nomenclature." Whether taxonomy *is* a method or *has* a method depended on a global conception that the young Piaget was still elaborating.

In spite of his doubts, Piaget clearly asserted a radical evolutionary nominalism: "I believe that the specific unit is a utopia . . . You think that there is some reality in present-day differences among species, without suspecting that you observe matter for just an instant" or realizing that species cannot be defined "on the basis of a minute part of an evolution that has never stopped, and never will" (ibid., 99). Since evolutionary time is not naturally divisible, science interrupts it artificially, thus retrieving mere fragments of it. Such a time is "duration," the basic concept of Bergson's philosophy, and the cornerstone of his critique of science.

In *Creative Evolution* Bergson contrasts life, defined as duration, evolution, and constant creation, to matter, characterized as inert and as an obstacle to the *élan vital*. Duration is for him the substance of life both in the universe and in the individual's mind.

Two modes of knowledge correspond to life and matter: to life, intuition, the method of Bergsonian metaphysics, a "direct vision" capable of appre-hending duration and evolution "from the inside," as totalities, without parti-tioning them through spatial analogies or the tools of mathematics; to matter, analysis, the method of science, aimed at breaking into segments the continu-ous flow of reality. By means of intuition, Bergson said, it is possible to "place oneself within duration and apprehend reality through the mobility that con-stitutes its essence"; "a truly intuitive metaphysics . . . would follow the undu-lations of the real" (Bergson, 1934, 1272). Knowledge of life thus proceeds from a communion with it, from a "sympathy" made possible by the identity of *durée* at the psychological and the evolutionary levels.

Bergson's considerations on the common essence of human psychology and organic evolution tie in with his insight that a theory of knowledge and a the-ory of life are inseparable. "A theory of life that is not accompanied by a criti-cism of knowledge is obliged to accept, as they stand, the concepts which the understanding puts at its disposal . . . It thus obtains a symbolism which is convenient, perhaps even necessary to positive science, but not a direct vision of its object. On the other hand, a theory of knowledge that does not replace the intellect in the general evolution of life will teach us neither how the frames of knowledge have been constructed nor how we can enlarge or go beyond them" (Bergson, 1907, xiii). Adoption of this Bergsonian perspective was the starting point of Piaget's epistemological project.

Piaget addressed his audience in dynamic images of Bergsonian inspiration:

> Imagine a straight line on which the points A, B, C, D, E, F are spread out. If you throw a ball along this line, you will find it impossible to say that the ball is at A, at B, at C. Right when you say it, it is no longer true; it is thus just as superficial to segment the flux of life, as Bergson says; and human analysis is no more than a procedure, a method, and rests on nothing. You believe that the matter which flows, slowly pushed by life, is more stable than the ball that goes from A to F. But how can you prove it, poor creatures of one moment? What is the minute abscissae of human science in the immense evolution that goes from $-\infty$ to $+\infty$? . . . Please tell me, what difference is there between fifty generations of ephemera studying a human individual, and fifty generations of men studying a species? (1912a, 99)

Piaget had initially written "arrow" instead of "ball," a word that would have more clearly revealed his debt to Bergson's analysis of Zeno's arguments against motion. Bergson examined those arguments in several works; in *Creative Evolution* he focused on the arrow paradox alone.

Zeno of Elea, a pupil of Parmenides, claimed that motion at a continuous straight line is impossible, since an object that is motionless at each point of its course is necessarily motionless during all the time that it is supposed to be moving. Bergson obviously did not concur with Zeno's conclusion, but saw in it an expression of the basic illusions of human intelligence, the assumption "that the arrow can ever *be* in a point of its course" (Bergson, 1907, 308). The course of the arrow, on the contrary, is like the extension of an elastic stretched from A to B: "To suppose that the moving body *is* at a point of its course," therefore, "is to cut the course in two by a snip of the scissors at this point" (ibid., 309). It was for the purpose of making a Bergsonian argument that Piaget asked his audience to imagine a straight line along which a ball is thrown.

Piaget further formulated the central point of his defense of nominalism by combining the image of an immense flow of evolving life with a familiar sophism:

> If the species is not immutable, where does it begin? How is it to be delimited in the flux of evolution? Where can the invariable characteristics be found? Or, if all are variable, in what lapse of time should they be considered? If you proceed thus, from analysis to synthesis, you will rapidly conclude that there are only two things on earth, life and matter. Nevertheless, if, as Bergson says, such a method [synthesis] has to be followed to penetrate the secret of life, on the contrary, only analysis is effective to arrive at a complete knowledge of matter. This has led the human genius to establish a whole system of nomenclature, an admirable system if you will, but a system anyway, that is, something essentially abstract, purely artificial, and therefore without any intrinsic value. (1912a, 100–101)

As in Bergsonian epistemology, scientific analysis is the instrument for knowing matter, but not life. Patterning his argument after Bergson's, Piaget went from considering life as duration, to the critical notion that science is incapable of adequately apprehending duration, and therefore, of understanding life.

Piaget, however, did not mention intuition, Bergson's method for the study of life, but spoke of proceeding "from analysis to synthesis." To the extent that synthesis allows one to penetrate the "secret of life," it must be made to stand for intuition. This reading, which is supported by Piaget's later characterization of intuition as a "*synthesis* of intelligence and instinct" (1918a, 50; emphasis added), confirms his dissatisfaction with Bergson's elusive methodology.

In *Recherche*, Piaget presents Sebastian as thinking that intuition is either a nonlogical incommunicable "vision" (and the intuitive philosopher, a mystic) or merely a "broadening of reason" (1918a, 50). Duration appears to him a self-destructive notion: for if no two instants are identical, then duration is nothing at all; if there is no duration outside the mind, then the mind itself could cease to last, or at least hope to do without time (ibid., 52, 53). In short, "Sebastian, who had always been enthusiastic about Bergsonism, did not admit any of its particular theses, while believing that he continued it in accordance with its underlying logic. He was Bergsonian without duration" (ibid., 53). While Piaget never used the term *intuition* in Bergson's sense, and reserved *duration* for use as a metaphysical rendering of geological time, his biological thought of the years 1912–1914 returns incessantly to the *logique profonde* of Bergsonian philosophy.

Mimicry

One of Piaget's first papers at the Club of the Friends of Nature consisted of observations on the mimicry of Neuchâtel mollusks (1911d). It was in addressing this topic that Piaget first dealt with adaptation and evolution outside the framework of taxonomy. From 1911 to 1914, his treatment of the subject changed significantly. In 1911 Piaget approached theories negatively, as something to be mistrusted. Three years later, the interest of mimicry would reside entirely in its import for theories of evolution and adaptation. Such a development is closely related to Piaget's discovery of Bergson. At the time, mimicry was still a favorite illustration of the Darwinian theory of natural selection; it thus provided the perfect opportunity for advocating a countertheory based on the biological epistemology of creative evolution.

During the second half of the nineteenth century, mimicry became an ideal testing ground for evolutionary biology. In 1861 the British entomologist Henry Walter Bates (1825–1892), on the basis of extensive research on butterflies of the Amazon valley, demonstrated that mimicry could be explained by the theory of natural selection. The species whose form, odor, or taste least resembled those of species protected by those features were gradually eliminated by predators; the species that deceived predators through similitude with protected species survived. Several other naturalists, including Bates's friend and codiscoverer of natural selection, Alfred Russel Wallace (1823–1913), further elaborated the subject of mimicry as a demonstration of Darwinian evolutionary mechanisms. (See Blaisdell, 1992.) Although natural selection was not the only explanation of mimicry, it was the favorite theory, even among French Lamarckians (Conry, 1974).

The main challenge to the selectionist explanation of mimicry came from the emerging field of genetics and the theory of mutations (Kimler, 1983). For Darwinism, mimetic similarity resulted from the gradual accumulation of small variations under the effect of natural selection. For mutationism, it was the outcome of a sudden mutation, and only its conservation was due to natural selection.

Piaget's discussions of mimicry show no awareness of the (then very new) mutationist alternative. In 1911 he listed different ways in which an organism effected mimicry: by adaptation to the environment's color; by addition of foreign objects (for example, of pebbles to the surface of a shell); by the use of natural secretions; by similarity with other animals' form or attitude. The source given was an article from *La grande encyclopédie,* one of the Friends' favorite references, by Edouard-Louis Trouessart (1842–1927), professor at the Paris Museum of Natural History, who admitted the explanation of mimicry by natural selection.

Thus, even if briefly, Piaget was acquainted with the most widely accepted theory of mimicry. Nevertheless, instead of borrowing from the theoretical section of Trouessart's article, he referred to it only to issue a warning: "We must remember that the ideas presented are only human theories, based on very few facts, and that, for mollusks in particular, there are very few observations, or none at all. We must therefore beware of drawing conclusions too quickly" (1911d, 3). Piaget's focus on facts was typical of his early papers. But the case of mimicry was special because it lent support to the Darwinian theory. Piaget's Lamarckian preferences prescribed exceptional prudence and influenced even his questions about the phenomenon: "Do the nature and color of the bottom [of the lake] influence *Limnaea*'s color and shell to the same degree that they influence the shell's form and thickness? . . . Very wonderful theories about mimicry have been developed, but one should not misuse them, and in particular not jump to conclusions. I will therefore limit myself to ascertaining facts" (1911a, 317). Since the "wonderful theories" were Darwinian, they could only give rise to suspicion; and it is indicative of Piaget's education that they would do so at the very beginning of his precocious career.

The 1911 "Observations" (1911d) focused on the convergence between the colors of the environment and the organisms. Piaget established a rule according to which species that live in the shade are dark, whereas those that live under the sun are light. Like variation in general, mimicry was assumed to be a direct adaptation of the organism to the environment. But what exactly did Piaget mean by "adaptation"?

Piaget's descriptions often suggest that the notion of will entered into his understanding of adaptation. Expressions from his earliest papers, such as that certain mollusks "adopt the color" of certain leaves or that others "hide themselves in the midst of dry herbs whose shadows resemble their streaks" (1911d, 4) are perhaps best understood as figures of speech. The metaphorical interpretation, however, is less applicable to the texts that followed his Bergsonian initiation.

After finding a shell under small lumps of dry mud, Piaget wrote that it "presents a good example of mimicry by addition—albeit involuntary!—of foreign objects" (1913c, 85). He used the same language in other contexts: one species "chooses residence where the physical conditions are satisfactory" (1914a, 113); another arrives at the bottom of the lake "by the power of factors independent of [its] will" (1914d, 1, 6); yet others "are obliged to be very shrewd in their choice of habitat" (1916b, 15) or "profit from the slightest advantage" (1916a, 77). A 1913 article on mimicry in marine mollusks demonstrates that Piaget did not mean to imply the existence of a true will of mollusks, but rather to highlight the active role played by organisms in their adaptation to the environment.

Probably because mimicry seemed to lend such strong support to the theory of natural selection, Piaget chose not to enter the theoretical debate right away. In his 1913 article on the subject he accepted natural selection but minimized its evolutionary significance. Thus, he warned that mimicry "has become a sort of deus ex machina in all kinds of biological problems," and that it was therefore necessary to give up "philosophical imagination" and stick to observation alone (1913h, 127). In fact Piaget's warning was just the opening of a critique of Darwinian mechanisms largely inspired by Bergsonian philosophy.

From the beginning of his text, Piaget revealed his orientation by saying that mimicry "doubtless should not be considered as a quest or tendency of every living being, but as an entirely passive consequence of adaptation" (ibid.). The examples he gave (protective coloration, similarity between animals and plants, stones, or other animals) were all "passive" results of natural selection and the "struggle for life" (ibid., 133). Thus,

> a *Dixipus morosus,* an Oriental insect that resembles a piece of wood, will not choose its residence among twigs and branches because it knows it resembles them. On the contrary, it must be admitted that much more polymorphous *Dixipus* were formerly scattered everywhere, but that, in the struggle for life, all were destroyed except those that resembled dry wood and lived precisely in that environment, and were thus protected without the assistance of their will. In other words, these animals' evolution has been directed by the force of things to the point where we see it today, and we are tempted to consider [it] as the result of a mimetic t e n d e n c y. (Ibid., 128)[1]

Not only morphological characters but also defensive habits develop "by the same passive means of natural selection . . . independently of the animal's will or instinct" (ibid., 132–133).

Piaget emphasized that "all those results are purely passive," claimed to know only one case "in which the nervous system of the animal plays some role," and thought mimicry could be understood by observing "the conditions into which, so to say, the current of evolution was channeled"—it "must be studied as a result, and not as a tendency" (ibid., 129).

Piaget attributed a limited role to Darwinian evolutionary mechanisms. It is not obvious whether he thought of Darwinism or spoke figuratively when he wrote, for example, that certain species "were forced to high regions by climatic modification, or by competition from recent animal invasions" (1914a, 107; see also 1914k, 135). The core of his thinking was expressed in comments such as: "As to the ultimate reason that determines . . . the difference between resistant and weaker forms, it remains absolutely enigmatic. Neither selection nor the struggle for life will enable us to understand such facts" (1914i, 253). Mimicry, then, was for Piaget a purely passive and foreseeable result of natural selection—one of those factors with which external conditions may restrain the evolutionary current. Much more interesting for him were the unpredictable, and therefore creative, adaptations that depended on the instincts and the will, and thus expressed true evolutionary tendencies.

The dichotomy between active and passive adaptation was consistent with neo-Lamarckism, and could conceivably be an echo of Le Dantec's (1899b) distinction between two types of resemblance: "imitation," obtained with some participation of the will, and mimicry, which was completely involuntary. Piaget's vocabulary, however, manifests above all a debt to Bergson's philosophy.

In the philosophy of creative evolution, the *élan vital* is a tendency toward differentiation, toward the perpetual realization of life's potentialities against the obstacle of matter. Bergson writes, for example, that "everything bears out the belief that vegetable and animal are descended from a common ancestor which united the *tendencies* of both in a rudimentary state"; "the same impetus that has led the animal to give itself nerves and nervous centers must have ended in the plant, in the chlorophyllian function" (Bergson, 1907, 113, 114; emphasis added). Like Bergson, Piaget did not think that the mechanistic theory of natural selection was false. It applied to certain natural phenomena (mimicry), but it was insufficient to explain more elaborate adaptations or the formation of new species.

The contrast between passive and active adaptation is purely Bergsonian. In *Creative Evolution* Bergson (ibid., 70) distinguished two senses of adaptation. One designates the "gradual complication of a form which is being better and better adapted to the mold of outward circumstances," in which case "matter merely receives an imprint." The other implies that "the increasingly complex structure of an instrument [such as the eye] . . . derives more and more advantage from these circumstances," in which case matter "reacts positively, it solves a problem." "Obviously," Bergson remarks, "it is this second sense of the word 'adapt' that is used when one says that the eye has become better and better adapted to the influence of light." But the ambiguity of the word may give rise to confusion: "one passes more or less unconsciously from this sense to the other, and a purely mechanistic biology will strive to make the *passive* adaptation of an inert matter, which submits to the influence of its environment, mean the same as the active adaptation of an organism which derives from this influence an advantage it can appropriate." In his 1913 discussion of mimicry, Piaget was clearly thinking in terms of the Bergsonian dichotomy between passive and active adaptation; and that is where we ought to see the roots of one of the main themes of his mature thought.

As for the role of will and instinct, Bergson maintained that an organism's life was an "effort" to obtain something from inert matter; instinct and intelligence were for him two different modes of action on matter. Neo-Lamarckism was to be preferred to other sorts of evolutionary theory because it was "the only one capable of admitting an internal and psychological principle of development" (ibid., 77), that is, an "effort" to adapt to the environment—the will and instincts Piaget could not find in mimicry—and an internal tendency to evolve in a certain direction.

"The Vanity of Nomenclature" illustrates how Piaget transformed his instrumental taxonomic nominalism into a radical evolutionary nominalism of Bergsonian inspiration. Similarly, his work on mimicry shows how, while abandoning neither empirical research nor the norms of scientific style (not once is Bergson mentioned in his zoological publications), Piaget introduced a whole philosophy into his scientific concerns. Like other Lamarckians, he undertook to explain mimicry by natural selection, but highlighted the exceptional character of the case. His position, however, was unusual in that it set against natural selection an alternative directly inspired by the philosophy of creative evolution and *élan vital*; indeed, it was unique, since it has now been convincingly demonstrated that Bergson did not play a major role in the resistance of French biologists to either Darwinism or genetics (Burian et al., 1988).

Isolation

Piaget asserted that only an adaptation that persisted a long time in conditions of geographic isolation could lead to the formation of new species. He thus adopted a clear position vis-à-vis contemporary evolutionary debates; once again, he did so simultaneously as an experienced naturalist and as a Bergsonian, and sought to apply the philosophy of creative evolution to concrete scientific questions.

In his catalogs, Piaget approached evolution by simply declaring that it had taken place in a particular case, or by cursorily explaining it in terms of adaptation. Although he was well acquainted with mollusk paleontology and zoogeography, he did not elucidate and justify the evolutionary relations whose existence he sometimes affirmed. Not until his 1918 dissertation did he ask whether the morphological continuity between two species could be taken for granted as a sign of phyletic relationship between those species (1921a, 28). Such uncertainty was typical of Piaget's dissertation: a solid traditional catalog introduced by doubts about the value of catalogs and purely descriptive taxonomy.

Piaget's statements on the conditions of speciation are quite clear. In a 1913 lecture on life in deep waters, he explained that lakes were isolated environments, but that they were too recent to include new species: "because of their youth, our waters have not yet produced many novelties resulting from this isolation" (1913i, 19). In conformity with the idea that variations are nascent species, he wrote: "It is only in the long run that nascent adaptations . . . will become hereditary," that is, genuine species (1914d, 13).

By attributing to geographic isolation a key evolutionary role, Piaget adopted a precise point of view in one of the most important debates in early evolutionary theory. In *Origin*, Darwin considered that a morphologically well-defined variety could be considered as a nascent species. For him, geographic isolation helped increase the likelihood of a variety's transformation into a species. Isolation hindered crossbreeding and migration, thus enabling natural selection to act for a long time on the isolated variety (Darwin, 1859, 104–105 and chaps. 11 and 12). Natural selection was the main evolutionary agent.

Several post-Darwinian evolutionists gave more weight to isolation. Darwin's protégé George John Romanes (1848–1894) went so far as to assert that "heredity and variability given, the whole theory of organic evolution becomes a theory of the causes and conditions which lead to isolation" (1897, 145). Geographic and reproductive isolation were confounded. The former consists of a physical barrier extrinsic to the isolated organisms, whereas the latter prevented crossbreeding by means of biological or behavioral mechanisms. For the neo-Darwinian "modern synthesis," speciation requires the acquisition of such mechanisms: a new species evolves when a geographically isolated population acquires characters that guarantee its reproductive isolation, even without external barriers.

Piaget's thought in the 1910s illustrates the amalgamation of the two notions of isolation. For example, while trying to demonstrate the geographic isolation of deep-water *Limnaea,* he commented: "This isolation is the natural consequence of different bathymetric distributions [that is, geographic isolation] that prevent crossbreeding, and also of the fact that the fertile periods are different in surface and deep-water species" (1914j, 331). As we shall see in Chapter 7, geographic, not reproductive isolation, played a key role in Piaget's arguments. Of concern here is his insistence on duration. Piaget's repeated assertion that isolation must last to be effective derives from his blending geological time with Bergsonian duration.

The example of isolation that Piaget knew best, and which he cited several times, was that of sea fauna in isolated regions of salt water: "In large ponds progressively separated from the sea, brackish water forms develop, and differentiate themselves little by little from the corresponding marine species . . . But if the pond remains autonomous, and becomes l i t t l e b y l i t t l e . . . a freshwater lake, its fauna evolves slowly, as paleontology shows, and produces absolutely authentic and hereditary species" (1914j, 330). Another case was that of insular populations, whose evolution, Piaget said, could not be understood in the absence of isolation. On cavernicolous animals, he wrote that "the relatively great isolation of caves produces . . . variations that are at first fluctuating, then hereditary, and even generically distinct" (ibid., 331).

In advocating the role of isolation, Piaget referred to the German naturalist Moritz Wagner (1813–1887), the only evolutionary theorist ever mentioned in his many articles of the years 1911–1914. For Wagner, natural selection could act only on a population that, through migration, had become completely isolated from the original species. He thought that this *Separationstheorie* was an essential complement to Darwin's theory. Darwin acknowledged the importance of migration and isolation but did not consider them indispensable to speciation. (See Sulloway, 1979, 49–58; Mayr, 1976, chaps. 10 and 11.)

Wagner's "law of the formation of species by separation" was actually more Lamarckian than Darwinian. Once migrant individuals had been isolated from the original species, two processes then accounted for their transformation into a new species: the adaptation to new living conditions, and the transmission and development of adaptive modifications in their descendants.

Wagner (1882, 71) declared that, without isolation, natural selection was incapable of acting, or that at least its role was severely limited. The "struggle for existence," he thought, might precipitate migration; its influence, however, was indirect, and isolation was "the most active" evolutionary factor (ibid., 18–19). Time was also essential for speciation to take place; an insufficiently lengthy isolation would lead to the formation of ill-defined species, with numerous transitions. In contrast, a formed species underwent no funda-mental morphological changes as long as it remained isolated in the same en-vironment.

Piaget's position was like Wagner's in that he correlated environmental changes and hereditary modifications induced by direct adaptation in condi-tions of isolation. He claimed, for example, that a population's "evolution" might be "retarded by the scarcity of variations in the environment" it inhab-ited (1914d, 14). Like Wagner, moreover, Piaget thought that duration was responsible for the efficacy of isolation. He emphasized that insular faunas "have become i n t h e l o n g r u n absolutely autonomous" (1914j, 330). The duration of isolation determined the transformation of varieties into gen-uine species. Thus, the significance of Wagner's ideas for Piaget's evolutionary thinking is beyond question. It is worthwhile, however, to examine their lan-guage in detail.

Both employ the word *duration*. Wagner (1882, 16) mentions the conse-quences of "an insufficient duration of isolation"; Piaget (1914d, 14) claims that "only duration will have a real effect." Both likewise use the word *ten-dency*. Wagner (1882, 44) explains that the new living conditions of the iso-lated populations reinforce "the tendency of their organization to vary in a certain direction," and determine the development of a new species; Piaget writes that "a new species is not from the start characterized by its properties, its acquired characteristics, but by its t e n d e n c i e s" (1914d, 14). Whereas for Wagner *duration* and *tendency* were solely geological and biological con-cepts, for Piaget they were also philosophical terms.

After saying that a nascent species is characterized by its "tendencies," Piaget unequivocally alluded to Bergson: "as more than one philosopher has pointed out." For Bergson, the sciences may apprehend a succession of instants, "ab-stract time" but not "concrete duration"; they are concerned with "an instan-taneous present that is always being renewed." "But, in time thus conceived," he asked, "how could evolution, which is the very essence of life, ever take place? Evolution implies a real persistence of the past in the present which is, as it were, a hyphen, a connecting link" (Bergson, 1907, 22). The continuity of the "flux of life" that Piaget had appealed to in his nominalistic argument about the vanity of nomenclature was no more a purely biological or geologi-cal factor than it was Bergsonian duration; and the same must be said for the duration necessary for speciation to take place in the conditions of geographic isolation.

The distinction between scientific time and Bergsonian duration is again ap-parent in the notion of tendency. An organism's tendency to vary and adapt in accordance with its biological makeup is not the same thing as the tendency of life to act on inert matter by virtue of its "original *élan.*" In accordance with Bergson's view that "vital properties are never entirely realized, though always on the way to become so; they are not so much *states* as *tendencies*" (ibid., 13), Piaget discerned no tendencies in mimicry, but discovered them in evolving species. Thus, when geographic isolation facilitated the heritability of acquired characteristics, it favored the realization of the primary tendency of life to manifest itself as creative evolution.

Conclusion

In 1911 Piaget was Paul Godet's brilliant disciple. A nominalistic attitude toward taxonomic categories was the norm in the field of malacological taxonomy. By 1912 Piaget was combining this practical nominalism and his taxonomic practice with a radical evolutionary nominalism of Bergsonian inspiration. Taking up Bergson's idea (1907, 13) that "[a] perfect definition applies only to a *completed* reality," Piaget tried to be consistent with his vision of the "flux of life."

At fifteen, when Piaget dealt for the first time with mimicry, his approach was cautiously descriptive. At eighteen, he focused on theory. He explained mimicry by natural selection rather than by Lamarckian processes, but he underlined the exceptional character of the case and contrasted the "passive" adaptation that results from Darwinian mechanisms with the "active" adaptation that follows the tendencies of the vital impulse.

Piaget had learned that isolation was one of the conditions of speciation, since it makes the action of the environment last long enough for direct adaptations to become hereditary. Nevertheless, by 1913 at the latest, he considered that the length of isolation involved Bergsonian duration rather than the spatialized numerical time of science. Speciation thus manifested the creative tendency of vital evolution; isolation favored the actualization of such a tendency.

In no case were the Bergsonian and the scientific points of view incompatible. On the contrary, Piaget's Bergsonism cannot be separated from his science. Philosophy became a constitutive part of his scientific practice, materializing most often in connection with problems in taxonomy. It was in that context that Piaget initially used a Bergsonian vocabulary, including "duration," "tendency," "current," "flux," "canalization," "flow," and diverse dynamic images. Bergson thus guided him from a descriptive and classificatory natural history to properly biological concerns about life, evolution, and adaptation. The philosopher's magnum opus was filled with scientific references and discussions of the latest biological theories. Piaget became a "biologist" at the same time that he became Bergsonian; his initiation to modern biology did not take place in nature, and even less in a laboratory or a classroom, but through the pages of *Creative Evolution*.

7

At the Threshold of Biology

The Piaget-Roszkowski Debate

From 1912 to 1914 Piaget was involved in a debate about the classification of deep-water *Limnaea* from Lake Geneva. Ultimately, however, the object of the debate was the definition of the zoological species. Wacław Roszkowski (1886–1944), a Polish doctoral student at the University of Lausanne, sought to define species by constant and hereditary characteristics. He thus claimed that external shell morphology had no systematic value, and replaced it by characteristics of the internal anatomy. His viewpoint was close to the recent theory of mutation, according to which a new species resulted from a sudden and discontinuous large-scale variation, the mutation, and was hereditary and stable from the beginning.

Piaget, on the contrary, advocated a classification based on conchological characteristics, and defended a gradualist viewpoint according to which an isolated variety could in the long run become a hereditary species. He concluded that if a variety manifested a tendency to become a species, then it could be classified as such right away. The detection of such a tendency became for him the basic criterion of species definition.

Piaget's choice was borrowed directly from *Creative Evolution*. According to Bergson, clear-cut, "static" definitions may be good for the mathematical and physical sciences; but distinctions in the life sciences (between the vegetable and the animal realms, for example) must be "dynamic"—that is, they must take into account how, in the course of a group's evolution, certain latent or potential characteristics are "emphasized." A group, wrote the philosopher, "must be defined not by the possession of certain characteristics, but by its tendency to emphasize them" (Bergson, 1907, 106).

The debate got started the day one of Piaget's scientific correspondents pointed out to him an article on Lake Geneva's abyssal *Limnaea* including "interesting anatomical details."[1] The article reported a presentation by Roszkowski's supervisor on his graduate work, and summarized his reclassification of *Limnaea* on an anatomical basis (Anon., 1912; Roszkowski, 1912; Blanc, 1913). Evidently after reading it, Piaget sent Roszkowski his paper on the *Limnaea* of the lakes of the Neuchâtel region (1911a). The latter reciprocated by sending the printed version of his critique of *Limnaea* taxonomy (Roszkowski, 1912), and commented: "I must confess that I am not annoyed by the fact that the difference between our methods of investigation led us to opposite results; it is rather a stroke of good luck to meet, even as an adversary, a distinguished disciple of the eminent master in conchology Professor Paul Godet" (Roszkowski, ms. 1912). Soon Piaget (1912c) questioned Roszkowski's classifications and went on to study (1913e) diverse technical aspects of the question. Roszkowski (1913) replied by highlighting the theoretical differences between himself and Piaget, who rejoined with a theoretical article (1914j) that elicited no direct response. Roszkowski remarked on the debate in his final monograph on the *Limnaea* of Lake Geneva (1914) and in papers published in Poland (1915 and 1922). Piaget alluded to it later on; and in December 1913, two months before finishing his theoretical paper (1914j), he elaborated on its background in a presentation at the Club of the Friends of Nature. The debate was attentively and impartially followed in the Parisian *Journal de conchyliologie*.[2] Like others later (J. Favre, 1927; Hubendick, 1951), Piaget came to recognize the superiority of Roszkowski's arguments. He even showed considerable disdain for the "novelties" dared in his own 1912–1914 articles, which he described as written "by a simple high school student" and totally lacking in "biological culture" (1929, 489).

Roszkowski's Argument

Roszkowski's supervisor at the Zoological Laboratory of the University of Lausanne was the zoologist Henri Blanc (1859–1930). Blanc's specialty was abyssal faunas and hydrobiology. He had studied with August Weismann and kept up with the most recent developments in biology. Although he is said to have "oriented his students as much toward descriptive zoology and systematics as toward experimentation" (Carl, 1932, 7), his own work showed a clear preference for experimental and anatomical studies—the methodological options followed by Roszkowski (see also Murisier, 1930).

In an article published in the summer of 1912, Roszkowski proposed to revise the taxonomy of Lake Geneva's deep-water *Limnaea*. This group was divided into three species, defined on the basis of shell morphology, *Limnaea abyssicola, L. profunda*, and *L. Foreli*. These species were considered to be descendants of three shallow-water species, *L. palustris, L. stagnalis*, and *L. auricularia*, respectively. By means of the method of continuous series, *L. auricularia* was sometimes lumped with another littoral species, *L. ovata*. Roszkowski brought to this classification two radical modifications resulting directly from his anatomical and experimental methodology.

In the first place, Roszkowski turned to internal morphology to discover characteristics that would be more stable than the shell. He chose the genital apparatus (hermaphrodite in the species considered), with a focus on the seminal receptacle. He acknowledged that *L. auricularia* and *L. ovata* were connected by conchologically intermediate forms; yet, he observed, their internal anatomies were sufficiently different to rank them as distinct species. As he concluded: "Each form, difficult to define on the basis of the shell, can be unequivocally identified by the anatomy of the seminal receptacle" (Roszkowski, 1912, 377).

Always on the basis of internal anatomy, Roszkowski challenged the very distinction between abyssal and littoral species. He noted that *Limnaea profunda* and *L. Foreli* differed from *L. ovata* only by the shell, and that the same applied to *L. abyssicola, L. stagnalis*, and *L. auricularia*. Consequently, he lumped *L. profunda* and *L. Foreli* into a single variety, called *profunda*, of *L. ovata*, and reclassified the species *L. abyssicola* as a variety of *L. palustris*. In short, he ranked as distinct species two littoral varieties that were linked by conchologically continuous series yet differed greatly in genital anatomy (*L. auricularia* and *L. ovata*); and transformed abyssal species into varieties of the littoral species with the same genital anatomy.

One novelty of Roszkowski's approach consisted in the use of comparative anatomy. Problems of determination were resolved on the basis of anatomical considerations. According to Blanc (1913, 188), his student's work demonstrated "how cautious one must be when studying certain animal forms." Roszkowski himself (1914, 523) claimed to have shown that, given the shell's sensitivity to environmental conditions, conchological characteristics were practically useless for systematics. "I was able to arrive at certain reliable results," he wrote, "because, from the beginning of my research, I learned not to believe in the absolute value of the characters of the shell of mollusks" (ibid., 527). Such caution was exceptional among malacological taxonomists of the 1910s.

Roszkowski's work was also original in its use of laboratory techniques. He tested his taxonomic decisions by breeding deep-water *Limnaea* in an aquarium that reproduced littoral conditions. He found that, from the first generation, the shell of the offspring of abyssal specimens tended to resemble the shell of littoral species. He then concluded that conchological characteristics were not hereditary, but transient adaptations to the deep-water environment, and should therefore not be used to define species (Roszkowski, 1912, 379). This result also vindicated his choice of internal anatomical traits.

In order to decide which of the two lumped groups would be the species and which its variety, Roszkowski made use of Forel's theory that abyssal populations were born from littoral specimens that continually migrated to the bottom of the lake: "The littoral specimens that migrate to the bottom of the lake adapt imperfectly to the conditions of their new environment, stay there several generations, and end up disappearing and being replaced by new arrivals" (Roszkowski, 1912, 379). The abyssal fauna would thus be composed of constantly renewed migrants from shallow waters. Roszkowski's formulation, which became the crucial technical issue in the debate, significantly modified Forel's original idea.

Forel's theory was indeed centered on migration. "The deep-water fauna," he argued, "descend from littoral animals that arrived at the bottom [of the lake] . . . and adapted there to the environmental conditions" (Forel, 1885, 154). He thought that migrations took place every year, and that the "arrivals" of littoral animals were probably "very frequent" (ibid., 157). Nevertheless (and contrary to Roszkowski's interpretation), he also believed that the abyssal population was permanently established in its milieu, independently of migrations, that "it lives quite normally in the lake's great depths, and has become regularly acclimatized" (Forel, 1873, 146).

Forel classified as species "every type [from shallow waters] that has adapted to deep-water conditions, provided it has attained the definitive form that it should attain after an infinite number of generations spent in that environment" (Forel, 1885, 184). That is why, even though he asserted that "abyssal fauna is merely a modified littoral fauna" (Forel, 1873, 15), he considered deep-water *Limnaea* as species, whereas Roszkowski ranked them as varieties. At the same time, Forel highlighted the gap between theoretical definitions and taxonomic practice. Since he was a gradualist who thought of varieties as nascent species, he pointed out that the bottom of the lake could be inhabited by "all the degrees of transformation," from the recent migrant of littoral appearance to the "totally modified species," an outcome of the adaptation of several generations to the abyssal milieu (Forel, 1885, 185).

Forel, in sum, did not reduce abyssal populations to constantly renewed, partly adapted migrants from shallow waters. Unlike Roszkowski, he advocated evolutionary nominalism; taxonomic categories, in his view, expressed only "more or less close degrees of morphological differentiation"; "absolute precision" was neither possible nor necessary (Forel, 1885, 183). As for evolutionary mechanisms, Forel was a Lamarckian: abyssal species evolved by the direct adaptation of littoral specimens to deep waters, and by the gradual acquisition (and eventual heritability) of the adaptive characteristics over a large number of generations.

Roszkowski's rendering of Forel's hypothesis betrays a theoretical position that is contrary both to taxonomic nominalism and to a gradualist and Lamarckian theory of speciation. His point of view required continuous migration. Moreover, his classification of abyssal *Limnaea* was based on a choice of anatomical characteristics sheltered from environmental influence. This choice was itself governed by the principle that only strictly hereditary characteristics are useful to define a species, and that there is therefore no continuity between variations and species. As he wrote:

> Hereditary characteristics make it possible to define a species, to the exclusion of the characteristics called fluctuating. As a consequence of an environmental change, the latter can appear, and differentiate between individuals endowed with the same hereditary makeup; but a return to the normal environment leads to a return to the species type. The appearance of such fluctuations, produced by the influence of the environment, in no way alters the hereditary makeup, and does not permit the definition of a new species. (Roszkowski, 1913, 89–90)

Contrary to Forel, Piaget, and most other malacological taxonomists, Roszkowski asserted that a characteristic was either hereditary or fluctuating. In consequence, the existence of abyssal *Limnaea* could be explained only by a continuous migration from shallow waters; and such an explanation justified ranking abyssal populations as varieties.

Roszkowski's argument was based on the unquestionable fact that shell features were fluctuating. Against him, two things were necessary to maintain abyssal groups as species. Theoretically, a species concept had to be substantiated that allowed for continuity between fluctuating and hereditary characteristics. Empirically, the continuous migration hypothesis had to be invalidated. In Roszkowski's argument, this hypothesis merely lent further support to a classification founded on a redefinition of the species concept itself. But from the gradualist point of view, if the hypothesis was true, then it sufficed to justify Roszkowski's lumping of abyssal and littoral groups. Piaget *had* to prove it wrong; and he tried to do so by arguing that abyssal populations were isolated in their environment.

Piaget's Argument

Piaget's basic claim was that "nothing proves . . . that today's abyssal forms derive from today's littoral forms, or the other way around" (1912c, 206). Against the continuous migration hypothesis, he argued that present-day *Limnaea* originated in "ancestral *Limnaea*" that evolved separately in their own environments, abyssal or littoral (ibid.). The seminal receptacle, identical in abyssal and littoral populations, was for him an ancestral feature that, unlike the shell, had not been altered by the environment (ibid., 206–207).

Piaget thus affirmed exactly the opposite of continuous migration; the common origin of abyssal and littoral *Limnaea* (suggested by anatomical resemblances) was likely only if the two populations were isolated from each other. He therefore focused on demonstrating isolation, without questioning Roszkowski's choice of the seminal receptacle or contrasting it to his own choice of conchological characteristics. To the extent that he believed that varieties were nascent species, his use of variable characteristics was compatible with the morphological species concept. He went as far as creating a new abyssal species *(Limnaea Yungi)* and a new variety (*L. limosa* [var.] *sublittoralis*), both on the basis of external shell morphology (1912c, 209–211 and 220–221). (Roszkowski [1913] retorted by lumping *L. Yungi* with *L. profunda*, *L. Foreli*, and *L. ovata*.)

Piaget's creation of the *sublittoralis* variety is highly significant. We have seen that, for him, species evolved through the combined action of time and environmental influence, and that specific characteristics could never be absolutely and definitively stable. In his first reply to Roszkowski, Piaget maintained that abyssal *Limnaea* were more stable and more similar to one another than littoral species because they were "subject to very uniform environmental action" (1912c, 207). "The surface [littoral] forms," he explained, "exist under very variable external influences, and have thus produced species that are much more variable, but also more unstable"; they are "very polymorphous, and offer numerous intermediates," whereas abyssal species "have less divergent and better defined characteristics" (ibid.). Such observations were consistent with Forel's. For Roszkowski, in contrast, the idea that a species could be anything but constant was necessarily the epitome of paradox or incoherence.

Piaget's *sublittoralis* embodied the gradualist notion of continuity between varieties and species. Piaget recognized that the new variety was not endowed with very distinct characteristics. Yet he chose to differentiate it "under a special name, because it is not conceivable, at a depth of 30 to 50 meters, for the animal not to have followed the laws of adaptation to the environment" (1912c, 221). According to Forel (for example, 1873, 149–150), deep-water fauna could be found at depths ranging from 20 to over 300 meters. The name "sublittoral" comes from the fact that the variety lived in the upper zones of the abyssal region.

For Piaget, the most important element to justify the creation of the *sublittoralis* variety was its potential adaptation to an environment different from the littoral milieu. The organism *must* have adapted to its milieu; "consequently," Piaget professed, "this *Limnaea* must have a less colorful integument . . . and an aerial breathing system that is becoming an aquatic one" (1912c, 221). Piaget's language is clear: the adaptations described are the most probable ones, and they are conceptualized as taking place. Thus, Piaget created a new taxonomic group on the basis of tendencies, the formative processes he supposed to be under way; the group did not yet exist as separate species, but it necessarily would if isolation and environmental action lasted long enough. As empirical as this sounds, it is all a direct application of Bergson's ideas.

Piaget's justification for the *sublittoralis* required geographic isolation. When he defined the new variety and invented the term *sublittoral fauna,* he argued that this fauna did "not constitute an imperceptible transition" between littoral and abyssal populations (1913d, 616), that it was not the trace of a continuous vertical migration from surface to bottom. Morphologically, it was indeed "intermediate"; but it was not "the passage followed by shallow-water mollusks to produce deep-water species" (ibid., 624).

To prove his point, Piaget first sought to demonstrate the rarity of sublittoral forms (1913b, 157, 160, 162; 1913d, 616). If the continuous migration hypothesis were true, vertical draggings (carried out at different depths in the same area) should retrieve littoral, sublittoral, and abyssal specimens together. This, according to Piaget, was not the case (for example, 1913b, 162).

In the second place, Piaget made use of all his paleontological and limnological knowledge to suggest the ancient origin of abyssal *Limnaea*. He hypothesized that at least some deep-water species had arrived at the bottom of the lake when water levels rose at the end of glaciations, and would thus be vestiges of the ice age (1913d, 623–624; 1913g). Against the idea that littoral species were pushed downward by water currents, Piaget observed that the only river mouth on Lake Neuchâtel was far from the region where abyssal *Limnaea* were found. He concluded that if these *Limnaea* were indeed driven downward by that river, then an ancient origin alone could explain their distance from its point of entrance into the lake (1913b, 158–162). As a comparative illustration of the processes that might have formed abyssal *Limnaea*, Piaget enumerated cases where geographic isolation played a key role in speciation (1913f, 1914d, 1914j).

Finally, Piaget examined biological factors. On the one hand, he remarked the decline of the littoral *Limnaea*'s "vital power." The "difficulty of their existence," he speculated, "makes it unlikely" that they have "persevered in a descending migration" (1913d, 263). On the other hand, he replicated Roszkowski's finding that first-generation offspring of abyssal specimens resembled the littoral "original type." But whereas for Roszkowski the notion of "original type" denoted littoral *Limnaea*, for Piaget it designated a hypothetical phylogenetic ancestor; "the direct return to the type . . . seems to confirm the theory according to which sublittoral fauna formed independently" (1914d, 11). He emphasized that, "in conformity with Forel's experiments," his specimens did not return entirely to the type, and that, according to Roszkowski himself, total regression took place only after several generations.

In sum, Piaget offered three arguments for ranking deep-water *Limnaea* as species. First, he defined a sublittoral fauna bathymetrically separate from littoral and abyssal populations. This discontinuity was reinforced by the absence of water currents susceptible of driving littoral specimens toward the bottom of the lake. Second, Piaget examined different paleontological factors that suggested the glacial origins of the abyssal groups. Third, he interpreted the experimental regression of abyssal *Limnaea* to the littoral "type" without intermediates as yet another proof of their discontinuity. The technical goal of these three arguments was to prove the geographic isolation of abyssal *Limnaea*, and thus to invalidate the hypothesis of the continuous migration of littoral specimens.

The Theoretical Disagreement

Piaget believed that he had proved the validity of his classification: for him, both littoral and abyssal *Limnaea* deserved to be ranked as species. Each of his hypotheses presupposed the adequacy of using shell characteristics to define the species; Piaget never examined this assumption critically, even though it was directly questioned by Roszkowski. Piaget certainly displayed great knowledge of zoogeography, paleontology, and limnology—but always as a naturalist concerned above all with description and classification. Roszkowski's work, in contrast, illustrated the methodological developments that eventually resulted in Hubendick's (1951) global revision of *Limnaea* systematics. He criticized taxonomic decisions based on external shell morphology; and he was the first to notice that he and Piaget were "far from understanding each other" because they had "entirely different conceptions of the species" (Roszkowski, 1913, 89).

The real issue of the debate indeed was the concept of species itself. Each author's choices followed from incompatible theoretical frameworks. Piaget held a morphological and gradualist species concept, according to which both varieties and species were defined on the basis of shell characters, varieties could evolve into species, and variable characteristics could become hereditary. Roszkowski defined species on the basis of stable characteristics of the internal anatomy, a choice determined by the postulate that species should be based exclusively on constant hereditary characteristics. For him, fluctuating, or variable, characters were discontinuous with hereditary ones; varieties and species differed in their very nature, and not just in their degree of constancy. The opposition between the two naturalists echoes a central debate of turn-of-the-century biology: Roszkowski (1913, 89) remarked that Piaget's approach was "no longer in conformity with the ideas that are presently accepted in biology"; and Piaget (1914j, 328) characterized his rival as "a distinguished disciple of the Mendelian school." (For historical background see Dunn, 1965; Carlson, 1966; Allen, 1978).

By the 1890s, Darwin's (1859, 95) idea that natural selection acted by "the preservation and accumulation of infinitesimally small inherited modifications" was being questioned. William Bateson (1861–1926), for example, observed that environmental gradations were not always correlated with gradations in the species characteristics of the organisms inhabiting that environment. He argued that the variations that gave rise to discontinuities between species were determined not by external agents (environment or natural selection), but by heredity. Bateson's conclusion undermined the gradualist notion of species. If, as he wrote (Bateson, 1894, 568), "the Discontinuity of Species results from the Discontinuity of Variation," then, contrary to Darwin, speciation was not a continuous process. Abundant materials from the study of variation and geographic distribution seemed to suggest that only large-scale discontinuous variations were inherited, and that small continuous "Darwinian" variations were temporary effects of environmental influence. Natural selection would thus act on discontinuous variations, but did not determine their becoming the inherited traits of a particular species.

Toward 1900, when Mendel's laws were "rediscovered," the debate on the gradual or discontinuous nature of speciation had become the most important controversy in the domain of evolutionism. Since the Mendelian theory of heredity postulated the existence of distinct "factors" that could vary independently of each other, it lent support to the discontinuous view of evolution. The fact that certain characteristics that were absent in one generation could suddenly reappear in another justified interpreting Mendel's laws as a theory of discontinuous variation. The study of these laws was carried out in many different domains of biology, and the idea of discontinuity rapidly became bound up with the idea of Mendelian heredity.

The publication in 1901–1903 of the theory of mutations by the Dutch botanist Hugo de Vries (1848–1935) was a culminating point in the debate on the nature of speciation. For de Vries, species could arise by the occurrence of a "mutation," a discontinuous variation that falls outside the organism's normal range of variation, and that is hereditary and stable from the beginning. They could also appear by other means (for example, intercrossing or extinction of intermediate forms), but hereditary characteristics could arise only by mutation. Mutation was therefore the primary mechanism of evolution and speciation.

The theory of mutations provided systematics with a theoretically based natural criterion for differentiating species (defined by hereditary characteristics) from varieties (defined by fluctuating characteristics). The distinction between mutations and fluctuations implied that only strictly hereditary characteristics defined species, and that fluctuations might serve at the most to define varieties. As de Vries (1906, ix) announced, "The work now demanding our attention is manifestly that of the experimental observation and control of the origin of species." The future of biology seemed to rest with the study of heredity, the genotype, and Mendel's laws.

Piaget was correct in calling his adversary a disciple of the "Mendelian school." Roszkowski tried to discover hereditary characters by means of anatomy and breeding experiments, and studied the Mendelian transmission of color in *Limnaea* (1912, 381). For all we know, in fact, Piaget might have even first heard of the "Mendelian school" from Roszkowski himself, who in a letter to Piaget dated 17 May 1913 mentioned Mendelism's main features and basic idea (Roszkowski, ms. 1913a; see Vidal, 1992, 118, n. 16). A few days later he endeavored to tell the young naturalist why it was wrong not to distinguish between hereditary and fluctuating variations: "It is precisely the philosophical reasoning upon facts, demonstrated by the Mendelian school, that led us to differentiate them: hereditary variations originate in the disappearance or appearance of a 'genetic factor' . . . or 'genes' . . . whereas fluctuating variations consist of a more or less large external manifestation of an already existing 'factor'" (Roszkowski, ms. 1913b). Roszkowski's approach in malacological taxonomy was virtually unique at the time; until the 1920s he was one of very few *Limnaea* taxonomists to study internal anatomy and to criticize the traditional use of conchological characteristics.

Piaget, Critic of Mendelism

Piaget's efforts to prove the geographic isolation of abyssal *Limnaea* are not only part of a technical argument against continuous migration, but also the starting point of a theoretical reply to Roszkowski's so-called Mendelism. Be-

cause Mendel's laws were routinely interpreted as laws of discontinuous variation, adherents of Mendelism commonly supported mutationism. But in fact
what Piaget criticized under that name was the theory of mutations.

The debate took a theoretical turn after the initial exchange of letters, when,
toward the end of 1913, Roszkowski pointed out that his conception of species
was totally different from Piaget's, and that species ought to be defined exclusively on the basis of hereditary characteristics. Earlier he had submitted to
Piaget specimens of three generations bred from abyssal specimens in littoral
conditions; Piaget acknowledged that they had to be classified as littoral, but
considered it "very natural 'that a form living at a depth of 100 meters, whatever its origin, gives birth, in an aquarium, to descendants radically transformed by the complete change of [environmental] conditions'" (letter quoted
by Roszkowski, 1913, 89). Roszkowski replied that, "though very natural," the
transformation demonstrated "that the conchological characteristics Piaget
uses to define species vary under the influence of the environment, and are
therefore not hereditary" (ibid.).

Nothing in Piaget's training really prevented him from giving up such variable characteristics as a basis for species. He knew that Godet had placed another mollusk, *Anodonta anatina,* in the environment of *A. rostrata,* observed
that it acquired the latter's particular features, and consequently rejected those
features as useless for defining species (Godet, 1874, 47). Given the alternative,
however, Piaget could not abandon the use of variable characteristics without
at the same time renouncing his nascent Bergsonian vision.

Piaget apprehended that the main idea of the "Mendelian school" was the
distinction between hereditary and fluctuating characteristics, but he did not
understand that hereditary characteristics were of purely internal origin. He
believed that whereas fluctuating variations resulted from a change in the intensity of an existing environmental factor, hereditary characteristics originated in the appearance of a new environmental factor:

> Everything happens as if the appearance of a new factor, [such as] darkness in
> abyssal waters, produced the hereditary variation as long as the [environmen-
> tal] factor remains active. But the factor's suppression also suppresses hered-
> ity. The eye is again what it was before, with the same structure and function.
> Moreover, it is not the appearance of a new factor, in this case light, that
> could at once craft an organ as complicated [as the eye], and as similar to
> what it was, or to what it would have been without interruption if the factor
> of obscurity had not intervened.   (1914d, 12)

Piaget's summary of the basic idea of the Mendelian school was even more
straightforward:

there exists a fundamental difference between hereditary variations and variations called fluctuating. The former are determined by the appearance of a new factor in the habitat of the species, while the latter are only the result of the intensity of factors already present. The former alone are specific, while the latter are the property of simple varieties. (1914j, 328)

In sum, Piaget mistakenly attributed an environmental nature to the "factors" postulated by Mendel's laws. Thus in a December 1913 presentation titled "The Notion of the Species according to the Mendelian School," he declared: "The distinction between fluctuating and hereditary variations is obviously very logical and verifiable. But what is a new factor as opposed to an already existing factor? Cold and hot? Clearly not, [since] there are all the transitions [between the two]. Obscurity and light? Neither. Altitude, depth? What do I know, everything is relative. Frankly, I am incapable of figuring it out" (1913f, 129). Piaget's perplexity echoes Roszkowski's words; his vocabulary ("appearance," "already existing factor") is Roszkowski's; and his argument is a direct and immediate reply to the latter's explanations.

Although in 1913 Piaget could have hardly been acquainted with the most recent developments of early genetics, he could have understood that Mendelian factors were not environmental. In spite of the resistance of French biology to Mendelian genetics, reliable up-to-date information was readily available in French (Delage, 1903; Delage and Goldsmith, 1909). A sheet of paper left inside the manuscript of Piaget's paper, probably written by Gustave Juvet, contained an accurate if awkward formulation of Mendel's laws (see Vidal, 1992, 117–118, n. 15). Roszkowski's explanations were brief but not unclear. By July 1914 Piaget knew about chromosomes—though nothing he wished to say in a scientific paper.[3]

Yet Piaget's misunderstanding is comprehensible. By 1913 his whole way of thinking about evolution excluded discontinuity and the action of independent factors. He thus distorted Mendelian theory in the direction of Lamarckism and Bergsonism, which furnished the basis of his theoretical alternative to Mendelism. His strategy consisted of accepting the validity of the distinction between hereditary and fluctuating variations, and simultaneously questioning its "absolute" character. In "The Notion of the Species" he claimed that "demonstrating the existence of species of purely fluctuating origin amounts to refuting Mendel's law" (1913f, 129). His published articles were less assertive, but said basically the same thing. The key idea always is that varieties may become genuine species if they remain under the influence of the same environment for a long period, and under conditions of isolation that prevent migration and crossbreeding. Isolation is therefore "a more important factor than (Mendelian) heredity" (1914j, 330; compare 1913f).

Piaget also argued that forms accepted as being specifically or even generically distinct might be linked by intermediate forms without losing their autonomy. According to him, if the Mendelian conception were always true, "there would only be fluctuating variations in nature" (1914j, 329–330)—and would, therefore, be always false. As Gruber and Vonèche (1977, 5) point out, Piaget's reasoning is a *reductio ad absurdum* aimed at demonstrating that the distinction between hereditary and fluctuating variations is not absolute.

To the extent that abyssal *Limnaea* were isolated from littoral and sublittoral populations, they could be considered genuine species. "Nevertheless," Piaget observed, "they are still in a period of formation, and their evolution has in addition been retarded by the scarcity of variations in their environment" (1914d, 14). It was only "as long as abyssal *Limnaea* remain isolated from littoral forms" that they might be considered as different species (1914j, 331).

Thus, for Piaget, species and heredity were relative. Fluctuating variations were not necessarily fluctuating forever; they could become hereditary, and only that "becoming" really counted. Piaget wrote: "If those factors [of geographic isolation] stay the same, it is permissible to predict that some day the *Limnaea* in question, already very stable in their environment, will be hereditary even outside their milieu, that is, will have acquired the fundamental character of the Mendelian species" (1914j, 331). The taxonomic consequence of such a reasoning was that "in practice" nothing prevented abyssal *Limnaea* from being classified as species "characterized by several particular features that are hereditary in deep waters" (1914d, 12).

Piaget took the rather unusual decision of classifying abyssal *Limnaea* as species because of the probability that they would become species. His approach was legitimized by his Bergsonian view of evolution. In his view, the main defect of the Mendelian school indeed was that "it is close to those radical mechanistic doctrines so well criticized today" (1914d, 12). By Bergsonian standards, the Mendelian species concept was "static," Piaget's, "dynamic."

Piaget reasoned entirely in terms of the Bergsonian critique of "mechanistic" science, that is, the science that, like Mendelism and mutationism, partitioned the flux of life and missed its creative impulse. Such a critique reinforced the naturalist's typical objection to the experimentalist: "Mr. Roszkowski's experiments," Piaget remarked, "are obviously very convincing, but they are carried out outside the natural environment of abyssal *Limnaea*" (1914j, 331). In classification as much as in philosophy, it was for him indispensable to stay close to life and nature to apprehend their true functioning.

Regardless of its misconceptions about Mendelism, Piaget's critique is most significant in revealing his Bergsonism. One same phrase manifests both his confusion in the field of biology and his certainties in the domain of philosophy: "it is not the [environmental factors] that must be new, but the totality of those factors, their r e l a t i o n, their s y n t h e s i s." "In other words," he concluded, "a new species is not from the beginning characterized by its properties, its acquired characteristics, but by its t e n d e n c i e s, as more than one philosopher has remarked" (1914d, 14). This allusion to Bergson summarizes the young Piaget's view: a new species is defined by its becoming, by its evolutionary tendencies, by none of the features revealed by the analytic methods of mechanistic science. Piaget thus conceived of a Bergsonian realism: species are defined by their actual or probable evolution, and, in the domain of life, nothing could be more real than evolution itself. As Bergson (1907, 106) explained, a group must be defined by its tendency to emphasize certain characteristics; only such a definition, he said, "befits the sciences of life."

Nominalism, Realism, and the Science of Genera

In practice, Piaget remained a nominalist because species constantly evolved, and because the partitioning of evolution for the purposes of classification implied the establishment of artificial boundaries. More fundamentally, however, he was a realist because he believed that species could be defined by the very fact that they were constantly evolving. By 1914 his initial assimilation of Bergsonism into systematics had led to the project of constructing a natural science that, in Bergson's words (1907, 272, 273), would see "in duration the very stuff of reality" and would deal with "the true evolution, the radical becoming." Thus it is not surprising that he did not contrast his nominalism to Roszkowski's realism, since he himself proposed a radically different, but equally realist, conception of species.

The passage from nominalism to realism was the high point of Piaget's philosophical thinking in the years 1912–1914. In his autobiographical writings Piaget does not mention the debate with Roszkowski, emphasizing instead the transformation he underwent when he realized that the problem of species could be treated in logical terms: only at that point he ceased to be "antimathematician," and understood the union of the biological and the logical. Before that conversion, he explains, "I believed, under Bergson's influence, that vital processes were irreducible to logico-mathematical structures" (1961, 144, n. 1).

Piaget further remembers how "Bergson's pages on the disappearance of the problem of *genera* in modern thought, dominated by the problem of *laws*," persuaded him of the antagonism between "the biological spirit and the logico-mathematical spirit" (1959b, 45). He also says: "Very impressed by Bergson's pages on the opposition of genera and laws, I dream[ed] of a specifically biological science of genera" (1959a, 9). And elsewhere:

> I had been struck by a remark of Bergson that appeared to give me a guiding thread for the start of my philosophico-biological studies. This was his surprise at the disappearance of the problem of "genera" in modern philosophy in favor of the problem of laws . . . While continuing my articles on malacology . . . I began to write "my" philosophy . . . After having read [William] James, I produced an "Outline of a Neo-Pragmatism," which took account of the rationalist criticism of Reymond, but remained under Bergson's influence, and in which I tried to show that there exists a logic of action distinct from mathematical logic. Then, turning to the problem of "genera," I wrote a tome . . . on "Realism and Nominalism in the Life-Sciences," in which I put forward a kind of holism, or philosophy of wholes: the reality of species, genera, etc., and, of course, of the individual as an organized system. My original intention was to create a science of genera—neither more nor less—which would be distinct from science as a lawlike endeavor, and would thus justify the Bergsonian dualism between the vital and the mathematical, a dualism in which I still believed. (1965, 6)

The texts mentioned by Piaget have not yet been found, and a reconstruction of the earliest form of his "science of genera" remains to be attempted (but see Chapman, 1988, 412–415).

Piaget (1959a, 9) recalled that "Realism and Nominalism" was written "in connection with a lesson on universals" given at the gymnasium by his philosophy teacher Arnold Reymond. Piaget was a student of Reymond's from 1913 to 1915. If the program of studies was followed even approximately, then the problem of universals was treated in 1914–15 (see *Programme*, 1914–15, 10). In 1915, already at the university, Piaget received for his paper a prize from the Academic Society of Neuchâtel (1959a, 10; Reymond, 1950, 153). But the inception of his project must be set earlier. In July 1914, when Piaget submitted to Reymond a paper on "moral conscience according to Cresson," his teacher commented: "In my view, what you call the passage from nominalism to realism is what is most original in your paper, and it would be worthwhile focusing entirely on that point" (Reymond, ms. 1914)—which is what Piaget eventually must have done in the lost "Realism and Nominalism."

The question of genera and laws as conceptualized by Bergson fits with Piaget's arguments against Roszkowski's Mendelism. In *Creative Evolution*, Bergson explained (1907, 227) that ancient philosophers "did not ask why nature submits to laws, but why it is ordered according to genera." For instance, according to Aristotelian physical law, when a stone falls, it reaches the "natural place" of all stones, and thereby realizes the essence of the genus "stone." Ancient philosophy thus attributed to physical bodies the same individuality as to living organisms; "the laws of the physical universe," Bergson wrote, "would express relations of real kinship between real genera" (ibid., 228). Consequently, ancient science seemed to him confined "to a more or less clumsy interpretation of the physical in terms of the vital" (ibid.).

For Bergson (ibid., 229–230), modern philosophy also confounded genera and laws, but inverted the relationship. "Our theory of knowledge," he observed, "turns almost entirely on the question of laws." Since laws express relations between things or facts, they have "objective reality only for an intelligence that represents to itself several terms at the same time." "The idea of a science and of an experience entirely relative to the understanding," he concluded, "is therefore implicitly contained in the conception of a science one and integral, composed of laws." For Bergson, both the "relativism of the moderns" and the "dogmatism of the ancients" originated in the confusion between genera and laws, that is, between the vital and the physico-geometric orders.

A Bergsonian science of genera, then, implied a clear distinction between the vital order (genera) and the geometrical order (laws). The confusion of the two orders originated in the fact that the vital order, "which is essentially creation," appears to our intelligence under the form of accidents that "imitate" the geometric order of repetitions that make lawlike generalization possible (ibid., 231). A science of genera is a science of the vital order, and is therefore biological. Thus, for Bergson, the idea of genus corresponded "to an objective reality in the domain of life, where it expresses an unquestionable fact, heredity" (ibid., 227). In heredity, however, there is not only repetition, but also *élan vital*. For the philosopher, the "unceasing transformation" that constituted life could take place only by means of the reproduction of living creatures. Heredity, he claimed, "does not transmit only characteristics; it transmits also the impetus in virtue of which the characteristics are modified, and this impetus is vitality itself" (ibid., 231). Repetition may be essential in the "physical order," but it is "accidental in the vital order" (ibid.). In such a perspective, Roszkowski's experimental Mendelism was confined to the physical and geometric order, whereas Piaget's definition of species in terms of tendencies fitted into a biological science of genera.

Piaget's 1914 Bergsonian realism is consistent with the two other elements of his thinking. One is his nominalism, which started by being purely instrumental and taxonomic, and became Bergsonian and evolutionary in 1912. The second one is his Lamarckism. It too began as a practical presupposition, taken for granted in Piaget's numerous early remarks on evolution and adaptation. It became explicit and more refined only in a Bergsonian framework, initially when Piaget distinguished between passive and active adaptation (in his discussion of mimicry), and later when he emphasized the importance of geographic isolation. But there was more.

In *Creative Evolution*, Bergson made his Lamarckism perfectly clear. He considered that one of its "most solid positions" was its resorting to a psychological factor, which he characterized as "effort." For him, a hereditary change "in a definite direction" must be related to "an effort common to most representatives of the same species, inherent in the germs they bear" (Bergson, 1907, 86, 87). Such an "effort," independent of circumstances and transmitted from generation to generation, is the vital impulse itself. Piaget incorporated the idea into his scientific discourse in a remarkably discreet manner. During the debate with Roszkowski, while discussing geographically isolated populations, he mentioned the "psychological moment" of the "formation" of new species (1914j, 330). He then explained that if the environment remains autonomous and changes "little by little," then "its fauna evolves slowly . . . and produces absolutely authentic and hereditary species" (ibid.). The "psychological moment" is evolution itself being made through the gradual transformation of an adaptive change into a hereditary characteristic. It is "psychological" because, according to the Bergsonian conception, it represents the inner "effort" of a species that changes by realizing its evolutionary "tendency" under circumstances facilitating the action of "duration" and making possible the organism's "active adaptation." The young Piaget's science of genera is therefore not only biological but also, at least implicitly, psychological. This happens to be the case in two ways: first, as we just saw, speciation is partly a psychological phenomenon; second, it follows, from the Bergsonian premise that duration is essential to both life and mind, that the mental function of generalization is akin to the biological process of the formation of species and genera.

In *Creative Evolution*, Bergson briefly explained how the confusion of genera and laws was intimately related to human psychology. Genera are composed of individuals. Now, when perception "cuts inert matter into distinct bodies," it is guided "by the interests of action, by the nascent reactions our body indicates"; these are "the potential genera that are trying to gain existence" (Bergson, 1907, 227). Genera and individuals, he concluded, "determine one another by a semi-artificial operation entirely relative to our future action on things" (ibid.). The justification of these remarks is to be found in the sections of *Matter and Memory* where Bergson (1896, 296–301) examines the formation of categories or "general ideas." For the philosopher, generalization does not start, as currently assumed, with the perception of individual objects, but with an unclear feeling of resemblance, intermediate between "fully conceived generality and clearly perceived individuality" (ibid., 299). This responds to the utilitarian origin of perception: the herbivore is attracted to "grass *in general*"; the individual differences brought out through memory against this background of generality are secondary to its purpose (ibid.). Through the combined action of memory and understanding, human beings rise from the mechanical idea of generality ("awareness of an identity of attitude in a diversity of situations") to the general idea of the genus (ibid., 301). Once again, the theory of knowledge and the theory of life are inseparable.

In spite of its predominantly critical role, *Recherche* confirms our reconstruction of the earliest form of Piaget's science of genera. After stating that Sebastian was a Bergsonian who did not admit any of the specific theses of Bergsonism, Piaget adds that he

> delighted above all in the manner in which this philosophy had sketched a possible rehabilitation of the Greek [notion of] genera. Indeed, Bergson had brilliantly understood that the moment had come to reintroduce genera in modern science. All his psychology showed the effects of this ulterior motive. His biology, which remained quite superficial and verbal, was compatible with the same interpretation.
>
> Only Bergson had not defined the genus, and one cannot see how he could have done it without altering his system quite seriously. All the work thus remained to be done, and moreover, it was much more of a scientific than of a philosophical nature. Aristotle, the genius of genera, was a biologist: the edifice had to be built through biology. (1918a, 53)

The theories presented in *Recherche* reach well beyond biology, but they pivot on the notion of genus. Sebastian's theory of living organisms as an equilibrium between general and partial qualities explicitly extends his notion of the species (1918a, 98). Piaget's focus (in the closing essay of *Recherche*) on the relations between parts and wholes prolongs the concern with the relations between generality and individuality that characterized the problem of species and the conceptualization of genus.

Piaget at the Threshold of Biology

In 1912, shortly after the beginning of his debate with Roszkowski, Piaget communicated to the Friends of Nature his ideas on "the vanity of nomenclature." The radical evolutionary nominalism he then elaborated was Bergsonian: Piaget's adherence to Bergson's critique of "mechanistic" science inspired his conclusion that it was "superficial to partition the flux of life," and that "human analysis" was abstract and artificial. In no way did this nominalism contradict the principles that governed his scientific practice.

Piaget's confrontation with the Mendelian species concept led him to introduce an alternative realist criterion into his own practice of classification. His hypothesis concerning the geographic isolation of abyssal *Limnaea* reinforced reproductive isolation as a criterion of species. Nevertheless, morphological resemblance lingered on as the chief criterion; for Piaget classification remained based on the description and comparison of external forms. That is why, in 1914, he reached only the threshold of biology. His outlook was "biological" in a very different sense from that of the comparative anatomist or the geneticist.

The young naturalist's taxonomic nominalism was the restrictive consequence of the idea that life was characterized by evolution. Realism was its constructive outcome: for while it was impossible to attribute absolute limits to a species, it was feasible to define it by its "tendencies." Piaget acknowledged that abyssal *Limnaea* were still evolving and that their conchological characteristics were still variable; yet he maintained that they deserved to be ranked as species because, given their isolation, they manifested a "tendency" to become stable and hereditary. Through the formulation and practical application of such Bergsonian realism Piaget reconciled realism and nominalism; and from them emerged the project of a "specifically biological science of genera."

A Bergsonian science of genera could only aim at apprehending the vital order without partitioning, quantifying, or spatializing it. It should not deal with repetition, essential in the geometric order but accidental in the order of life. Its object was "vitality," the force creative of forms. The "logico-mathematical structures" that Piaget contrasted in his autobiography with "vital processes" were no "structures" at all, but a 1950s manner of referring retrospectively to Bergson's "geometric order" and the methods of "mechanistic" science. The adjective "biological" that he applied to the science of genera is much more immediately related to the project of studying life *qua* creative evolution and *élan vital* than to the scientific discipline of biology.

The young Piaget's project was not only "biological" but also "psychological" from the start. The point of departure certainly was the question of zoological categories, and we have seen how Piaget treated it in the years 1912–1914. To the extent that he was a Bergsonian "without duration" (1918a, 53), we may wonder whether he was at all Bergsonian. As the philosopher wrote in a 1915 letter, the "intuition of duration" was "the very center of [his] doctrine" (Bergson, 1972, 1148). For Piaget, however, Bergsonism was contained in the vision of a universal and continuous creative evolution, and in the postulate of an essential identity of life and mind. This is confirmed by the range of application attributed to the theory of equilibrium elaborated in *Recherche*, which Piaget sums up as "an advanced Bergsonism" (1918a, 161). Yet it is also clear that in 1912–1914 Piaget did not yet see psychology as his future realm of specialization.

Piaget's autobiography situates at the time of his discovery of Bergson the intuition that between "biology and the analysis of knowledge" he needed something other than philosophy: "I believe it was at that moment that I discovered a need that could be satisfied only by psychology" (1952, 240). While such a need fits perfectly well with Piaget's adoption of a Bergsonian perspective, it is only considerably later that psychology emerged as a professional option. In *Recherche*, psychological questions are central, but not psychology as a science. Piaget later confirmed that at the time he wrote the book (September 1916–January 1917), "There was as yet no question of choosing between philosophy and psychology, but only of deciding whether it was necessary for a serious study of epistemology to spend several semesters studying psychology" (1965, 9). We shall return to this question in the Epilogue.

Up to now we have been concerned with how Piaget intertwined natural history and the philosophy of creative evolution. We have seen that it was at the very heart of his scientific practice that the young Piaget introduced "duration" and the "vital impulse." The more involved he got in the elaboration of a science of genera, the more he withdrew from natural history. His scientific production decreased significantly starting in 1914: four articles in 1912, eight in 1913, fourteen in 1914—then one in 1915, two in 1916. His 1918 doctoral dissertation, a traditional malacological taxonomy, went so far as to question the validity of its own methods.

World War I upset everything. As Piaget noted in *Recherche* (1918a, 98), the system constructed over four years (1912–1916) was marked by the times: "two years of peace during which he [Sebastian] worked for himself alone, and two years of war during which the sting of social suffering pursued him every day." As we shall see, this painful experience profoundly altered the form and content of Piaget's thinking.[4]

8

The Protestant Context

By 1914, Piaget had elaborated a Bergsonian view of religion; after the onset of World War I, his worldview was energized by what he later called "the sting of social suffering" (1918a, 98); as the continuation of the war led him to face the problem of evil and the question of the goodness of God, he lost faith in a transcendental deity; out of his spiritual and, more specifically, religious crisis emerged the immanentist and constructivist perspective that we may start recognizing as distinctly Piagetian.

Piaget's blend of philosophy, religion, and science is best understood in the context in which it evolved during World War I. Piaget was always recognized as an outstanding young man. But his concerns and thinking were consistent with those of Swiss-French Protestant intellectual circles, particularly of the Swiss Christian Students' Association. This was a milieu in which philosophy and the human sciences, as well as ethics, literature, and even political thought, were intimately linked to religion; theology was often hardly more than a sort of introspective psychology, and religious instruction was more moral and philosophical than dogmatic (see Chapter 9). This explains Piaget's comment about his discovery of Bergson: "It was the first time that I heard philosophy discussed by anyone not a theologian" (1952, 240). But it does not make his philosophical education any less religious or less shaped by what was felt as a specifically Swiss-French spiritual tradition.

Liberalism and Evangelicalism

The most essential component of the Swiss-French culture was a special combination of liberal and evangelical Protestantism—predominantly liberal from the doctrinal point of view, but expressed with the kind of affectivity more usually found in evangelical and revivalist circles.

The term *liberal Protestantism* does not designate a doctrine, but rather an attitude, perhaps best described as an effort to adapt religion and theology to secular developments in science, philosophy, and society. One consequence of this attitude is the diffusion of Christian dogma into morality and philosophy. The paradigmatic liberal method is "historico-critical." Although the Bible is studied as a purely human text, it is asserted that faith will remain intact whatever the results of historical analysis. Liberal Protestantism evolved out of the eighteenth-century humanization of Christian theology, its replacement of external authority by an appeal to individual conscience, and the elaboration of a religion deemed more reasonable and better adapted to human limitations and capacities.[1]

Immanuel Kant (1724–1804) was one of the direct sources of inspiration of liberal Protestantism. In Kant's system, religion was inseparable from morality. The existence of God, the immortality of the soul, and free will were postulates of practical reason that could be neither demonstrated nor invalidated; the believer's only guide was personal conscience. Kantian religious philosophy thus transformed transcendency into immanence, interpreted dogmas through a "pure religious faith," emphasized sincerity over adherence to a creed, and focused on the moral consequences of dogma rather than on dogmatic propositions. Friedrich Schleiermacher (1768–1834), the founder of hermeneutics, made experience and sentiment the foundations of theology. Like Kant, Schleiermacher received a Pietistic education. From it he retained a mystical inclination, a sharp distinction between doctrines and experience, and an idea of the church as a free association of believers. Unlike the Pietists, however, he questioned the dogmas of redemption and of Christ's divine nature.

While Schleiermacher's reading of Kant led him to understand religion in terms of ethics, his religiosity corresponded more to Romantic *Naturphilosophie* than to Kantian criticism. For him, the essence of religion was a feeling of absolute dependency on God, a feeling that was linked to an intuition of infinity. Thus, Jesus' divinity lay in his intuition of the universe, and Jesus was the intermediary through whom individuals established their relation to the Whole. Since Christians were defined as those individuals who based their religion on an intuition similar to Christ's, dogmas were only abstract expressions of religious intuitions. Schleiermacher's subjectivism and immanentism, his appeal to inner experience, feeling, and conscience, his fundamentally human Jesus, and his historical and psychological interpretation of dogmas became defining features of liberal Protestant theology.

Auguste Sabatier (1839–1901) was Schleiermacher's chief French-speaking successor. He argued that faith alone saves, and that dogmatic beliefs are constantly evolving symbolic expressions of an eternal spiritual truth. His *Outlines of a Philosophy of Religion Based on Psychology and History* (1897) sharply distinguished between the moral essence of Christianity (conscience and intuition) and its historical and symbolic expression (dogmas), thus implying that genuine faith is essentially a psychological phenomenon.

In a controversial article, Sabatier contended that the "psychological root" of Christ's "messianic vocation" was the feeling of being "a child of the Father"; consequently, it could be understood only as relating to the "inner development of his moral conscience" (Sabatier, 1880, col. 367). In the same vein, he observed the "psychological connection" between the apostle Paul's creed and his inner life (Sabatier, 1899, viii).

Sabatier advocated a "scientific" theology that would investigate religious experience and conscience by means of introspection and the study of documents. That is why he is generally considered a major liberal theologian. Yet he was also among those who revived evangelicalism and defended it against extreme versions of liberalism that evolved in France. He did not reject any fundamental Christian dogma, but rather insisted on the need to modernize their formulation.

Sabatier contrasted the "religions of authority" to the "religion of the spirit" and placed them in a historical sequence. Echoing Comte, he described the religious progress of humanity as involving three stages: the mythological (paganism), the dogmatic (Catholicism and orthodox Protestantism), and the psychological (liberal Protestantism). By the last stage, revelation has become the inner experience of God felt as immanent to the individual and the universe; "dogmas, doctrines, received belief, are nothing else than the intellectual expression of the common religious consciousness in a given society" (Sabatier, 1904, 357).

At the end of the nineteenth century, liberal Protestant theology had for the most part become the study of religious "phenomena." The psychology of religion developed rapidly; conversion, mysticism, and spiritualistic and "psychic" phenomena became fashionable subjects. The "Life of Jesus" became one of the new theology's favorite genres, with Christ variously portrayed as "a master of the Enlightenment, a romantic genius, a Kantian philosopher, a rather puritan moralist, a champion of social revolution" (Perrot, 1979, 55). In all cases, the historical and human Jesus displaced the Messiah. As a critic observed, Christ became "a figure designed by rationalism, endowed with life by liberalism, and clothed by modern theology in an historical garb" (Schweitzer, 1913, 398).

Strongly intellectualistic, yet at the same time based on the "heart" and "conscience," Christianity increasingly resembled a secular morality often judged as bourgeois and academic. At the turn of the century, some theologians began to revolt against a tradition according to which "A God without wrath brought men without sin into a kingdom without judgment through the ministrations of a Christ without a cross" (H. Richard Niebuhr, quoted in Reardon, 1968, 63). After World War I, the Swiss theologian Karl Barth (1886–1968) successfully led a dogmatic renewal that sought to reestablish a religion of transcendency irreducible to a subjective faith emanating from an individual's own conscience. For him, Schleiermacher was a "bad master in theology," and the object of theology was the "word of God" alone, independent of historical or psychological conditions (for example, Barth, 1922).

Parallel to the rise of liberal Protestant theology, and also in the wake of Romanticism, revival movements sprang up throughout Europe during the first half of the nineteenth century and recurred periodically; the most recent one at the time we are studying had taken place in Wales in 1904–1905.

A "revival" is an "awakening of consciences," a break with established order, a "new birth" supposed to open the way to personal salvation in a millenary and messianic perspective. Typically, the revivalist conversion takes place in an atmosphere of individual or collective emotional exaltation. Enthusiasm, fervor, the spiritual agony of the personal discovery of sin, and finally the exhilaration of an intimate revelation of the Savior are typical ingredients of all revivals and are also elements of the evangelical spirituality.

The common denominator of the diverse evangelical currents is their opposition to theological rationalism and liberalism and the claim to orthodoxy. For evangelicalism, the Bible as divinely inspired text is the source of all Christian truths, particularly of the doctrine of salvation by faith in the atoning death of Christ. Throughout the nineteenth century, the debate between liberalism and evangelicalism was mainly doctrinal, and centered on the problem of the church's official confession of faith. The two camps looked at the problem from entirely different points of view: "Orthodoxy [evangelicalism and revivalism] started from the idea of church, and declared that a church is the association of those who confess the same faith: it is therefore necessary to formulate such a faith. Liberals started from the idea of Protestantism, whose fundamental principle is for them the free examination of biblical teachings: it was thus impossible to formulate even a minimum of faith" (Maury, 1892, 1:510). In sum, the "orthodox" party adhered to the Apostles' Creed, particularly the dogmas of the Trinity, Christ's divine nature, expiation, and resurrection; the divinity of Christ was its fundamental doctrine. The liberals, in contrast, saw themselves as disciples of the historical Jesus and wished to follow him as a spiritual, moral, and social model free from dogmatic allegiances.

By the end of the nineteenth century, the attitudes of the orthodox and the liberal camps often coincided: both favored the secularization of public schools, included individuals who attacked and supported the separation of church and state, and promoted the involvement of Christianity with social questions. Both evangelists and liberals also subscribed to the primacy of the individual over institutions and believed that confessional boundaries were irrelevant to salvation. For both, individual "conscience" and "heart" were supreme arbiters in religious matters. The outcome of both orientations was to disincarnate and desacramentalize religion. And both had to face the cognitive and epistemological problem of reconciling an individual faith with a universal church, and a subjective belief with an objective religious truth. How to believe, and yet remain objective; how to be certain that one's faith corresponds to an eternal universal truth; how to reach the transcendent by means of the immanent—such were the great themes of the religious impulse that animated the Swiss-French Protestant tradition.

The Swiss-French Tradition

Questions about the existence of a specifically Swiss-French political and cultural identity are still debated (see Seiler and Knüsel, 1989). At the turn of the century they crystallized into the idea of a local "spirit" or "tradition," characterized by the omnipresence of its special brand of Protestantism (see Berchtold, 1963, especially 33–214).

At the time, a salient feature of Swiss-French culture was its close-knit social network of academics and intellectuals. In 1906 a group that included two of Piaget's mentors, Pierre Bovet and Arnold Reymond, started to hold informal annual meetings; in 1923, at the initiative of Piaget, Juvet, and their friend Jean de la Harpe (1892–1947), it was formalized as the Swiss-French Philosophical Society (Société Romande de Philosophie; see Miéville, 1956, 281). Most of its members were in close touch with the Swiss Christian Students' Association (Association Chrétienne Suisse d'Etudiants; ACSE), to which Piaget belonged; some of their most influential texts were delivered at Christian students' conferences and published by the ACSE itself. Their names are found in the chief cultural publications of the region: *Revue de théologie et de philosophie* (Journal of Theology and Philosophy, the main Swiss-French philosophical journal), *L'Essor* (a "social, moral, and religious" monthly whose name means "flight" or "blossoming"), *La semaine littéraire* (The Literary Week, a cultural chronicle), *Jeunesse* (Youth) and its *Cahiers,* later renamed *Cahiers protestants* (Protestant Notebooks), both published by the Young Men's Christian Association.

Theology

In the Swiss-French tradition, philosophy, psychology, pedagogy, literature, ethics, and even politics were colored by religious and theological concerns. Reciprocally, theology was largely a "psychological" discourse. Every domain manifested in its own way a Protestant individualism, as well as a characteristic oscillation between emotionality and rationality.

Piaget was fully aware of belonging to this tradition. In a 1917 letter to Romain Rolland, he said of himself: "Everyone is a metaphysician at eighteen, and in addition a theologian if one is Swiss-French" (1917a). Four years later, when he moved from Paris to Geneva to work at the Rousseau Institute, he asked: "what is the secret motive of Geneva's effort to apply psychological methods to education . . . if not the moral, and consequently religious motive, that led Frommel to look for the psychological roots of his faith, and Vinet always to start from man to explain Christianity?" (1921b, 410; see also remarks in 1942 and 1944).

Piaget's singling out of Vinet and Frommel is highly significant. Alexandre Vinet (1797–1847), a theologian from the canton of Vaud, was a leading advocate of Protestant individualism (a term that Vinet rejected in favor of "individuality," but which nevertheless persists in connection with his thought). His follower Gaston Frommel (1862–1906) stated the objective of Protestantism as "the increasingly total obedience to an increasingly internal authority" (Frommel, 1900, 177). Liberals and orthodox alike looked to both Vinet and Frommel as theological authorities.

For Vinet, true Christianity could emanate only from individual conscience. Sincerity was the most important aspect of religious experience. Faith had to be "living" and "personal" rather than based on prejudice, authority, habit, or logic. Freedom of conscience implied full religious freedom, as well as separation of church and state. Against state socialism, Vinet advocated a system of "solidarity" respectful of individual rights. (On Vinet, Rambert's 1875 biography remains essential; see most recently B. Reymond, 1990.)

Vinet's immediate spiritual descendant was Charles Secrétan (1815–1895), also from the canton of Vaud. Secrétan emphasized the conformity between the Gospel and man's "moral being." He saw "a burgeoning Christian in each man attentive to his conscience" (quoted in Grin, 1930, 157). Secrétan considered Kant one of his masters. He questioned, however, the possibility of deducing the object of moral obligation from pure forms of reason, claimed that man's duties could be ascertained through empirical knowledge of the world and humanity, and eventually elaborated a theology based on the analysis of conscience and religious and moral experience. Secrétan was a friend of Pierre Bovet's father, Félix, a committed Pietist.

Under diverse forms, Vinet's and Secrétan's basic tenets imbued Swiss-French Protestantism at the turn of the century. Theology was an exercise in inner observation. The Christian was the individual who remained attentive and loyal to his inner conscience and who tried to harmonize with it his reason, his experience, and his behavior.

Gaston Frommel was considered Vinet's closest follower. At the beginning of the twentieth century, he was one of the most influential figures of the Swiss Christian Students' Association. His theology was grounded on moral conscience and on each individual's inner conversion and spiritual experiences. Frommel (1915) described it as being "experimental," that is, experiential, proceeding inductively and descriptively from introspective observation. God was to be found in the personal sentiment of faith and a sense of duty. Only the "person," he said, is the ultimate foundation of religion. (On Frommel, see Berchtold, 1963, 97–115.)

Social Christianity and Christian Socialism

Late nineteenth-century Protestant bourgeoisie everywhere tended to pursue ideals of social improvement. Philanthropies, charities, and other "good works" were a traditional form of such commitment; members of the Swiss-French Protestant community also became *dreyfusards*[2] and militated against colonialism and for women's rights. Typically, neither political involvement nor practical humanitarianism implied a renunciation of individualism: the goal was to improve everybody's lot without diminishing each person's responsibility.

In Piaget's milieu, approaches to the widely discussed "social question," that is, the inequities that accompanied industrial capitalism, were dominated by two related doctrines, social Christianity and Christian socialism.[3] Their followers were known, respectively, as social Christians *(chrétiens sociaux)* and Christian socialists *(socialistes chrétiens)*. Although the distinction between the former, who wanted a better society, and the latter, who wanted a new society, was not always clear-cut, a formal division did take place.

In 1908 a Union of Christian Socialists (Union des Socialistes Chrétiens) was founded in France, with the motto "Socialists Because Christians" and a journal called *L'espoir du monde* (The Hope of the World). From 1910 to 1914, several groups were formed in French-speaking Switzerland, and a local Christian Socialist Federation (Fédération Romande des Socialistes Chrétiens) was established in March 1914. The war divided the French and the Swiss, the former supporting the principle of a just war and even insisting that German

Protestants admit their government's war responsibility, the latter remaining resolutely pacifist and nonviolent. In 1918 the Swiss Federation severed all links with the Union and launched its own journal, *Voies nouvelles* (New Ways).

Protestant social Christianity was very much alive among youth. The members of the Swiss Christian Students' Association often attended speeches on social problems and were encouraged to take part in their resolution. They heard, for example, the minister Paul Sublet (1871–1915) define "social conscience" as "personal conscience that moves ahead" and exhort them to enter the social arena (Sublet, 1914, 30–31; 1911, 25). Sublet, the social Christian leader in French-speaking Switzerland, was the founder of *L'Essor,* a periodical aimed at promoting a society that would be more in harmony with the Gospel's teachings. Social Christianity often appeared as a new revival, and its concerns and quite lyrical vocabulary permeated Christian students' groups.

According to Elie Gounelle (1865–1950), a French social Christian leader, it was first necessary to help the individual experience the "living Christ," since "the reform of inner life is the fundamental condition of universal social reform" (Gounelle, 1919, 7–8). Only then could it move to an initial social level, where it would follow Christ, "Holiness made man" (ibid., 8), by fighting alcoholism, prostitution, and other social evils. Gradually reform would extend to national and world politics. The social Christian enterprise was grounded on the belief that "the essential law of the universe is not competition, but cooperation"; the generalization of such a law "would be nothing other than a liberal and brotherly socialism" (ibid., 9–10). Gounelle's position exhibits the blurring of boundaries: while he was officially a social Christian, he participated in the elaboration of the Christian socialist platform (Baubérot, 1985, pt. 2, chap. 2).

A recurrent theme in social Christian writings (particularly in those with a socialist bent) was that the ultimate root of the social question was not poverty itself, but the conflict between capital and labor. Such socialism is best described as a form of "solidarism," a doctrine so named by the French sociologist Célestin Bouglé (1870–1940). Socialistic solidarity by no means implied equality, but only the free cooperation of distinct and responsible individuals. Piaget's godfather, Samuel Cornut, who sympathized with social Christianity and saw in the beehive a foreshadowing of the better world, optimistically believed that mutual aid had already started to replace the struggle for life (Cornut, 1910, 209–210).

Social Christianity in French-speaking Switzerland had clear socialist inclinations, even though of a very moderate kind. It rejected the idea of revolution and advocated gradual change. Its leaders were mainly bourgeois intellectual

ministers who, in conformity with the basic Christian principle that the transformation of the world starts with that of the human heart, insisted on the
formation of the individual.

One of the most fervent apologies of a conciliation between Christianity and
socialism was pronounced at the 1914 conference of the Swiss Christian
Students' Association by the French minister Wilfred Monod (1867–1943).
Monod was an old friend of Piaget's parents, and he would comment at length
on the manuscript of *The Mission of the Idea*. A year after his lecture to the
young Christians, he joined the French Socialist party. Monod explained that
Christ had been crucified "by the wealthy and the rulers," and because of his
ethics rather than because of his doctrine. If Christianity is based on Christ's
teachings, he concluded, "then the Gospel is essentially social" (Monod,
1914a, 32). Monod encouraged social Christians to supplement the study of
the Bible by that of the capitalist system, to become Christian socialists, and
thus to surmount the "dangerous and unacceptable antithesis" of the "two
great moral powers of our age, Socialism and Christianity" (ibid., 25).

In 1917 the minister Maurice Neeser (1883–1955), who would later teach
the psychology of religion at the University of Neuchâtel, championed the
"synthesis of the ideal of the Church and the International, both of which betray the Gospel if they refuse to combine with each other" (Neeser, 1917, 58).
His grand perspective on the future reverberated among young Christians:
"Outside socialism, outside the churches if necessary, men will march toward
the full Gospel; the realization of supreme syntheses is tomorrow's ideal"
(ibid., 63).

None of this made Protestants abandon their individualism. In true Reformation tradition, social Christians or Christian socialists found their truth in
the Gospel alone and oriented their faith and action according to Jesus' example and personality. Their rule of life did not come from a party program or a
church constitution, but from the Sermon on the Mount. In the words of
Leonhard Ragaz (1868–1945), the Christian socialist leader in German-speaking Switzerland, "We do not care to bind the Gospel to any economic order ...
We assert only that the economic goal of socialism seems in agreement with
the ideal of life that follows from the Gospel" (quoted in Léonard, 1964, 422).
The movement's ideal, in sum, was to Christianize the social order; and none
of its adherents would agree with the *Communist Manifesto*'s deadly epigram,
"Christian Socialism is but the holy water with which the priest consecrates the
heart-burnings of the aristocrat" (Marx and Engels, 1848, 89).

Psychology and Religion

As we noted earlier, Piaget was fully aware of the intimate relationship between
the distinctive features of the school of psychology he would himself exemplify

and the nature of Swiss-French Protestantism. The main figures of the Swiss-French psychological tradition that Piaget continued in the 1920s are Théodore Flournoy (1854–1920), his cousin Edouard Claparède (1873–1940), and their disciple and friend Pierre Bovet (1878–1965). In 1892 Flournoy founded the first experimental psychology laboratory at the University of Geneva's sciences department; in 1912 Claparède established the Jean-Jacques Rousseau Institute, which Bovet directed until 1933. The three were deeply committed Protestants, and much of their cognitive and moral universe overlapped with that of Piaget before he became Claparède's and Bovet's colleague at the Rousseau Institute in 1921.[4]

Flournoy and Bovet were militant Protestants, active in the Swiss Christian Students' Association. Bovet had been the ACSE's general secretary. Flournoy lectured frequently at its annual conference, and two of his lectures, on "religious genius" (1905) and William James (1911a), became classical references of local intellectuals. Claparède's militancy was more political, but it also derived from Protestant liberalism.

Claparède (1930, 83) defined liberalism as "a method of intellectual and moral loyalty." He described himself as "extremely attached to Protestantism, thanks to which this method of free inquiry was introduced into the world and the principle of toleration into religious matters." For him, religious belief could only be "the outcome of certain moral and emotional experiences that the individual feels called upon to interpret or explain" (ibid.). Liberalism, pragmatism, and Protestantism, he wrote, were to politics, philosophy, and religion what the empirical method was to science: "a method of truth, substituting the free study of facts for the coercion of dogma or the dead weight of prejudice" (ibid.). In such convictions, Claparède was Flournoy's disciple.

In 1902 Flournoy gave a series of lessons on religious psychology. At almost the same time his friend William James (1842–1910) delivered in Edinburgh the lectures that became *The Varieties of Religious Experience*. In Flournoy's vocabulary, the term *religious psychology* was shorthand for "psychology of religion or religious phenomena"—a fashionable and successful discipline from the 1880s until World War I (Berguer, 1914). For Flournoy (1903, 3, n. 1), this new science was neither religious nor antireligious. It was simply a "positive science" limited to the objective examination of "facts," and aimed at "detheologizing" and "psychologifying" the study of religion (ibid., 5, n. 2). Flournoy mentioned Frommel's theology as an enterprise animated by the same ambition.

Flournoy's first methodological principle was the "exclusion of transcendence": the question of the transcendent existence of spiritual entities was not within the competence of religious psychology. The second principle was the "biological interpretation" of religious phenomena: religion was a "vital function" to be investigated alongside the organic and psychological economy of the organism. Flournoy the psychologist, in consequence, was free to interpret reincarnations, the gift of tongues, and mediumistic states as "subliminal creations" resulting from "suggestibility" and "cryptomnesia," or to explain mystical ecstasy in terms of "erotogenesis" and "sublimation" (Flournoy, 1900 and 1915).

Yet Flournoy was convinced that psychological interpretations left the realm of belief unaffected. As he explained to a group of Christian students, religion was for him a "sentiment," of which dogmas were an "intellectual translation"; religion was therefore "undemonstrable by scientific procedures" (Flournoy, 1913a, 474, 478). Conversely, he affirmed that science "exists only in thought," "says nothing about the ultimate root of things," and "lets the ultimate mystery subsist" (ibid., 478). And he ended by citing approvingly his French contemporary, the mathematician Henri Poincaré (1854–1912), author of the 1902 classic *Science and Hypothesis*.

Flournoy's epistemology was indeed close to Poincaré's conventionalism, and both were akin to religious liberalism. This linkage was best exemplified in the Bergsonian Catholic Edouard Le Roy (1870–1954), for whom religious dogmas, like scientific concepts, were only practical rules for moral conduct (Le Roy, 1899–1900, 1907). Flournoy, a Protestant, was closest in style and spirit to James, who in a striking aphorism claimed, "God is real since he produces real effects" (James, 1902, 389).

Pragmatism and liberal Protestantism were committed to the sovereignty of individual experience and to the rejection of all forms of authority external to inner conscience. Flournoy (for example, ca. 1884) considered that both were essentially Kantian standpoints. Moreover, he saw in pragmatism the philosophical expression of the genuine Protestant attitude, since it "moves . . . the seat of authority in the same direction as the religious Reformation" (Flournoy, 1911a, 68). Following James, he called pragmatism a "philosophical Protestantism," consistent with the ideals of liberty, positive science, and democracy (ibid.; compare James, 1907, especially chaps. 2 and 8). Similar pronouncements can be found in Claparède's and Bovet's writings. They all shared what the French philosopher Emile Boutroux (1908, 345) called the "comfortable system of watertight compartments"—science in one, religion in the other.

Flournoy's influence on turn-of-the-century Swiss-French Protestant intellectuals came from what was perceived as a major achievement: to harmonize in one's personality the ideals of the scientist and the believer. Pierre Bovet (1920, 534), who was one of his most fervent disciples, observed that Flournoy managed to avoid both "theological rationalism" and "scientific dogmatism."

By means of publications, courses, public lectures, and private individual services as "physician of the soul," he demonstrated, to the satisfaction of his contemporaries, "the irreducible heterogeneity" between knowledge and belief. A thankful witness (who was a prominent conservative politician in Geneva) recalled that Flournoy's teachings "saved many from wasting their energy in the sterile conflict between science and faith." "It would be difficult," he noted, "to say how many students . . . have been grateful to the teacher who either delivered them from the distrust toward science that had been instilled by an orthodox and dogmatic religious instruction, or reassured them about the legitimacy of a spiritualistic faith shaken by the latest waves of materialistic monism" (Picot, 1920, 582–583).

The Writers' Malaise

Despite the rich diversity of *fin-de-siècle* Swiss-French literature (see Berchtold, 1963, 369–487), critics and historians agree that it was characterized by educational goals, civic commitment, and introspective roots. Didactically realist and sober, the Swiss-French writer seemed less concerned with polishing a style than with providing a useful firsthand testimony of the human condition. The personal diary was a genre by way of which numerous Protestants entered the realm of letters; and much of their writing reported a thinly disguised self-examination. The ubiquitous moralism of Swiss-French letters at the end of the nineteenth century was often nothing other than a dramatization of the main themes of liberal theology, social Christianity, and the conciliation between faith and science.

Protestant literary critics themselves considered that their literature was not very brilliant. Even the Neuchâtel writer Philippe Godet (1850–1922), who defended its "national and moral" character, attributed to the didactic and moralistic impulse "what has been sometimes called its mediocrity." His judgment is paradigmatic: "Nothing is further from the art-for-art's-sake aesthetics than our literature: it constantly aims at moral action; if not invariably grave and dogmatic, it is at least serious and chaste . . . Always and everywhere are asserted . . . a concern with great human interests, the authority of conscience, and the passion for usefulness. The Protestant soul expresses itself in this literature . . . it imposes upon itself the duty of being healthy and beneficial" (Ph. Godet, 1900, 335; see also idem, 1890; Rossel, 1903).

Philippe Godet's nephew, the Neuchâtel writer Charly Clerc (1882–1958), reported that before World War I his generation's literary preferences ran to texts in which an individual "narrated his spiritual odyssey" and scrutinized his own inner crises with a "Protestant voice" (Clerc, 1950, 52). He explained: "We liked . . . to be allowed to be doubters, without ceasing to be perfectly religious" (ibid., 53). The autobiographical novel was a favorite genre—and one to which Piaget contributed his 1918 *Recherche.*

Clerc placed Cornut among the writers appreciated by his contemporaries; and Cornut himself dreamt of a novel that would be recognized as Swiss-French not by picturesque details, but by the moral cast of the Protestant spirit.

The ambition to create a simultaneously Swiss and French literature embodies the tensions that, for Jean Starobinski, determine the Swiss-French writer. Placed at the intersection of two nations, within a culturally plural and multilingual country, Swiss-French writers refuse to be annexed by French literature yet want to be a part of it. They therefore adopt the attitude of the observer, of the marginal spectator. At least the great writers, Rousseau to begin with, artfully transform their marginality into "reflexive or poetic variations" on their own specificity, and they often do so under the form of two "extreme temptations," "critical vigilance" and a "lyrical withdrawal into inner experience" (Starobinski, 1970b, 397). Among nineteenth-century Swiss-French writers, these "temptations" tended to converge onto "a certain religious malaise" (Clerc, 1950) made up of doubt, anguish, and inner quest.

In 1852 Henri-Frédéric Amiel (1821–1881), a littérateur whose entire fame rests on an extraordinary, posthumously published diary, described Vinet in terms that remained valid fifty years later. Amiel called Vinet a "moralistic psychologist" and "the conscience-writer." The individualism that made Vinet's glory in theology was also "the cause of his weakness." As a writer, Vinet had no "grandeur" because he was constantly testing his thought; he was "too refined, subtle, analytic," and as a result his style conveyed a "feeling of scruple, anxiety, reserve." Thus, both his talent and his limitations were due to an "eternal suspicion of the self, a perpetual moral examination," an "excessively constant reflexivity" (Amiel, 1978, 320–321). A later critic diagnosed "the mania of analysis and abstraction" as the "almost incurable illness of the Swiss-French temper" (Weck, 1912, 15).

The Swiss Christian Students' Association

The Swiss Christian Students' Association was a major center of Swiss-French Protestantism, relaying the main themes of the local tradition by means of a discourse on youth's condition and mission. The Association contributed decisively to the formation of Piaget's identity as a young Christian intellectual, and to the elaboration of some of the central concerns of his work through the 1920s.

The ACSE belonged to the Universal Federation of Christian Students' Associations, established in 1895 by the American John Mott (1865–1955). Mott began his career as an itinerant secretary of the Young Men's Christian Association (YMCA), established in 1844 following the Great Awakening to bring young Christians together and organize them for evangelization. The ACSE's motto was "Make Jesus King"; its objective was to fight the "theoretical materialism" that had led to a "lack of ideals and sense of social responsibility" among students (Buscarlet, 1920, 5). Mott's triumphal tour of Swiss universities in 1911 was prepared through widely diffused pamphlets by his admirers Pierre Bovet (1911) and Théodore Flournoy (1911b).

The decision to found the ACSE (in 1897) was made at an 1895 YMCA conference held in the town of Sainte-Croix, in the Jura Mountains. The two groups were autonomous but maintained close relations. The ACSE was composed of local associations grouped in a German-speaking and a French-speaking branch. The latter held its annual meetings in Sainte-Croix. Composed of groups of university and gymnasium students, the ACSE organized meetings, administered student dormitories, and promoted missions. It published a monthly bulletin, *Nouvelles de l'Association Chrétienne Suisse d'Etudiants (ACSE News)*, and annual volumes summarizing the Sainte-Croix meeting and including in full some of the lectures presented there. It started accepting women in 1906.

The ACSE's self-proclaimed goal was to "bring together all those who sincerely search" and help them approach "the person of Christ as a *living personality*, and not as an object of theological argument" (Buscarlet, 1920, 8; see also *Statuts* and *Notre Association*). According to Charly Clerc, its raison d'être was "the development of *Christian individualities* among students" and the possibility of offering "to reserved and untamed souls its companionship . . . and its passion for free and open [spiritual] search" (quoted in Rougemont, 1921, 16, 17). The "Sainte-Croix community" seemed to him "the most complete manifestation of the spirit of the Reformation, which never ceases to search itself" (Clerc, 1923). But as he pointed out, "this tendency irritates."

> Whether in faith or politics, those long trials before taking sides for or against something; the serious flirt with diverse aspects of truth; the old way of approaching essential problems, too respectful and too individualistic; the taste for camping around a fire in the rain instead of staying by the stove, for running the dangers of the patrol instead of joining the main regiment—all that is no longer fashionable, it all recalls excessively the *Swiss-French tradition*, all that, as some begin to say more openly and contemptuously, is *Protestant*. (Ibid.)

Others characterized the Association diversely as "a seminar of psychological experiences," "a school of prophets," "a group of nice friends," "a place for the free development of religious personality," or a society aimed at "maintaining as close a contact as possible between Protestantism and modern culture" (Rougemont, 1921, 13–14). Its fundamental trait, however, was a certain "missionary spirit" (ibid., 15) that permeated the verbal and mental environment in which the young Christians evolved.

In *Recherche* Piaget portrayed the Association as a "fertile movement" (1918a, 38), characterized by flexibility. It had no creed and no political line, was neither liberal nor orthodox, and wished to reconcile everything. Its participants shared a need to search and create, and an "admirable common faith," which allowed them to discuss things "with a real independence" (ibid., 39). Sebastian, the novel's hero, is particularly attracted to the young Christians' religiosity: "Nothing compared to the life and majesty of their common religious service, when they joined their forces and their researches around a Christ stripped of all dogma. Each could commune with this Incarnation of the eternal value of the divine, since no intellectual translation dimmed this living contact" (ibid.). Such gatherings, where there was "a single silence, a single breadth, a single impulse toward God," were for Sebastian the best a "liberal religion" had to offer (ibid.). "The memory of those moments was enough for Sebastian to forgive Protestant youth for its incoherence" (ibid., 40).

The ACSE's conception of youth accorded closely with an emerging scientific and literary discourse (see Demos, 1972; Neubauer, 1992). Literature and science were in full agreement on the subject of youth. Thus one critic observed that Romain Rolland's *Jean-Christophe* presented such a "true" image of adolescent psychology that it seemed patterned after the table of contents of a "scientific" treatise (O'Brien, 1937, 205). In the same novel, the French pedagogue Gabriel Compayré (1843–1913) found passages that would have been inspired in G. Stanley Hall's "genetic psychology" (Compayré, 1909, 67). And for G. Stanley Hall (1846–1924), American pioneer of the psychologies of religion and adolescence, literary narratives were like "responses to questionnaires" sent to the past (Hall, 1904, 1:513). Scientific description accorded with personal experience and literary intuition.

Youth was described in terms of pure impulse and potential: the young man, wrote François Mauriac (1926, 10), "is a virgin force that no specialty monopolizes; he does not yet give up anything; all ways invite him." Youth was always depicted as passionate, full of dreams, hopes, and ideals, taking itself seriously, endowed with an emotional life in which energy, exhilaration, and ambition alternated with melancholy, insecurity, and dissatisfaction. Adolescence, Hall's age of *Sturm und Drang*, furnished the decisive impulse for humanity's major achievements.

Educators were unanimously concerned with adolescence, especially with channeling its multifarious energies and possibilities. Such was precisely the function of youth groups. The Club of the Friends of Nature appeared at about the same time as the major youth movements. Like Flournoy and Bovet (a promoter of the Boy Scouts), Hall took a keen interest in the Christian youth movements.

The Swiss Christian Students' Association proclaimed that there was an inherent link between religion and youth, and that the latter's mission was to regenerate Christianity and bring salvation to the world. The new psychological sciences seemed to validate such a belief. Hall (1904) thought that the Bible, especially the New Testament, was both the perfect psychological textbook and the reading matter best suited to the psychic makeup of youth. He saw religious conversion as a distinctively adolescent phenomenon. Christ was for him an exemplary case of adolescent psychology, and a model that educators should deliberately use. Hall's great treatise on adolescence (1904) and his psychological biography of Jesus were intrinsically related, for "Jesus' spirit was in some sense the consummation of that of adolescence" (Hall, 1917, 1:xviii). At Sainte-Croix, Flournoy told young Christians "that, of all the philosophies and religions, Jesus' religion is the one that offers most affinity with youth"; he emphasized "the special combination of features that, in Jesus' personality, speaks most to your hearts, and corresponds to the noblest aspirations of your age: heroism of the will, intellectual emancipation, and generosity of soul" (Flournoy, 1905, 46).

The Theme of Crisis

The ACSE's great leitmotif was the crisis that each believer was supposed to undergo in the progress toward genuine faith: "At a time when the student faces the most anguishing problems, those that shake the whole edifice of his childhood faith; when he is about to choose an orientation for his whole life and to prepare himself to struggle for the Good; and when, above all, he needs support and affection, he remains alone and abandoned" (Rougemont, n.d., 34). The ACSE would provide just what such a situation required. Former members recalled having lived "decisive hours," "found Christ," calmed their anguish, and found an environment for carrying on the "quest" in the company of their peers (see, for example, Margot, 1913; L. Schmidt, 1913; Galland, 1916).

According to one report, the members of the ACSE fell into three categories (Wyler, 1917, 68–69). The youngest (aged sixteen to nineteen) were high school students or had just entered the university. They were naive and enthusiastic, had received a religious education, and had already glimpsed the "higher values necessary to the flowering of their inner being." They did not yet know how to affirm those values; they found the churches "cold, static, amorphous," and joined the ACSE with the hope of being succored in their search for a personal religious life.

The second category consisted of university students "in the midst of a religious crisis," an event deemed "inevitable for all those who study seriously and passionately." They turned to the ACSE looking for support in that period "of doubt and, often, of suffering, when the personality creates itself and grows little by little."

The third category of members included students whose religious crisis had led either to a new and personal religion or to the annihilation of all religious life. Those who had acquired "certainties, perhaps minimal, but real," animated the Association's religious life and guided the younger members.

The spiritual crisis that was declared so essential for the life of young Christian intellectuals was also seen as an inherent condition of the ACSE as an institution. The Sainte-Croix meetings, it was said, demonstrated that no solution was perpetually valid, "that everything must always be started all over again, and that, in sum, the crisis rages" (Clerc, 1923). This endlessly repeated theme defined an age-related norm. Individual crises were lavishly prophesied to those who were about to enter the universities; they were placed by psychologists at the core of the adolescent experience, made prominent by writers, and thought by every religiously inclined educator to be an inescapable event in the life of every young Christian intellectual, for whom it was the only sure sign of the emergence of a genuine faith.

The Mission of Youth

The general mobilization in Europe in 1914 dramatically weakened all national Christian students' associations, and throughout the war the *ACSE News* reported the demise of one group after another as European youth was decimated. Reports about Austrian, French, or German casualties who had spent some time in Switzerland often also printed their letters, excerpts from their diaries, and recollections by surviving comrades. An analogous literature appeared in the publications of the YMCA.

In Switzerland, all men above the age of twenty were mobilized for the protection of national borders, although they did not participate in combat. Still, the Swiss situation was perceived as dramatic. The Association found itself in the privileged yet psychologically difficult position of being able to think about what was going on in the rest of Europe without losing its own members in the bloodbath.

The most persistent view of the wartime *ACSE News* and other publications of the Christian students' movement was that a new world would be born out of the war, and that Christian youth would play a crucial role in its construction (Dietrich, n.d.). Neutral countries, and the Swiss in particular, were widely perceived as having special responsibilities in preparing for the postwar era. In fact, however, the ACSE seemed consumed by malaise. In an atmosphere of anguished expectation, young Christians wondered "how to live" and how to participate in the "birth of the new world." Dominated by the painful and melancholy feeling that something would soon happen, they feared not being up to their redemptive task. The February 1915 report of the Neuchâtel ACSE group, to which Piaget belonged, is typical:

> As the echoes of the terrible tempest that rages in the distance reach us, we have, in tacit agreement, closed ranks, and we march more united than before, minds shaken by the same disappointments, hearts suffering from the same painful realities.
>
> Consciously or unconsciously, we have begun to create an atmosphere that will enable the mind to think freely, the heart and conscience to bloom, to experience, even if only for an instant, the realities we feel are true, and to speak freely, without the paralyzing fear of "not being understood."
>
> It is absurd to envision serious and fertile work as long as those who are called to make the common effort live separated from each other in watertight compartments. All we get is cold discussions of ideas or ingenious but perfectly sterile reasonings that barely touch our personalities, and only graze our lives.
>
> We have always suffered from that in Neuchâtel. This winter, we aspire to more intimacy and truth; we have only one desire: "more profound life" . . .
>
> The march is certainly slow and rough, but we do not lose courage, because we long for true communion. Only on such a basis have we the right to examine our moral and intellectual difficulties, with the desire to find the clue to life, and not selfish joys for our intelligence.
>
> Somebody said that a witness of the Christ is a man who *affirms, suffers,* and *acts* . . . This is how I would summarize [the needs] of Neuchâtel's Association:
>
> 1. An ever-stronger unity among the members;
> 2. A more pronounced spirit of consecration and prayer;
> 3. An ever-increasing sense of our responsibility.
>
> The members of our Association will then be able to be witnesses who affirm the realities of religious life because they have *experienced* them, who suffer because they love, because they feel deeply what they lack and what is missing from humanity . . . and who act because, in them, communion with God has become a power of life that must manifest itself. (L. Schmidt, 1915; see also Coulon, 1913)

For the young Christians of the ACSE, the war was a time of individual and

collective crises, full of painful moral and intellectual difficulties to be reconciled with the desire to "live" by enacting the model provided by Jesus. In
sum, the war was not just another topic of deliberation, but the occasion of
a new revival that would free youth from abstractions, guide them toward
a concrete Christian life, and thrust them forward in their redemptive mission.

Youth's "Anti-Intellectualism"

In 1916, to the question "What have been the effects of the War on your Movement?" the Swiss Christian Students' Association answered: "There seems to
be much more seriousness in the students' thought and life. Many of them feel
a strong desire to be rid of philosophical and theoretical discussions, and to
adopt a religion that allows them to believe without previous pondering . . . It
seems that religious needs are more clearly and more deeply felt" (Anon.,
1916a). Many personal testimonies and analyses of the contemporary situation emphasized the students' desire to root their spiritual life in the "living
reality" of God, and especially of Christ, to embody this "reality" in a personal
religion, and to make it the force that inspired their reconstruction of the
world after the war. Such a desire reflected a widespread opposition to "intellectualism."

Indeed, the generation of young intellectuals born about 1890 were united
in their rejection of the positivist, rationalist, and secularized universe of their
elders (Wohl, 1979). Bergsonian philosophy, facilely tagged "anti-intellectualist," attracted nationalists and internationalists, Catholics and Protestants,
"patriots" and pacifists. A 1916 synthesis of contemporary surveys of youth
concluded that young people were seduced by the Bergsonian emphasis on
spiritual activity, intuition, and instinct, as well as by its appeal to life, experience, and will (Dartigue, 1916, 291). Bergson's impact on the generation of
1914 is apparent not only in this generation's desire to "live" and be active but
also in the extensive literary glorification of the adolescent. As a critic of
Bergsonism noted, the literature of adolescence aimed at apprehending and
celebrating this age's élan vital, creatively advancing against the inertia of social
norms (Henri Massis in O'Brien, 1937, 59).

At the 1916 ACSE conference, a minister noticed that certain young people
were endowed with "more impulse, the firm intention of shaking off their self-
suspicion and the habits of unhealthy introspection . . . [and] a desire for practical achievements outside intellectual speculations" (Cuendet, 1916, 115). He
also underlined the discouragement and distress of young people who were
tired of "theological struggles" and the "unnerving conflict between science
and faith," who had emancipated themselves from positivism yet remained
troubled by Bergson's philosophy. Swiss-French Protestantism seemed to him

to suffer from an "illness of scruple" and doubt that prevented the "vital force" from flourishing. How to act, how to "enter into contact with reality and live it" so as to respond to postwar needs—such were the preoccupations of the group of young Protestant intellectuals to which Piaget belonged when he wrote *The Mission of the Idea.*

Sainte-Croix

From 1895 to 1922 the ACSE organized four-day meetings in late September or early October at Sainte-Croix. Participants included not only students but also theologians, ministers, writers, scientists, philosophers, psychologists, and other Christian intellectuals. Three generations, including Piaget's, considered it the most important spiritual moment of the year. The conference reports and the printed lectures became basic cultural references, and the meetings themselves were seen as a sensitive barometer of the region's philosophical and theological life.

The situation of the village of Sainte-Croix, at an altitude of about 1,000 meters in the Jura Mountains, with a view of the Alps on a clear day, inspired a discourse imbued with the symbolism of the mountain as the place where God communicates with man. In many ways the Sainte-Croix mystique is reminiscent of the conservative Catholic French writer Maurice Barrès's "sacred hill": "Places there are that arouse the soul from its torpor, places enveloped, bathed in mystery, and chosen eternally as the seat of religious emotion . . . In them we feel a sudden need for breaking our sultry bonds . . . and, on the two wings of prayer and poetry, we are launched into great affirmations" (Barrès, 1912, 1–2).

When going to Sainte-Croix, conference participants relived the mystical theme of ascension. It was common to speak of "up there" by contrasting the calm, hospitable, luminous, and purifying mountain with the plain to which one descended after unique moments of communion, illumination, and inner transformation. The "peace of the summits," the atmosphere of "harmony," "unity," "freedom," "sincerity," and "joy" encouraged the formation of friendships, the awakening of vocations, even "the vision of Christ." Only from high up was it possible to "glimpse tomorrow's ideal." (For the literary theme of Sainte-Croix, see the introduction to each annual conference report.)

Particularly during World War I, Sainte-Croix was perceived as the privileged place of a "quest." In the midst of their malaise and anguish, young people left the mountain invigorated, better prepared to carry out their mission in the agitated city environment. A report of the 1915 meeting states:

> One does not go to Sainte-Croix to see the students amuse themselves; I do not hesitate to say it: one goes there to see them suffer. The students . . . con-

centrate themselves to carry out their task, accept the anguishing problems, and offer themselves to God the better to serve Him among men. Never, not even on the occasion of revivals, have I attended such tragic and simple meetings of prayer, where one feels as much in contact with realities. Young people, in addition, are capable of a heroic seriousness that very few grownup men are able to sustain throughout their lives; they wish to see beyond darkness, they want to attain truth, and they want to serve truth . . .

Nevertheless, for the moral portrait of the conference to be accurate, it is still necessary to utter two more words: joy and trust; for true joy lies in suffering, and true trust is born from anguish.   (Jeannet, 1915, 2–3)

Sainte-Croix, in sum, was an often decisive experience and an engaging, somewhat mystical symbol that epitomized the mental outlook and the fundamental concerns of Swiss-French Protestants at the beginning of the twentieth century. But whereas in Barrès's "sacred hill" the self was invaded by pure religious emotion, the Sainte-Croix communion involved a lot of discussion. It was in lectures, religious services, and missionary or Bible sessions that young people were initiated to theology and philosophy, discovered social problems and the possible links between Christianity and socialism, searched for ways to resolve the conflict between religion and science, shared their agonizing spiritual quests, examined current events, and learned to see themselves as Christ's heirs, as apostles destined to pursue a redemptive mission in a world in crisis.

9

The Problem of Religion

According to Piaget's own account, by the time he discovered Bergson he "was already acutely aware of the conflict of science and religion." Such awareness was a result of having been "brought up in the Protestant faith by a believing mother, whereas my father was a nonbeliever" (1965, 5). "There was," he wrote, "the problem of religion":

> When I was about fifteen, my mother, being a devout Protestant, insisted on my taking what is called at Neuchâtel "religious instruction," that is, a six weeks' course on the fundamentals of Christian doctrine. My father, on the other hand, did not attend church, and I quickly sensed that for him the current faith and an honest historical criticism were incompatible. Accordingly I followed my "religious instruction" with lively interest but, at the same time, in the spirit of free thinking. Two things struck me at the time: on the one hand, the difficulty of reconciling a number of dogmas with biology, and on the other, the fragility of the "five proofs of the existence of God." We were taught five, and I even passed my examination in them! Though I would not even have dreamed of denying the existence of God, the fact that anyone should reason by such weak arguments (I recall only the proof by the finality of nature and the ontological proof) seemed to me all the more extraordinary since my pastor was an intelligent man, who himself dabbled in the natural sciences!
>
> At that time I had the good fortune to find in my father's library the *Philosophy of Religion Based on Psychology and History* by Auguste Sabatier. I devoured that book with immense delight. Dogmas reduced to the function of "symbols" necessarily inadequate, and above all the notion of an "evolution of dogmas"—there was a language which was much more understandable

and satisfactory to the mind. And now a new passion took possession of me: philosophy. (1952, 239–240)

The "second crisis" (ibid., 240), induced by the initiation to Bergson's philosophy, followed shortly thereafter.

Piaget's problem of religion has two aspects: the opposition between science and religion, presumably between the theory of evolution and the dogma of divine creation; and religion's apparent lack of solid foundations: the proofs of the existence of God seem to Piaget "weak arguments." Less apparent from Piaget's autobiographical comments is that the two dimensions of the problem were for him interdependent, and that the reconciliation of religion and science he aspired to realize was largely aimed at giving religion a more solid basis.

That is indeed the problem Piaget places at the beginning of his philosophical development when he writes that after his discovery of Bergson he decided to devote his life "to philosophy, whose central aim I saw as the reconciliation between science on the one hand, and religious values on the other" (1965, 5). According to the best-known autobiographical recollection, the encounter with Bergson inspired Piaget to consecrate his life to the "biological explanation of knowledge" (1952, 240). But the two accounts are not mutually incompatible. The conflict between science and religion in the young Piaget's life turns out to be much less a matter of contradiction between reason and dogma than a matter of handling the relations between subjective faith and objective knowledge as they were envisioned within the framework of Swiss-French Protestantism, and of elaborating a view of religion consistent with the Bergsonian critique of science.

The Family Constellation

Aside from Piaget's autobiography, there is little evidence available about the parts played by his parents in his religious formation. One sign confirms that Piaget reacted against his mother. In 1919, in the analysis of a dream that can be reliably attributed to him (Vidal, 1986a, 184–185), Piaget detected a "conflict" between the dreamer and his mother, as well as a "silent hostility" toward her. In the course of free association, Piaget reported that the conflict "recalls others, and witnesses to a hostility that has existed for a long time. The subject [dreamer] thinks about the moral crises during which he tried to free himself of the education imposed by his mother, and evolve in a more personal direction" (1920b, 21). Since, in his autobiography, Piaget mentions religious instruction in connection with his mother, it is plausible to consider such instruction as a factor in a larger conflict with maternal authority.

As for Arthur Piaget, he was an agnostic, but he was not indifferent to local religious affairs. This is attested by his participation in the 1906 campaign for the separation of church and state. Arthur Piaget advocated separation and signed, together with his more militant colleagues Philippe Godet and Pierre Bovet, an open letter defending the cause (see *La Séparation,* a periodical of "separatist citizens," 1 December 1906, 1). As an agnostic, he could only be on the separatist side, since separation implied the equality of all religious communities within a secular state that guaranteed the same freedom for all.

This is as much as we know about Piaget's family's position regarding religious matters. And psychologizing the problem of religion will not take us far beyond Piaget's attributing his adolescent crises "both to family conditions and to the intellectual curiosity characteristic of that productive age" (1952, 239). A crucial element in Piaget's religious development is provided by a context in which the conflict between science and religion was a virtually mandatory experience for all young Christian intellectuals, and in which the course of religious instruction was the standard procedure for ushering young people into such an experience.

Religious Instruction

Since 1874, Neuchâtel had had two churches. The National church was state supported; all citizens could participate in the election of its ministers, who were not obliged to submit to a confession of faith. The Independent church had been born from a concern with doctrinal unity, and therefore from the refusal to accept the law that prohibited the inclusion of a confession of faith in the church's constitution (Monvert, 1898). From the religious point of view, however, the two churches were essentially the same.

The first stage of religious education was the Sunday school, which children started attending at about age seven. One-hour lessons were given every week by a minister or a lay "monitor," usually a schoolteacher. In Piaget's youth, children from the two churches attended the same Sunday schools. The typical course presented chronologically arranged episodes from the New Testament, as well as parables and miracles, and was supposed to be delivered in a familiar and simple style. At the end of the nineteenth century, for a French-speaking Protestant population of 84,000, there were in the canton of Neuchâtel 145 Sunday schools, with about 11,700 pupils and 820 monitors (Joseph, 1896, 25).

Sunday school was the first step toward religious confirmation. From about ages twelve to fourteen, children participated in the "service of the young." From fourteen to sixteen, they attended a class of "preparatory religious instruction." In order to be confirmed, they ought to have attended for at least two years the youth's religious service and the preparatory instruction, and be sixteen years old. Finally, before confirmation, young people had to follow a course of catechism (the "religious instruction" Piaget mentions in his autobiography), which took place for two hours every day for six weeks. (See *L'instruction religieuse.*)

Piaget belonged to the parish of Neuchâtel's Collegiate church (the Collégiale), followed the six weeks of religious instruction with Charles-Daniel Junod, pastor of the Independent church, and was confirmed during Pentecost in May 1912.[1] Junod (1865–1941), a minister in Neuchâtel for almost forty years, was a well-known and esteemed local figure, concerned above all with social and moral improvement; he regarded the anti-alcohol campaign of the Blue Cross as "the church's true evangelization task" (quoted in Rt., 1941).

The religious instruction was colored by a certain revivalist spirit. The "six weeks" were considered as "solemn days," as a unique opportunity to "apprehend the eternal life." An official publication of the Swiss-French Independent Churches addressed to catechumens the following message:

> The six weeks of religious instruction go by fast, too fast. In a few weeks, in a few days, they will be over, and you will go back to your ordinary life, to your usual milieu, you will return to your daily occupations and to the concerns of your work. Will you ever again find an opportunity as the one that is offered to you now, to think about your soul, to examine the paths you follow, to explore your own heart and collect yourself before your Savior in order to hear his voice and listen to his promises of salvation? . . . This is the hour, you hear the voice of the divine friend; listen to it, do not harden your heart! (Joseph, 1915)

The message emphasized the individual's piety, conversion, and personal relation to Jesus. The "six weeks" were less focused on the transmission of dogma than on self-examination; catechumens were encouraged to abandon the faith of their childhood and to acquire a personal faith through the experience of conversion. The aim of this critical period was to induce a religious crisis supposed to be the starting point of the elaboration of a more genuine and individual faith (see also Vuilleumier, 1913).

In this context, the book whose discovery was Piaget's "good luck" (1952, 240), Auguste Sabatier's *Outlines of a Philosophy of Religion Based on Psychology and History,* played an indisputably crucial educational role.

Sabatier dedicated his *Outlines* to young people, with the goal of helping them resolve the "religious question," that is, the "mysterious problem" of destiny, which he thought to be the "most vital" of all (Sabatier, 1897, iv). He thought that the youth of each generation wondered about the sense and purpose of life "with a new passion, because it wants to live, because to live is to act, and because all action presupposes a faith" (ibid.). He was so convinced that youth necessarily ask the famous "question" that he defined it as the age group that imperiously felt the need of elaborating a personal faith in order to live.

The religious question was thus timelessly human, and inherent in the condition of being young. For each generation, however, its particular form was determined by historical contingencies. Sabatier wished to help the youth of his own time, for whom the question was embodied in the conflict between religion and science. He wrote:

> Our young people . . . are pushing bravely forward, marching between two high walls: on one side, modern science with its rigorous methods, which can no longer be given up; on the other, the dogmas and the customs of the religious institution in which they were reared, and to which they would, but cannot, sincerely return. The sages who have led them hitherto point to the impasse they have reached, and bid them take a part—either for science against religion, or for religion against science. They hesitate, with reason, in face of this alarming alternative. Must we then choose between pious ignorance and bare knowledge? Must we either continue to live a moral life belied by science, or set up a theory of things which our consciences condemn? Is there no issue to the dark and narrow valley which our anxious youth traverse? I think there is. (Ibid., v)

Sabatier found the solution of the dilemma in the "synthetic and pacificatory consciousness . . . of the universal and sovereign Being," or "sentiment of the presence of God" (ibid., 364).

Sabatier's "synthesis" is a sort of mystical communion leading to freedom and to a perpetually creative spiritual youth:

> Inward religion, sacred instinct of life, divine immortal force which necessarily appears at the first movement of the spirit, how they misunderstand thee who see in thee only the slavery of man! On the contrary, it is thou alone that breakest all the chains that Nature binds on him, that savest him from death and from extinction . . . it is thou that renderest his spontaneity creative, that renewest his forces, and that, plunging him into the fountain whence he issued, maintainest in him an eternal youth! (Ibid., 365–366)

As he explained in a less exalted tone, the individual feels God "to be active and present, in his thought under the form of logical law, in his will under the form of moral law. He is saved by faith in the *interior* God, in whom is realized the unity of his being" (ibid., 365).

For Sabatier, in sum, the conflict between science and religion was a constitutive part of youth's identity. Educators concurred. In 1913, for example, the high school group of the Swiss Christian Students' Association heard Théodore Flournoy (1913, 474) predict that the contrast between high school and university education would manifest itself as the antagonism "between traditional, childish religious faith and the new horizons created by scientific discoveries." Flournoy did not doubt that this tension, which echoed that of the Sunday school and the later religious instruction, would stimulate personal religious quests.

We do not know whether Piaget was present at Flournoy's talk; but he surely was one of those young men to whom Sabatier dedicated his influential book. Piaget's reading of the *Outlines* may have been haphazard, the outcome of deliberate research, or the result of a recommendation or a requirement. Whatever it was, Sabatier's views on the "religious question" functioned as a model through which, at least in part, Piaget discovered, adopted, formulated, and resolved the conflict between religion and science. Such process was consistent with Sabatier's aims, which coincided with those of the "six weeks": to lead young people to a personal faith by means of spiritual conversion rather than dogmatic learning.

What about the rational proofs of God's existence? Piaget recalls that Junod was interested in the natural sciences; a bent for natural theology and a preference for the physico-theological proof would have been unexceptional. Nevertheless, it is doubtful that the five proofs Piaget mentions were dogmatically held as a body of established truths to be adopted without discussion. Almost nothing would be more incompatible with Swiss-French Protestantism in general, and with what we know in particular about the prevalent catechism. Such proofs could be attributed no doctrinal significance in a religion largely inspired by Kant, who had concluded his critique of reason by a vigorous invalidation of all rational arguments in favor of God's existence (see *Critique of Pure Reason*, "Transcendental Dialectics," book 2, chap. 3, secs. 4–6).

Moreover, religious instruction was oriented toward moral edification. The readings recommended to catechumens were narratives of exemplary religious lives, advice to youth, and collections of spiritual thoughts; the few specifically theological texts that are to be found among those readings were closer to ethics than to dogmatics. Whatever catechisms were used (if they were used at all) naturally included the basis of evangelical doctrine, but were aimed at teaching young people the principles of the Christian way of life and at persuading them to follow the example of Christ.

The Christian socialist Wilfred Monod's catechism, for example, avoided theological vocabulary and consistently emphasized social issues. His commentary on "Thou shall not kill" reads: "Respect human life, do not impose exhausting labors on your fellow human beings, do not lead them toward weakening pleasures, do not provide them with unhealthy lodging or food, do not disseminate tuberculosis . . . Suicide, duel, war are all forms of murder" (Monod, 1908, 9). Christ demands not only the individual's "moral conversion" but also the transformation of society, since he "promulgates social laws that are unworkable in the present state of things"; the sacrifice on the Cross shows that he "preferred death to being the slave of a false social and religious ideal" (ibid., 44, 55).

In a message to the catechumens who would use his book, Monod (ibid., xiii) explained that the goal of religious instruction was to clarify, refine, and strengthen their intelligence, heart, and will so that they would be better prepared to face the difficulties of choosing Christ as a model and guide. This choice required a conversion experience, "the most important event of all human life, for one is not *born* a Christian—one *becomes* a Christian" (ibid., 76). A later catechism by Monod (1929) consists of biographies of individuals all of whom go through a spiritual conversion and regeneration, and turn themselves toward social issues.

Equally illustrative of the ultimate aim of religious instruction is the title of another, less socially oriented book, presented as a collection of "conversations of a minister with his catechumens." *Toward Life!* sought to help young people find "true happiness" through Christ (Amiet, Vincent, and Vuilleumier, 1922, dedication). The authors wanted to explore with youth the latter's "serious concerns." They did so by relating biblical phrases or episodes to subjects deemed interesting for youth (money, freedom, "life's difficulties") and by narrating Christ's exemplary life. The last "conversation" treats of "God's family" and encourages catechumens by telling them that they now know which road to follow in life.

In sum, the existing documentation indicates that the six weeks of religious instruction in early twentieth-century Neuchâtel had little to do with a dogmatic approach based on learning systematic rational proofs. Naturally, this does not mean that Piaget did not have to learn them. He did, after all, have to study the fundamental Christian dogmas of redemption and the divinity of Christ, which he later rejected. Yet his religious instruction involved other, more essential spiritual dimensions. In his autobiography, Piaget recalled only that which fitted best the general orientation of his narrative. But we may venture an alternative, hypothetical but plausible.

In order to be admitted to the "six weeks," it was necessary to have followed religion classes for two years. Nothing suggests that Piaget was exempted from this rule. From fourteen to sixteen (1910 to 1912) he followed these classes and became familiar with the Bible. About three months before discovering Bergson, in April or May 1912, he went through the "six weeks." The problem of religion arose in that context—but not primarily as the inevitable outcome of an obvious contradiction between scientific culture and religious dogma. On the contrary, Piaget learned about the "conflict between science and religion" and came to feel it in himself as part of the process of religious instruction. Sabatier's *Outlines* fitted right in, however Piaget may have found it. The "six weeks" were therefore a success, since their goal was to induce a crisis, the resolution of which was the adoption of a faith rooted in the individual's feelings and conscience.

Such a scenario accords with Piaget's involvement with the Christian Students' Association starting in 1914. It is consistent with contemporary descriptions of the spiritual development of French-speaking Swiss intellectual Protestant youth. And it corresponds to Piaget's sister's recollections, according to which Junod was a very tolerant, liberal, understanding, and by no means dogmatic minister. According to the late Mme. Burger, her brother was very impressed by his religious education and, imbued with a deep Christian feeling, even thought of becoming a minister.

The Problem as Described in *Recherche*

Piaget's autobiographical novel, *Recherche,* confirms that the problem of religion must be understood in relation to the questions raised by the subjectivist and individualist character of Swiss-French Protestantism. The conflict between scientific findings and certain Christian dogmas might have sparked Piaget's interest, but no more than that. While no biographically relevant document deals with that conflict as such, all confirm Piaget's desire to give religion and morality an objective and universal foundation while maintaining the supremacy of individual conscience in matters of faith and value.

Recherche has the double function of criticizing the past and setting the stage for the future. Thus, if the conflict between religious dogmas and scientific findings described in Piaget's autobiography had been crucial to his early development, he would have examined it in his novel as a personally relevant issue. This is not the case.

There is no mention of the six weeks of religious instruction, and only a passing reference to Sabatier (1918a, 37); the problem of religion appears as emerging from the hero's spiritual quest, and in the context of his involvement with religious youth. This is not to say that there is no such thing in *Recherche* as a conflict between religion and science.

The autobiographical and the theoretical sections of *Recherche* share one fundamental idea. Near the beginning, the novel's hero, Sebastian, is said to have understood "the social meaning of the conciliation of science and faith, the problem that is at the origin of the entire present-day disequilibrium" (1918a, 21). The very last words of the book state that only Humanity (that is, the harmonious unity of individual diversity) will reconcile science and faith (ibid., 210). Piaget's was not a problem of *religion*, but of *faith*, that is, of a mode of knowledge (or of formulating knowledge-claims) that does not require the kind of proof and evidence science is supposed to furnish; and in *Recherche* it is related to the question of evil and to the goal of restoring individual and social "equilibrium."

Sebastian's initial understanding of the "disequilibrium" of his world came from mystically inclined Catholic youth and their difficulties with the notion of revelation. Science, Piaget explained, has invaded everything; philosophy has given up on one problem after another; youth has lost interest in both, and cultivated, partly under the spell of Charles Péguy, a mystical adherence to the authority of the Roman church (ibid., 14–16; allusion to Péguy, 17–18).

Sebastian perceived that, deep down, these young Catholics believed in the symbolic character of dogmas, and that such a belief made them suffer. The most sincere among them refused symbolism as an unworthy compromise and were torn between faith and rational doubt (1918a, 18–19). Sebastian's contact with Catholic youth led him to understand "the social meaning of the conciliation of science and faith": the Catholics' faith has been "paralyzed" by the doubt science fosters, and only an active faith is capable of carrying out the urgent task of saving the "social order" and the "world" (ibid., 21). Science is problematic because the reality it discloses combines "evil and good, disorder and order, life and death, ugliness and beauty"; existence is therefore "a mixture of values and nonvalues" (ibid., 22). Sebastian thus wanted to unite in his religion value and existence. He observed that the Catholics' predicament was rooted in the doctrine of divine revelation. A priest he talked to condemned the modernist and liberal movement for trying to understand grace rationally rather than merely accepting it (ibid., 27). But grace is a God-given privilege, and that was something Sebastian could not accept; in repudiating the divine "despot," he rejected the notion of a revealed and omnipotent God (ibid., 27, 29).

Sebastian then turned toward Protestantism. In both its liberal and orthodox forms, Protestantism appeared to him to be a compromise between the only two logically possible religions, Catholicism and absolute liberalism: "an inner revelation," he remarked, "is not a revelation" (1918a, 33). Something else had to be found. Sebastian shared his search with the Christian students. The question that tormented them all was, "How can we live when our faith is paralyzed by our thought, and when our thought is paralyzed by our faith? The quest for truth and the quest for value are two pursuits that destroy each other" (ibid., 41). This was the "agonizing problem of science and faith, the torment of the present generation" (ibid.).

10

From Catechism to Philosophy

The years 1912–1914 were decisive in Piaget's life. In March–April 1912 he received the six weeks of religious instruction. He read Sabatier at about that time and before his discovery of Bergson, which took place during the summer. He read at least the first long chapter of *Creative Evolution* sometime before September. At the end of that month he delivered his lecture "The Vanity of Nomenclature," which already incorporated Bergsonian elements. Toward the end of 1912 he inaugurated the debate with Roszkowski on the classification of deep-water *Limnaea*. The debate lasted until "Does the Mendelian Species Have an Absolute Value?" was written, in March or April 1914. "Bergson and Sabatier," Piaget's first article outside natural history, appeared in March 1914. From "The Vanity of Nomenclature" to "Bergson and Sabatier" Piaget developed a biological and philosophical system based on the ideas of *élan vital* and creative evolution. In between, he met Arnold Reymond, a philosopher who had a decisive influence on his thinking.

In 1913 Arnold Reymond (1874–1958) had just been named professor of philosophy at Neuchâtel's gymnasium and university. At the university he was a colleague of Piaget's father and a successor to their friend in common Pierre Bovet, who had just left for Geneva to direct the Rousseau Institute. Piaget always considered Reymond as one of his masters. After an initial period of disagreement, Reymond's demonstration that the problem of the biological species can be approached as a logical problem led Piaget, according to his own recollection, to abandon Bergsonism (1965, 6–7). On 18 April 1913 Piaget attended Reymond's inaugural lesson at the university, titled "Mr. Bergson's Philosophy and the Problem of Reason" (ibid., 6; Reymond, 1913a). At that time he was in his first year at the gymnasium. Since Reymond taught only the two upper classes, he was officially Piaget's philosophy teacher from September 1913 to July 1915.

As in the realm of natural history, Piaget's philosophical education took place in a friendly atmosphere under the direction of a master, and was therefore closer to an apprenticeship than to a formal schooling process. Piaget met Reymond at the same time as two of his best friends, Gustave Juvet and Rolin Wavre, students in the scientific section of the gymnasium and both future mathematicians. The philosopher later said that he could not have wished for "better working companions" for his beginnings in the world of teaching (Reymond, 1945, 25).

Piaget has emphasized the significance of their personal relationship. Of Reymond's gymnasium class, he recalled "the unforgettable experience of a small-group initiation to philosophy, with all the spontaneous questions and dialogues it involves, in addition to the lessons themselves" (1959b, 44). The philosopher's "courses were only one aspect of our philosophical formation, and it was often during walks with one of us, or during visits which he always encouraged, that Mr. Reymond revealed his thinking. He even managed to read entirely the often voluminous papers we submitted to him. He annotated each page of those embryonic essays, constantly referring to reliable bibliographic sources; above all, he manifested his respect for our thought in the way he discussed, as with equals, the point of view of simple beginners" (1945a, 18). This "spirit of respect and reciprocity" also obtained outside the classroom:

> The most surprising aspect of his contact with his students was that he succeeded in giving them the impression of having the need to meet them outside class. Already at the gymnasium, I often visited him at his successive addresses outside town [Neuchâtel] . . . He received you as if he had all the time, and often proposed a walk. While walking, he started asking you about your readings and your work. He then thought aloud, and ended up telling you about his own concerns and problems. He recounted the article he was writing, and summarized his projects. After getting back, he ended up thanking you as if your listening to him had stimulated or encouraged him. And he asked you to come again, pretending to deplore the solitude of the true philosopher, he who was the most sociable and humane of philosophers! (1959b, 45)

The relationship between the master and the disciple was rapidly established. Piaget's "Bergson and Sabatier" (March 1914) not only echoes some of Reymond's ideas but also includes an acknowledgment "for his valuable advice" (1914l, 194).

Reymond was tied to the Swiss-French tradition in many ways. He was a former minister and theologian, having given up a pastoral career in 1904 when the Free Church of the canton of Vaud established a compulsory confession of faith. He then devoted himself to his longtime interests, epistemology and the history of exact sciences. At the time he met Piaget, he was still quite absorbed in figuring out the relationship between science and faith, which he formulated as the epistemological question of the relationship between scientific and religious knowledge. (On Reymond, see Virieux-Reymond et al., 1956.)

Reymond had left the church to profess freedom of conscience. Since he viewed the Protestant "principle of authority" as "internal," the only admissible confession of faith was for him religious rather than theological and had to unite believers on the "grounds of inner experience" alone (Reymond and Guisan, 1902, 1904; Reymond, 1919). Reymond opposed the idea, defended by his mentor, Théodore Flournoy, that faith and science were irreducibly heterogeneous. He considered that, in spite of its purely internal and personal foundation, religious authority possessed a certain kind of objectivity.

As a theology student, Reymond (1900) sought to "forgo [the] subjectivism" characteristic of the liberal Protestant tradition. He pursued the project in several talks at the Swiss Christian Students' Association (Reymond, 1903, 1913b, 1913c, 1918a, 1921). His thesis was that, to the extent that scientific laws do not cover the whole of reality, God and providence are possibilities the Christian believer has the right to assert as real (see also Reymond, 1905, 1910).

Reymond (for example, 1908, 1914) affirmed the possibility of a transcendental world on the basis of his philosophical and historical study of mathematics. The objectivity of science, he observed, took the form of laws, whereas the objectivity of religion manifested itself in the historical and mental permanence of religious phenomena. Thus, history and psychology established the objective existence of spiritual realities by showing that beliefs, "in spite of their diversity, manifest an ideal value that remains identical through the ages" (Reymond, 1918a, 24). Upon his return from Paris in 1921, Piaget (1921b, 412) characterized Reymond's theses as the "moral and intellectual catechism" of Swiss-French Christian intellectuals. In 1913, however, his relationship with Reymond centered on Bergson's philosophy.

In his inaugural lecture of April 1913, Reymond denounced what he saw as the Bergsonian solution to the "problem of reason," that is, the problem of knowing what reason is and how it appeared in the course of evolution. In Reymond's rendering, Bergson's solution was to argue that, contrary to intuition, intelligence and reason were not capable of "truly knowing." His explanation shows that he misinterpreted the French philosopher. He believed, for instance, that he could refute the Bergsonian notion of duration by pointing out that scientists did not actually think of time as a juxtaposition of spatially imagined instants (Reymond, 1913a, 10). He thus ignored Bergson's distinction between *élan vital* and matter and misconstrued his view on the limits and possibilities of intelligence.

Furthermore, Reymond attributed to Bergson the idea that reason "is forever incapable of knowing anything beyond the superficial elements of reality" (ibid., 15). For Bergson, however, intelligence was capable of knowing matter, the part of reality that was its own and to which it had to limit itself. That is why it was irrelevant to attack him by pointing out that natural discontinuities, such as can be observed in the formation of crystals, appear to occur "in accordance with laws that are invariable and independent of our will" (ibid.). In short, for Reymond, Bergson's philosophy left "intact and unresolved the great problems of the nature of being, and of the origins of matter and life" and did not surmount "the dualism inherent to all metaphysics" (ibid., 16–17). That was the critical point on which Piaget in 1913 differed most from his future teacher.

Some passages of "Bergson and Sabatier" certainly echo Reymond's lecture. Like Reymond (1913a, 11), Piaget (1914l, 195) mentions the fuzziness of the notion of *élan vital*. Reymond (1913a, 11) declares it "strange . . . to see how Mr. Bergson, after having established . . . that logic is forever incapable of apprehending concrete reality, relies precisely on the contradictions of logic" to show that nothingness is unthinkable. In turn, Piaget (1914l, 197) wonders "why the intellect would be capable of deciding whether or not nothingness and immutability exist given that, according to the author [Bergson] himself, our present-day faculties are hesitant and limited in the search for the metaphysical Absolute."

But Piaget's agreement with Reymond is a minor element in the context of his generally Bergsonian outlook. The following is Reymond's characterization of the "metaphysical dualism" he thought Bergson did not surmount:

> You proclaim . . . that in reality there exist only discontinuous elements, atoms, electrons, or even living organisms; and your assertion is invalidated by the existence of continuity, becoming, and change that are to be found in nature. If, on the contrary, you claim that the only real thing is the fluid and incessant mobility typical of the life of the universe, you are hampered by the inverse problem, since what is permanent, stable, and immobile cannot be derived from becoming and change posed as unique reality. Such a dualism is in the facts, and seems irreducible. (Reymond, 1913a, 17)

Reymond overlooked Bergson's premise that the vital impetus coexists with matter, and is therefore not the "unique reality."

In contrast, for Piaget, who wished to approach life by means of a Bergsonian science of genera, it was possible to assert the absolute continuity of biological evolution and at the same time conventionally to define stable units. In science, the dualism of continuity (duration) and discontinuity (matter) was overcome thanks to the double point of view, realist as far as evolution is concerned, nominalist with respect to the divisions of organisms into natural species. Recalling Reymond's 1913 lecture, Piaget mentioned his adherence to Bergson's "biologism" against "the logical and mathematical spirit" of his future teacher (1959b, 44) and described himself as "anti-intellectualist and above all anti-mathematician" (1959a, 9; also 1965, 6). Piaget's "anti-mathematical" orientation, however, was not an opposition to mathematics or logic as such, but a constructive Bergsonian commitment.

Piaget, Bergson, and Sabatier

In his autobiography, Piaget (1952, 240) recalled that Sabatier's interpretation of dogmas was for him "much more understandable and satisfactory" than dogmatic theology. In *Recherche* (1918a, 36–37), he remarked that youth had been unknowingly inspired by Sabatier's "risky but fertile" conception of symbolism and by the antidogmatism of the French educator Ferdinand Buisson (1841–1932).[1] Young people, he explained, described themselves as "Bergsonian and pragmatist. But this Protestant Bergsonism and this Latin [as opposed to American] pragmatism had been anticipated in Sabatier's *Outlines* and Buisson's lectures."

Piaget's "Bergson and Sabatier" elaborates a Protestant Bergsonism. Sabatier (1897, vi, vii) wished to "study all phenomena in their natural succession," to "observe each fact as it appears," and by order of appearance, since this order determined their truth and value. Nevertheless, his assumption that "evolution" was only "a study procedure, a method" (ibid., vi) was necessarily unacceptable to Piaget. Only the discovery of *Creative Evolution* led Piaget to "the certainty that God is Life, under the form of the *élan vital*," and to the project of studying creative evolution in the "small sector of study" furnished by his "biological interests" (1965, 5). What Piaget does not mention in his autobiography is that he extended Bergsonism to theology by reducing the evolution of dogmas to an aspect of creative evolution. This he did in "Bergson and Sabatier," an eight-page article published in March 1914.

"Bergson and Sabatier" appeared in the *Revue chrétienne,* a Paris journal founded in 1854 to fight extreme liberalism. The *Revue* was the main publication of French Protestant moderate intellectuals; it advocated a "theology of conscience" which it characterized as being simultaneously "evangelical and liberal," and as descending directly from Friedrich Schleiermacher and Alexandre Vinet (Encrevé, 1985, 102–103). Auguste Sabatier had been one of its main contributors.

Piaget's goal in "Bergson and Sabatier" is to demonstrate that the *Outlines of a Philosophy of Religion Based on Philosophy and History* contain the "germs" of certain fundamental concepts of *Creative Evolution*. In pursuing this goal, Piaget offers a Bergsonian interpretation of Sabatier's evolutionism.

Piaget opens his article with an abstract of the "most important points" of Bergson's philosophy (1914l, 193). Thereafter he adopts a comparative method, first naming or succinctly explaining a Bergsonian concept, then juxtaposing quotations of Sabatier's text.

Early in the article Piaget asserts that "the religious evolution studied by Sabatier is a limited aspect of vital evolution, and moral conscience may be considered as one of the purest and highest forms of Bergsonian intuition" (1914l, 192–193). Intuition, he explains, represents "the faculty of life to understand its inner nature and to apprehend the Absolute that is in itself. Now, it is striking to compare this to [Sabatier's] definition of consciousness: 'What we call the religious consciousness of a man is the feeling of the relation in which he stands . . . to the universal principle on which he knows he depends, and with the universe in which he sees himself as a part of one great whole' [Sabatier, 1897, 183]" (ibid., 193). From the start, therefore, Sabatier's "evolutionism" is considered as a special case of Bergson's philosophy, the evolution of dogmas as a "limited aspect" of creative evolution, and the feeling of universal communion that Sabatier called "religious conscience" as a form of Bergsonian intuition. The subsequent comparisons fit Sabatier's theology into the Bergsonian mold.

The first comparison concerns duration, the key concept of Bergson's philosophy. Duration is a universal reality that can be directly known by means of intuition because, as Piaget explains, it is also "psychological time." For Piaget, Sabatier's observation that the individual perpetuates older dogmas while putting in them "new contents" is close to Bergsonian duration, insofar as the historical transformations of dogmas are linked to a certain "continuity of inner evolution" (ibid., 194–195). In other words, psychological time (or inner duration) is to individual religious consciousness what outer duration is to the historical evolution of dogmas.

Piaget also detects the characteristics Bergson attributes to the *élan vital* in Sabatier's idea of life as "a force, ideal in its essence, real in its manifestations," that incarnates itself in living organisms (Sabatier, 1897, 204). The creative nature of the vital impulse manifests itself in the perpetual renewal of dogmas: for Piaget, that is what Sabatier meant when he designated "God's word" and "inner religion" as "creative" (1914l, 196).

In *Creative Evolution*, Bergson (1907, 273) held that the idea of immutability is an illusion: since our intelligence is unable to perceive "the true evolution, the radical becoming," we suppose that "we can think the unstable by means of the stable, the moving by means of the immobile." According to Piaget (1914l, 197), the demonstration of that illusion could be deduced from Sabatier's evolutionism; ultimately, for him, the theologian's symbolism was based on a theory of knowledge akin to Bergson's.

Similar reasoning applies to Bergson's critique of finalism and conception of progress. To the claims of "mechanistic" biology, the philosopher opposed the "hypothesis of an original *élan*," or "internal push that has carried life, by more and more complex forms, to higher and higher destinies" (Bergson, 1907, 102). For Bergson, such a hypothesis did not imply teleology, since progress is only "a continual advance in the general direction determined by a first impulsion," a "creation that goes on for ever in virtue of an initial movement," without a goal to be attained or a plan whose accomplishment would mark an end (ibid., 104, 105).

Piaget finds an analogous idea of progress in Sabatier's assertion that religious perfection (embodied in Christ) is to be found at the beginning rather than at the end of Christianity. Sabatier (1897, 182) explained that a "germ" was needed for organic life to arise, "and that this germ was a sort of positive perfection in relation to all inorganic matter." For Piaget, Christ is to Christianity what the "original impulse" (Bergson) or the already perfect "germ" (Sabatier) was to evolution as a whole.

Finally, Piaget writes, "Sabatier thinks that religion is one of the manifestations of the *élan vital*, and that moral conscience is above all the link *(religio)* between the individual and the universal Principle" (1914l, 197); thus, Bergson's "apparently so original" idea, that the problem of knowledge and the problem of life were inseparable, had already been elaborated by Sabatier.

Not only does Piaget compare; he also criticizes. Bergson's notion of psychological time, he asserts, was "not very clearly" defined, and the concept of *élan vital* "unfortunately remains in a thick obscurity" (ibid., 195). The philosopher's reasoning on immutability strikes him as singularly limited, since it showed only that immutability is unthinkable. Following Reymond, Piaget wonders why, if according to Bergson our intellect is "limited" in the quest of the Absolute, it should "be capable of deciding whether or not nothingness and immutability exist" (ibid., 197). These criticisms are minor compared to the article's most extensive and elaborate critical comment, prominently placed (in the conclusion) and focused on the fundamental tenets of Sabatier's thought.

The theologian's "evolution," Piaget points out, is a purely methodological notion, and it "is quite superficial, reconstructed after the event with fragments of what has already evolved"; it is "merely a series of juxtaposed states, in which one perceives no current, no slow transformation advancing with the regularity of time" (ibid., 199). Piaget then presents a proposal for a Bergsonian evolutionism of dogmas:

> We feel that a process is perpetually taking place in ourselves, with or without external influence, which makes our conceptions vary constantly . . . but in a continuous progression. External factors may intervene, but they are immediately transformed in our own way, assimilated in a certain conscious synthesis, then repressed into the subconscious, where they germinate before they emerge vivified and rejuvenated. Such is the true evolution of dogma; in my opinion, Sabatier has not insisted enough on the striking parallelism that exists between this inner work of each individual and the collective work of humanity.
>
> On such points, Bergson is incomparable, and has succeeded in logically equilibrating the few glimmers of evolution that we have found in the *Outlines.* (Ibid.)

The "true evolution of dogmas" depends on duration as a psychological process. In Bergsonian terms, it takes place in the "inner" or "fundamental self," that is, in the self that is not subdivided into heterogeneous instants.

By the time "Bergson and Sabatier" was published, Piaget had taken Arnold Reymond's psychology course, given during the second year at the gymnasium. The vocabulary of Piaget's article ("synthesis," "subconscious," "repressed") is not exclusively Bergsonian. Nevertheless, the emphasis on an inner "continuous progression" refers directly to a psychology that, in Bergson's words, "intends to reason about facts as they are being accomplished" rather than about accomplished facts (Bergson, 1889, 92). Such is the metaphysical and epistemological core of Piaget's argument.

"Bergson and Sabatier" not only "Bergsonizes" the French theologian but also necessarily "theologizes" Bergson. For Sabatier, religious experience was individual and psychological, and it was grounded in humankind's feeling of being related to a "universal principle" (which he called God) and of belonging to the universe as a part belongs to a whole. This sentiment was for Piaget a form of Bergsonian intuition. The essence of religion, therefore, was the experience of communion with creative evolution; and to know God was to have an intuition of duration. Thus, as the French Thomist Jacques Maritain (1882–1973) acutely perceived, Bergsonism implied that dogmas are "the transitory and indefinitely improvable expression of a certain religious feeling that is itself in evolution" (Maritain, 1913, 167).

God is conceptualized accordingly. For Bergson (1907, 248), the idea of creation was unintelligible "if we think of *things* which are created and a *thing* which creates"; "things and states are only views, taken by our mind, of becoming." "There are no things," he wrote; "there are only actions." Vital and cosmic creation "represent the action that is making itself" out of a "center" that Bergson characterized as a "continuity of shooting out." God, for him, was such a "center." And "God thus defined has nothing of the already made; He is unceasing life, action, freedom."

Such conceptions of God and religion illuminate Piaget's ecstatic "identification of God with Life itself," and his perceiving "in biology the explanation of all things and of the mind itself" (1952, 240). The religion of "Bergson and Sabatier" is the counterpart of his contemporary Bergsonian biology. In both domains, Piaget was determined to pursue not the "phantom of duration," as Bergson would say, but duration itself.

Let us recall that Piaget attributed a central evolutionary role to "active" adaptation, and that the formation of a species was for him a "psychological moment" (1914j, 330)—"psychological" because duration is originally an individual mental reality. The species itself was defined not by external causes or any fixed condition, but by its evolutionary becoming, by the realization in duration of its "tendencies." Exactly the same view applied to the historical transformations of religious dogmas.

In both cases, Piaget's aim was to apprehend reality by way of the creative mobility that, in Bergson's perspective, was its true essence; to think in terms of "duration" rather than in terms of states or instants; to introduce the idea of creative evolution into the practice and theory of biology and religion; in short, to construct a radical evolutionism whose object would be the "perpetual becoming" where, as Bergson said (1907, 272), reality "makes itself or unmakes itself, but it is never something made."

11

The Mission of the Idea

In December 1915 Piaget published *The Mission of the Idea,* a prose poem in which he chastised everything that "betrayed Christianity," and proclaimed that the mission of youth was to follow Jesus and to commit themselves to "the new birth of Christianity." But *Mission* is not just a poetic cry of revolt; it actually includes Piaget's first metaphysical system. This system, in turn, is inseparable from his life project: to reconcile in himself the thinker and the believer, and to work toward the renewal of Christianity and the creation of a better world out of the ruins of the war.

Piaget completed *Mission* before May 1915 and amended it in accordance with the suggestions of Wilfred Monod (ms. 1915). A letter from the secretary of the Swiss Christian Students' Association reveals that Piaget wanted the ACSE to publish his text as a self-contained brochure, and that he also considered submitting it to the *Cahiers vaudois,* an avant-garde literary review published in Lausanne; but the Association could not afford a separate publication, and Piaget realized that the readership of the *Cahiers* was not the most appropriate audience for his poem (Rougemont, ms. 1915). *Mission* appeared in December 1915 as a double issue of the *ACSE News,* and subsequently as a "special edition," with a cover dated 1916 and no mention of the Association.

The Mission of the Idea reveals a young Piaget radically different from the one presented in his autobiography. In a commentary to their abridged translation, Howard Gruber and Jacques Vonèche offer an excellent introduction to the poem:

> *The Mission of the Idea* is a long prose poem written at the height of the First World War to castigate a Europe afflicted with a conservative spirit, nation-

alism, egoism, pride and inertia. These are the evils seen as killing the Idea. As the work progresses, the identity of the Idea seems to change, or rather, the particulars chosen to exemplify it: justice, equality, women's rights, free expression of the human spirit in all its diversity, faith in Jesus, faith in the people, self-discipline, struggle for the good, peace, socialism, and so on. The Idea is all these things, and above all, the never-ending movement of thought towards them. The author expresses over and over his belief in the power of ideas, they "lead the world," govern action. If we must sum up his message in a few words, we can call it the outcry of youth against the smug hypocrisy of the Church and the bourgeoisie during the long suffering of the war, and a romantic, moralistic belief in Christian socialism. (Gruber and Vonèche, 1977, 26)

Unfortunately, as Gruber and Vonèche acknowledge, their abridgment deprives *Mission* of much of its poetic character and religious tone—two features that are essential to an understanding of the text.

The Mission of the Idea (1915a) is divided into five parts, each containing several sections: "Hymn to the Idea" (§§I–IX, pp. 3–15), "Nineteen Fourteen" (§§X–XX, pp. 16–31), "The Betrayal of Christianity" (§§XXI–XXX, pp. 31–46), "The New Birth" (§§XXXI–XXXVIII, pp. 46–59), and "The Idea and the People" (§§XXXIX–XLVI, pp. 60–68). "Hymn to the Idea" characterizes the "life for [that is, devoted to] the idea." "Nineteen Fourteen" elaborates on the postulate that the cause of the war is "everything that has fettered the idea." "The Betrayal of Christianity" accuses the churches of having "betrayed Christ." "The New Birth" is an appeal to spiritual conversion. "The Idea and the People" claims that the churches have betrayed the people. The end of the poem formulates the wish "that the tears shed during the war bear this beautiful fruit: the new birth of Christianity." (In the rest of this chapter, numbers in parentheses refer to pages of *The Mission of the Idea* [Piaget, 1915a].)

Metaphysics

The Mission of the Idea states Piaget's earliest metaphysics. It is within the context of the "system of the Idea" (as I will call it) that Piaget asserts his religious and social outlook and formulates projects for his own identity and future life. The "mission of the idea" is "the new birth of Christianity" (68). The pursuit of this "mission" is youth's inherent duty and does not follow from historical contingencies but from the metaphysical principles of the system of the Idea. The same can be said about the poem's political, social, and religious statements. Yet the doctrine of the Idea is not expounded systematically. In *Mis-*

sion, philosophical thought tends to be conveyed by stylistic features rather than by theoretical discourse.

Piaget points to the foundation of his metaphysics by distinguishing between "idea" and "Idea." His system consists of a hierarchy of three levels: the Idea, an absolute, transcendent, and ineffable principle; specific ideas (for example, fatherland, justice, liberty), collectively singularized as "idea"; and the human expressions or "formulas" (5) of the ideas.

"Idea" is reserved to emphasize the grandiosity of an event or the enormity of a crime. Thus, the church's disavowal of Jesus' wish to save the world "through the people and for the people" is described as an attack on the Idea (60); the Bible, a book "inspired by the Idea," becomes in the church "intangible" and "dead" (36). The Idea is also the ultimate cause of the "new birth" and the source of all hope. Christianity, Piaget says, "has sunk in the darkness of death"; but it contains "in itself latent forces that will save the world. The Idea is that hidden germ" (47–48). Regarding the dogma of atonement, Piaget writes that it is "only one interpretation" of Jesus' death, a "particular idea that by no means exhausts the living and true Idea" (35). Each idea "is merely a fragmentary and temporary view of the whole" (12).

History—that is, progress toward the Idea—is animated by the ideas themselves. For Piaget, "the idea leads the world" (10); it "is the motor of life" (47). This "idea" signifies the ensemble of ideas (love, charity, justice, freedom, fatherland, and so on), the pursuit of which will bring humanity closer to the Idea. As mediator between the Idea and the human world, "Jesus is the idea made flesh" (8).

"Hymn to the Idea" introduces the conceptual and stylistic leitmotifs of the entire text and formulates the principles on which all later propositions are based. Here Piaget makes extensive use of "successive approximations," the formulation of several nonsynonymous terms to designate an object that remains beyond expressive or cognitive reach; and he highlights the Idea's inaccessibility by focusing on the idea.

Piaget first approaches the idea in highly visual terms of what it is *not.* Thus, "The idea is not a dried-up plant stranded in the dust" (3) implies that it is endowed with the features of a living organism. Similarly, "The idea is not . . . the dull reflection of colorful and living realities, the skeleton stripped of flesh, or the bark that contains the creative germ" (3) suggests that it is a vital principle. Piaget goes on to compare the church's official beliefs to a "bark," a "dead shell" that must be broken so that the "kernel"—that is, the Idea—may germinate (48). Like life, the idea is creative. Jesus was an "innovator," a "creator" who "opened new directions for life" (44). But priests are "instruments . . . of the struggle against life, against the idea, against the new and the better";

conservatives oppose the "movement of innovating and moral life" (37). In accordance with a Bergsonian vision, the essence of life and the idea is their being creative. "The idea is an organism," and "the dogma is a dead idea" (4).

When Piaget writes, "The idea is not to be found in books" (3), he formulates the key metaphysical and religious principles of his poem. As he explains, the idea "emerges from the innermost depths of our being, from . . . that vital center, the emanations of which surge only under the sway of the sublime: the night on the ocean, an autumn sunset, or the august silence of two friends' hearts" (3). The innermost regions of the self are "mysterious" but "fertile" (3); this and the setting of the "sublime" are Romantic commonplaces and distant echoes of *Naturphilosophie*.

Indeed, *Mission* postulates a correspondence between universal processes and the individual's inner experiences. The cosmic "great whole" is for Piaget a "symphony" that leaves a "resonance" or a "chord" vibrating in each soul; the idea, he adds, "is this kernel of life" (4).

The musical metaphor designates the intuition of the cosmos and a sense of human limits. In the mountains, Piaget says, you may feel the "grandiose and powerful harmony" that fills nature; but you manage to seize only a phrase or two of this music: "Thus, faced with the immeasurable richness of life, we understand one or two melodies alone. And one of those rhythms is the moral sentiment" (17).

The "great whole" is not only metaphysical but also social and moral; it is "the ideal and absolute Humanity that we construct above our souls" (23). The individual must become "a harmonious note" within the grand composition: "No, Humanity is not a sum of individuals; it is the superior whole that extends beyond and coordinates the manifold resonances" (22).

The construction of this "future Humanity" (26) corresponds to the movement of morality, progress, and life itself, conducted by the idea: "Launched into the world, it [the idea] passes like a hurricane, overthrows kings and priests alike, stirs up the masses, dictates life and death, decides the outcome of battles, creates people's strength, and guides the whole of humanity" (4). In short, the idea "leads the world" (10) and is the motor of history. Yet it is itself "launched by Jesus" (34). Consequently, only those who launch ideas become saviors. "Action," Piaget proclaims, "is the servant of the idea"; it is "beautiful and good," but it perverts the idea by apprehending "only one of its aspects, thus destroying the beauty of the whole" (10). Progress "comes from the sages' brains, not from the arms of men of action"; the French Revolution was carried out "in Rousseau's walks . . . The future Republic will be created by idealists' visions" (10–11).

The idea "is not to be found in books"; it emerges "from the innermost depths of our being as an echo of the cosmic symphony"; but it resonates in particular within the thinker. The movement of history toward "absolute Humanity" begins when thinkers "launch" the idea. Moreover, history is cyclical: "Everything is idea, comes out of the idea, and goes back into the idea" (4). "The idea renews itself constantly," under the form of ideas that succeed one another (4); but this succession is in fact a return to the origins: "In the beginning was the Idea, say the mysterious words of the Christian cosmogony" (4).

This statement completes the foundation of the system of the Idea. "In the beginning was the Idea" is an adaptation of John 1:1. The Idea replaces the Word, and therefore stands for the Logos, the Reason that governs the cosmos; it thus embodies the essential underlying unity of what human intelligence perceives as a multiplicity.

In sum, "In the beginning . . ." deals with the origins of the world but does not elaborate on its functioning. "Everything is idea . . ." characterizes history as a circuit going from the Idea to the Idea through the idea. "In the beginning . . ." defines the Idea as the demiurgic composer of the "symphony" whose "stream of melodies" is life, and whose echoes are the ideas, "fractions of the great whole" (4). This "whole" is also the end of the cosmic evolution that starts in the Idea. The idea's *élan* "will unite in a supreme synthesis the diverse tendencies that tear the world apart" (67), thus rejoining the Idea and attaining the end of history. World War I appears as an omen, a cataclysm that enables Piaget to glimpse the future: "At the end of time," he writes, "only those who lived by the idea will find themselves together, since together they will remain within the current of life" (7). Metaphysics belongs in such a life.

Metaphysics is for Piaget "the supreme manifestation of the idea" (54). As he wrote in *Recherche,* Sebastian "believed in metaphysics, and believed that it had the power of someday uniting in itself being and value, science and faith"; as he discovered with despair "the relativity of a science to which he had devoted himself," he came to believe that he would know "how to build by himself a metaphysics that would give him back his center of gravity" (1918a, 23, 96).

Piaget identifies his metaphysics with a precise philosophical tradition. Only four books are mentioned in *The Mission of the Idea:* the Bible, Plato's *Phaedo,* Plotinus' *Enneads,* and Pascal's *Pensées*—all "books inspired by the Idea, but of divine inspiration" (36). Piaget espouses Pascal's confidence in the heart as the seat of faith. From the *Phaedo* he retains the aristocratic inclination of those who consider themselves true lovers of knowledge, and whose reasons never coincide with those of the crowd. The doctrine of the immortality of the soul, which occupies a large portion of Plato's dialogue, is less present in *Mission* than a certain "philosophical" attitude toward Truth and a belief in the purifying virtues of the quest for the world of Ideas.

Piaget's metaphysical system is closest to Plotinus' neo-Platonism. In the Plotinian doctrine, the world of the Ideas is organized as a hierarchy of hypostases: the Idea (or the One, or the Good) is at the top, just above the Intellect and the Soul. Each hypostasis "emanates" from the preceding one. The Soul may "descend" into individual material bodies; this descent or "procession" is an alienation, a break away from the One, as well as the source of moral evil. The ontological hierarchy of *Mission* represents different degrees of differentiation of the One (the Idea). The return of the manifold to the One (the Plotinian "conversion") takes place along the same path. Human potentialities originate in the soul's original union with the Idea; this union is to be re-effected by means of an ascetic life leading to the contemplation of ideas and, ultimately, to absorption into the Idea.

Piaget's thinking is not alien to the Pauline statement that in the end, God will be "all in all" (1 Cor. 15:28). Yet it is rather the idealist tradition that gives full meaning to the musical metaphor, reminiscent of the Pythagorean conception of music as a microcosm of universal harmony and as a means of relating to it. The idea, echo of the cosmic symphony, continues to "palpitate" in accordance with the original "harmony"; the human soul, in spite of its vicissitudes, is essentially identical with the World Soul, and acts as the microcosmic sound box of the Cosmos. The microcosm is ontologically weaker than the "great whole" because the ideas are only "fractions," resonances of the symphony.

The neo-Platonism of *The Mission of the Idea* combines naturally with Bergsonian metaphysics. The philosophy of creative evolution embraces the Plotinian theme of a "descent" into matter: the potentialities of the original vital impulse realize themselves in particular material forms, while the individual may unite with the One, with "duration," by means of intuition. Metaphysical knowledge itself appears as a means of elevation to the One and to absolute Humanity. (On Plotinus and Bergson, see Mossé-Bastide, 1959.)

A whole section of *The Mission of the Idea* is devoted to metaphysics (§XXXVI). Piaget compares "the nature of metaphysics" to the child's experience when his parents reveal to him "the secrets of his birth"; though troubled, the child feels "the pure and noble joy of true knowledge, and a grateful adoration for the beautiful truth," and "raises himself to the sublime of human quest, to the point where knowing and feeling merge in one religious act" (54).

Although metaphysics must remain "living sympathy and not a dry ratiocination" (54–55), it does not consist in the mere exercise of feelings. Its goal is rather to unite "reason" and "practical faith." Far from annihilating the "true life," intellectual understanding adds to it "a strength of synthesis" that sustains the march toward the "great goal" (55). The "quest for rational truth," Piaget writes, possesses "a superior truth that is almost religion" (54); it is a "holy quest" (55). He claims that metaphysics "will pull religion out of its present torpor, since in speculation the Christian learns the value of truth, even when this truth is opposed to his individual interests" (55).

Metaphysics involves both faith and doubt. The metaphysical quest starts with the effort to "apprehend" the Christ "without going through the symbols of the brain" (52). When the individual reaches "a sympathetic understanding of divine realities," he may "doubt through thought," without fearing that the "brain's anguish" will destroy "the soul's impulse"; he may examine beliefs, reject whatever seems an affront to reason or morality, "and try to reconstruct the house that crumbles" (48). This is a clear allusion to Jesus' comparison of two men, one who hears his words and acts upon them, the other who does not, with men who build their house, respectively, on rock and on sand (Matthew 7:24–27).

Piaget contrasts the attitude of the seeker to the believer's in an apologue probably modeled upon the Gospel's parable of the two children (Matthew 21:28–31). Two children are lost in a forest. One, frightened, "worshiped," then went on along the forest paths, convinced that they "were a wise work whose unknown laws would prevent him from getting lost"; he finished by giving up. This child represents faith. The other "doubted, pondered, and only then worshiped"; he "climbed a tree and examined the depths of the forest" before getting under way. He represents "sincere doubt." For Piaget, faith and doubt complete each other. In the realm of thought, faith is "an abdication"; doubt, in contrast, "is the painful condition of the birth of the idea . . . It is the motor of research, and research is the driving force of progress" (49–51). In sum, metaphysics is the activity in which humankind unites faith and reason, feeling and knowing, worship and speculation.

Piaget proceeds in a manner that may be called Bergsonian. The characteristic successive approximations are a means of apprehending and expressing an absolute reality capable of adopting any number of concrete forms. No definitive formulation may be given of this reality; it is therefore akin to life in a Bergsonian perspective: both are unknowable through "mechanistic" science, and inexpressible by means of its analytic discourse. Bergson himself said that imagery sometimes conveys a literal meaning, while abstract language expresses itself figuratively. "In the spiritual realm, the image, if it merely seeks to suggest, may give us the direct vision, while the abstract term . . . most frequently leaves us in the metaphor" (Bergson, 1934, 1285).

In spite of the numerous explanations that weaken its poetic dimension, *The Mission of the Idea* is an attempt at philosophizing by "figures." Thus, Piaget associates the "idea" with images, akin to Sabatier's and Bergson's, related to movement, vegetable parts, or the life cycle. The idea is not explicitly identified with life. But the fact that those images apply to life highlights the relationship between the idea and life, between the "march" of the idea and the *élan vital*. The whole metaphysics of *Mission* is embodied in metaphors that are easily grouped into paired opposites: the living versus the inert; movement versus immobility or, more accurately, obstacles to movement (Gilbert, 1988).

The poetical and metaphorical style of metaphysics in *Mission* is inherent in the metaphysics itself, which is elaborated more by "sympathy" than by analysis. Piaget characterizes the poet as the man who tries to apprehend the idea. His conception corresponds to the Romantic view of the poet who participates in the eternal, the infinite, and the One: "The poet feels in himself a superior beauty, which his verses cannot depict and which they partly kill" (10). He is like the man endowed with true faith, "who communes without understanding . . . has felt the ineffable and has become imbued with the incomprehensible" (37–38). In *Recherche,* while recounting the "joy of systematizing" Sebastian felt when he began to speculate, Piaget (1918a, 97) speaks of the "[d]ivine joy of creating, experienced by the scientist and the philosopher as well as by the poet and the musician." As metaphysics lost for Piaget its cognitive validity, poetry later lost its value as a vehicle of philosophical thinking. Yet, as documented by two 1918 sonnets, poetry remained for him a valid means of expressing feeling, particularly in connection with nature (1918b).

Religion

The religion of *The Mission of the Idea* is rooted in the individual's heart and based entirely on faith in Christ. It is secular and Christocentric, and gives more chances of salvation to "atheists" and to "free-thinkers" than to priests (33, 34). It defines itself *against* dogma and the church, characterized as the antithesis of genuine religious truth.

For Piaget, the church is the worst enemy of the idea and of "true" Christianity. *Recherche* shows that he was perfectly aware of the dismal role national churches played during the war: "Each believer had identified his God to the endangered Fatherland"—and this included the Catholic priests and the Protestant ministers who blessed their country's armies and claimed that God was on their side (1918a, 74). *The Mission of the Idea* emphasizes the problem of dogmatism. As he recalled in *Recherche,* Protestant churches were animated not by a spirit of "quest," but by the certainty of possessing the truth (1918a, pt. I, chap. 4); the apostle Paul was a "Protestant Christ" who invented sin to serve as basis for dogmatic theology (ibid., 30).

Dogma is for Piaget the instrument of the church's domination over humanity. The doctrine of salvation is the worst, since it leads straight to egoism and, therefore, to war; the churches' support of war originates in "the egoism of individual salvation" (33–34).

The church interprets Christ's teachings according to its own "selfish plan," which is contrary to "the good and life" (63); it has thus "become the worst center of conservatism, the wound that putrefies the whole organism" (61); it manifests the "conservative spirit . . . incarnation of those vilest of tendencies, egoism and pride" (30).

The church is also socially irresponsible: it has "ignored everything, and has withdrawn into a scandalous optimism" (62). "Christian egoism has refused all just concessions to science, at the same time that it has refused to the people its most necessary good"; that is why science and the people will end up uniting "without the church" (63). Although he condemns the church violently for social, doctrinal, moral, and historical reasons, Piaget believes that it can be saved if it "sees its faults" (64).

The new birth of Christianity largely depends on the church's regeneration. Piaget dreams of a universal and invisible church based on a common faith that each believer would express with different symbols. "Tomorrow's church will no longer be the church" (66), but a communion of human beings sharing faith in Christ. Thus, when Jesus preached, "all listened to him, and among them was woven the invisible tissue of moral harmony. Ignorant or knowledgeable, they communed through the soul because no creed divided them . . . Such will be the church . . . when it is true life instead of external dogma" (66). Piaget's future church will realize the utopia of a primitive community, bound only by pure faith, animated by the principle that "the idea is not to be found in books." Dogma, "always immutable and false, empty and authoritarian" (37), hinders the rebirth of Christianity. Rational explanations do not matter. What counts, Piaget writes in typically liberal vocabulary, is the "fact" of Christ's redemptive advent: "the interpretation of the fact is not religion, and if we possess the fact, we are brothers in Christ" (49). "Dogma," he asserts, "has killed the Idea of Christianity" (34). The "richness of true religion" will be found only through the constant replacement of dogmas and explanations; "such is the law of life" (35). As Piaget emphasizes in *Recherche,* the core of religion is not symbolism itself, but an "ardent assertion of the value of life" (1918a, 20); and this assertion is grounded on a conversion experience.

Piaget exhorts his reader to believe "in conversion, in life" (35). Human beings advance toward the idea through conversion; the life for the idea is akin to the crisis that leads them to a spiritual "new birth." To live as a Christian is to relive the Passion: "Most painful of all, the life for the idea is the most fertile, since to suffer is truly to live" (14). This life of "struggle, renunciation, and agony" is for Piaget "normal existence" (9).

The Sainte-Croix conferences and the local meetings at which young Christians affirmed their desire to live the "true life" in spite of their tormenting doubts are part of the renewed church's form of worship. For Piaget, the war demonstrated that "true worship arises from the solitude of sacrifice, from the anguishes of the common struggle, from the calm of infirmaries; from the torments of the soul, from limitless charity, from love in the midst of action" (43). This worship "in spirit and truth," which the church has tried to empty of its substance, is "painful in its perpetual struggle toward the distant idea, tragic like all life devoted to the idea" (36).

To characterize such a life, Piaget resorts to the image of a lonely traveler passing through a snow-covered countryside: "Night was falling. A vague anxiety took hold of him and grew gradually." The traveler then oscillated between a "mystical impulse" and a melancholy feeling of "void." He felt united to the falling snow by an "immense sympathy," and saw in it the image of the "inner convulsions" of his soul. The mass of snow heaping on the ground encouraged him: "We fear the vanity of our efforts . . . We do not see the ideal, but we construct it nevertheless" (13–14). The traveler's intuitions are a step toward the full conversion experience. For Piaget, conversion consists in "confidence in Christ, a self-forgetfulness that suppresses the anguish of the hereafter so that we can better work in the struggle for the good" (38). Above all, it implies the rejection of dogma. "Let us apprehend through feeling the reality of our evil nature . . . Let us then make the living experience of the conversion in Christ . . . In a word, let us follow the teachings of Jesus, and only of Jesus" (49).

A stormy night depicted at the opening of the section "The New Birth" is Piaget's image for the experience of conversion. A "lost man" wanders through "the solitude of the night." He trembles, the atmosphere is terrifying. He is anxious; he runs, and collapses. At dawn, when the "phantoms of night" dissipate and an "immense hope" illuminates the plain, the man gets up, worships, and keeps going; in the same way, "Christianity will be entirely born again" after the war (47). For all this to happen, Piaget claims, "a revival is necessary"; the church must repent, hasten to meet Christ, "shed her old skin," and renew its concepts and beliefs (47). The same applies to the individual.

The convert's "first duty" is to present his new faith to his reason; "the ensuing struggle is the field of the Idea" (51). Thus, conversion inaugurates metaphysical research; it gives a general direction to the heart but does not lay out straight roads or define conceptual frameworks. After their new birth, individuals still have to find for themselves explanations and symbols that suit them and enable them to remain loyal to Christ.

Piaget's main youthful texts include narratives of conversion and always relate conversion to a mystical experience. It is to recounting such an experience that *Mission* limits the use of the first person. Most of the text is written in the third person. But at two critical moments, "I" is used. In the first (§XXVII), the narrator discovers the church's treason and the emptiness of its form of worship. The revelation takes place during a cryptic "great year," at dawn, as bells toll and believers fill the churches. Outside the churches, "men wander about, alone, opening themselves to the idea." While the believers are seeking to secure eternal salvation, the "lonely men" advocate "self-forgetfulness" and announce a new "birth"; "and I understood," the narrator says, "the sepulchral emptiness of the church's rites, and the beauty of the life for the idea. And I understood the abdication of Christianity, whose mute lips had vainly moved during twenty centuries to honor the Lord, and the goodness of God, whose unrecognized love bled over our misfortunes"(43).

The second episode of illumination (§XXXVIII) takes place "during the war," on the occasion of a Requiem mass: "I experienced the terrors of the orthodox before God's anger, better afterward to apprehend the beauty of nascent ideas" (57). The "passionate music" elicits a sort of trance, with terror, tears, and tremor (57). The narrator listens to the *Dies Irae,* the Catholic prayer for the dead, which he incorporates in the text. After an "hour of anguish" and new "inner convulsions," he hears the "sweet and pleasant voice . . . of the God of forgiveness," glimpses the beauty of "tomorrow's ideal," and asks: "When will the God of love and pity destroy the 'holy' God of vengeance?" (59).

In *Recherche,* Piaget later emphasizes the essential link between mysticism and metaphysics in his hero's development. Sebastian's hope that metaphysics would give him a "center of gravity" expressed itself "as an acute mysticism" (1918a, 96). While praying alone in his room (depicted as a sort of monastic cell), Sebastian was filled with a "sacred emotion" as he

> received the divine mission of reconciling through his life science and religion. He felt God, was possessed by him without seeing him, but heard an august music that stirred the depths of his being, and drove out unknown forces and a supernatural enthusiasm.
>
> And, his eyes filled with tears, he interrupted his prayer to sit down at his table and, innocently, noted the first certainties of his philosophy. (Ibid.)

Among these certainties was the rejection of the church's conception of God.

For Piaget, God sets the idea in motion (43), and man is brought back to God by his "moral conscience" (19), that is, by an intuition of the idea. "We think we act in the void, but we weave . . . the invisible tissue that links us to God" (14). When all believers are united in the same march toward the ideal, "God will be all in all, interpreted by each in a different way, until death reveals to good men the unique perspective on the absolute" (67). God and Idea stand for the absolute toward which history advances. When evil "pollutes" the Idea, it also "veils" God (40). The church corrupted the relationship between God and humanity, to the point that His suffering may consist in seeing what the church does with His love (57). The church rendered God "simultaneously merciless and omnipotent" (56) in order to be able to use Him as a tool to dominate humanity; without the church-imposed fear of a vengeful God, "men would have found the loving God by themselves" (39). The church thus attributes to God "the decrees of its pride" and even justifies evil through the "simple barbarity of the God-Fatherland" (55–56).

What disturbs Piaget most is the notion of a retributive justice administered by the "terrible Justiciary" (43), the "Just God" whose anger turns man into a "hard" and "rapacious" being (33). One of the great tasks of those who struggle for the idea is to rediscover God as a friend of humanity. The doctrines of punishment and expiation must be suppressed. The former is absurd: for how could Christ preach forgiveness, while man deprives God of charity and of the power to forgive (52)? The latter is "a bloody drama" in which God "needs fresh flesh and cries of distress to rouse and take care of men" (52). The church teaches Christians to forget "that man's salvation is perhaps not God's goal, and that Jesus must be sought in sacrifice, love, and self-forgetfulness" (34). That is why "the atheist, who worked without hope, and served God without asking anything from Him," has more chances to be saved than alleged believers (33).

The discovery of the "true God [who] transcends the church's God" (59) is the theme of the two conversion narratives. The first contrasts the believers who crowd the churches and the men who "wander alone" discovering the idea: "God cries with us, thought the lonely ones, and an immense love filled their hearts" (43).

The second conversion narrative declares the convert's revolt against the irate God of the orthodox and celebrates the "God of action" who launches the idea, and the "forgiving God" who suffers with humankind (58).

In sum, the God of *The Mission of the Idea* has three complementary meanings. As beginning and end of history, He may be identified with the "great whole" and the Idea. But He also represents a belief subject to the laws of symbolic evolution. Finally, the evolution of this belief progresses toward a precise goal: the notion of a good, loving, merciful, and forgiving God. This notion is related to Piaget's view of Jesus and Christ.

In *Mission,* Jesus is the definitive model for every individual who wishes to live for the idea; Christ is a more abstract, more purely spiritual, theological, or metaphysical being. Piaget writes, for example, that "Jesus died for us," and a few lines below urges: "Let us respect the ultimate reality of the facts of Christianity, believe in Christ, in his salvation, in his action upon us, in man's sin, in conversion, in life; let us follow Jesus in everything he has established, since his teaching is neither theoretical nor authoritarian, but purely practical, and made up of feeling. And let us deny to the disciples and Paul of Tarsus the right of imposing their verdicts" (35–36). The distinction is traditional: the individual who traveled through Palestine preaching a new morality and a new relation to faith and God before dying on the cross is the historical Jesus each Christian must try to imitate; Christ is the Messiah, the expression of eschatological hopes and expectations.

Christ represents true doctrine; Jesus, true life. For example, while Christ created the Pater Noster and was a source of faith and belief, Jesus, in his own life, incarnated the prayer's authentic spirit (41–42) and "was an idealist, an innovator, a rebel" (44).

The individual who follows Jesus by rejecting the church's conservatism returns to the authentic Christ (45). The experience of conversion is "nothing other than confidence in Christ" (38); it is the condition of a life in the service of the idea; and such a life is an imitation of Jesus: "Jesus is the idea made flesh" (8), and "Only Jesus has realized the idea" (9). He was not God's son, endowed with a divine nature. Rather, he was a man capable of "gigantic impulses" that made him feel the ineffable and find God (8–9). His "sacrifice was superhuman" only because it enabled him to reach God (9). Thus, Jesus became the sole "fixed point" of humanity's march toward the Idea, since only he "elevated himself to the moral absolute" (51). In the midst of a perpetual flux of beliefs and symbols, Jesus is for Piaget the unchangeable reference, the perfect model of moral and spiritual life that persists under historically contingent and individually determined appearances.

Morality

The Mission of the Idea includes an ethical doctrine that identifies the good with the idea. Their identification structures Piaget's universe of values, imbues his attitudes toward war and social reform, and shapes his efforts to come to terms with the problem of evil. Since Piaget also identifies the idea with life, life and the good are the same thing. He thus transforms a "biological" notion into an ethical concept and incorporates a moral doctrine into his Bergsonian and anti-Darwinian view of evolution. As he writes, "The Good is life" (17). Life is a force "of altruism and union"; the good "is the free action of this force" (18), or "the free blooming of life" (16).

The good and the "blooming of life" imply "the unlimited development of consciousness and the whole soul" (16).[1] The good coincides with the perpetual creation of novelty characteristic of Bergsonian evolution: the idea is essentially "creative" (49), whereas the conservative spirit works against "the movement of innovating and moral life" (37). The philosophy of creative evolution thus acquires a moral dimension.

When Piaget proclaims that life "is a force, an impulse, a current of consciousness that, by penetrating matter, organizes it and introduces into it harmony and love" (17), he adds to Bergson's definition of life the idea that the *élan vital* creates morality out of matter. Consciousness, which in *Creative Evolution* "is synonymous with invention and freedom" (Bergson, 1907, 264), and consists in emancipation from the constraints of matter and instinct in the domains of thought and choice, becomes in *Mission* a moralizing agent. This extension in the meaning of *conscience* derives from the theology of "Bergson and Sabatier."

In a similar way Piaget assimilates Bergson's distinction between instinct and intelligence. For the philosopher, those two modes of knowledge completed each other and were equally useful as long as each limited itself to its proper realm. The intellect seemed to him "characterized by a natural inability to comprehend life," whereas instinct "is molded on the very form of life" (Bergson, 1907, 165).

In "Bergson and Sabatier" (1914l, 192–193), Piaget defined moral or religious consciousness as "one of the purest and highest forms" of intuition. In Bergson's philosophy, however, intuition belonged in the same evolutionary line as instinct; it was "instinct that has become disinterested, self-conscious, capable of reflecting upon its object and of enlarging it indefinitely" (Bergson, 1907, 176). Naturally, then, instinct was close to both metaphysics (whose method was intuition) and religion (whose foundation was moral consciousness).

In about June 1915 Piaget presented to the Neuchâtel group of the Swiss Christian Students' Association a paper on the "empirical genesis of consciousness and its conciliation with religion" (Anon., 1915). Piaget's text has not been found. Yet, in the light of "Bergson and Sabatier" and *The Mission of the Idea,* we may guess that the "genesis of consciousness" consisted for him in the development of intelligence on the one hand, and of instinct and intuition on the other. Its "conciliation with religion" was founded on the idea that instinct was the evolutionary ancestor of moral and religious *conscience.*

As we have already seen, in 1914, when the debate with Roszkowski forced Piaget to examine the Mendelian species concept, he used the notion of chromosome in a discussion of moral conscience, probably in connection with the question of the relation between the individual and society. In *Mission,* however, specifically biological ideas remain subsidiary to Piaget's Bergsonism and to the system of the Idea. Thus, his interpretation of the Fall and of the subsequent history of humanity derives from the relationship among life, instinct, and intelligence. "Life," he writes, "is good; the individual makes it bad" (18). Each "living being" is engaged in the "great impulse" and places "above itself an ideal . . . to the realization of which tend all the efforts of its obscure instincts."

When intelligence appears, it first opens up "unknown regions" to humanity; later, however, it suffocates instinct, convinces the individual "that his interest is not that of his species," and thus leads him to live for himself, without regard for the group. "Life was menaced: the injured instinct recovered fast, and reappeared as the sacred sentiment that reinstates man on his original way and brings him back to God: moral conscience" (19). Yet humanity remained torn between self-interest and renunciation: "Such is the sense of the Fall" (20). By bringing humankind back into communion with life, instinct and intuition will return people to the good.

The identification of life with the idea implies the supremacy of change. In the first paragraph of *Mission*, Piaget affirms that the idea "is an organism" that lives, dies, and "constantly renews itself" (4). Later he asserts: "To be is to change, and when life changes, it marches toward progress" (26). Progress, or humanity's drive toward the idea, is a "blooming," a "development," an "evolution."

In *Mission*, "evolution" must be understood in two different ways. On the one hand, it refers to the historical transformation of dogma and belief. Piaget declares that only Jesus attained the moral absolute and adds: "All that is not this absolute must change. The characteristic of this evolution is that the good varies with men's conceptions, in harmony with the development of human reason" (51–52). On the other hand, evolution refers to progress toward the "moral absolute" by way of mechanisms that are themselves moral:

> The evolution of life and the goal of morality coincide entirely. The struggle for life is not of the essence of evolution: it does not result from vital action, but from the encroachment of individuals or societies upon the force of solidarity itself. The struggle for life is determined by that which is the specific characteristic of evil: the misappropriation of life by those who consider themselves its goal.
>
> To hasten evolution is to do the moral good. (18)

Piaget here extends the identification of life and the good to the mechanisms of evolution, thus moving from an ethical postulate to a biological statement.

The contrast between solidarity and vital action on the one hand, and egoism and the struggle for life on the other, completes Piaget's earlier critique of Darwinian evolutionary mechanisms. In 1913 he conceded that mimicry resulted from natural selection and the "struggle for life," but he also emphasized that it was a merely "passive" adaptation, and that evolution proceeded from "tendencies" and activities. In *Mission,* the opposition to natural selection is largely based on a literal interpretation of the metaphor of the "struggle for life." To the extent that "life brings harmony [and] solidarity" (18), its evolution could not take place by means of competition and egoism. *Struggle* and *natural selection* become antonyms of *life.*

By considering evolution as a moral concept, Piaget entered contemporary debates. In 1915, discussions about the moral meaning of Darwinism (often reduced to the "struggle for life") were nothing new. World War I, however, gave them a new topicality. Some authors, such as the German general Friedrich von Bernhardi in *Germany in the Next War* and *Britain as Germany's Vassal,* argued that war was a biological necessity, and that the "law" of the struggle for existence applied to the human species. Others, such as the Russian anarchist prince Peter Kropotkin in his famous *Mutual Aid: A Factor of Evolution,* claimed that "mutual aid" was a main evolutionary mechanism, and that in any case the "struggle" could be neither an explanation of nor a justification for the war (Crook, 1989; La Vergata, 1985, in press).

Piaget's adoption of a clear position within that debate is a crucial moment in his intellectual development. On the one hand, it strengthens his rejection of Darwinism by adding moral reasons to previously formulated philosophical (Bergsonian) and biological (Lamarckian) arguments. On the other hand, starting with *The Mission of the Idea,* Piaget's moral thinking is based on the identification of evolution with the good. Moral progress is thus immanent to development; evil keeps coming up only because humanity is not evolved enough.

Piaget later tried to provide evolutionary ethics with scientific foundations. The metaphysical and mystical dimensions of *Mission* disappeared, but the global point of view remained the same. In *Recherche,* he asserted that "evolutionary moralities have proved that the good is life itself, and that evil is everything that hinders the flourishing of this life" (1918a, 173–174). Elsewhere he wrote: "To struggle against war is . . . to act according to the logic of life against the logic of things, and that is the whole of morality" (1918c, 380). At the beginning of the 1930s, Piaget (for example, 1931) concluded that nationalism and the arms race are less a consequence of economic and social circumstances than of the fact that, from the international point of view, man is still a primitive or a child.

Piaget stands clearly against the war; he sees it as a consequence of conservatism and orthodoxy (17, 31, 45); setting the idea in motion and following life is for him the means of preventing a new world crisis (16). Yet his view of moral progress compels him to find the good in every historical development, and this includes the war. Like revolutions, wars are "heroic hours" during which "everything that opposes the march of the idea is annihilated" (6). Piaget proclaims that after the war Christianity will be reborn (47). It was "during the war" that the narrator met the "true" and "forgiving" God in a dramatic moment of illumination.

"The war itself is a sign of progress" (25), a catalyst of greater consciousness. Thus, when Piaget represents soldiers in a trench, he depicts them all suffering from the same "anguish" and realizing that their enemies are brothers who also struggle "for humanity, for God" (23). The soldiers' brotherhood suggests the moral potential of the idea of fatherland.

Conservatives, Piaget explains, consider the fatherland as a mere "interest of the army" (16). Nevertheless, as the idea advances, only the "ungodly" will dare speak "of a country's empire, of a nation's honor, of fatherland's interests" (66). As a social unit "larger" than (and therefore superior to) the family, the clan, the tribe, and the ethnic group, the fatherland may be a step toward "the great soul of Humanity" (25). This process is for Piaget illustrated by Belgium's "heroism," portrayed as a "sign of progress" (27).

The choice of Belgium reveals Piaget's position, which he had to attenuate. Piaget suppressed from *Mission* his most openly anti-German statements at the behest of the secretary of the Swiss Christian Students' Association, who wrote to him: "I would personally like not to issue in the *Nouvelles,* which circulates throughout the world and officially represents our Association, phrases that may render tomorrow's reconstruction more difficult" (Rougemont, ms. 1915). This approach was of course consistent with Piaget's own views.

Without the conservative spirit, Piaget claims, "people would not have remained in misery . . . and would not have encountered the obstinacy of a bourgeoisie that ignores its own duties"; without it, "woman would be an equal to man" (17).

Piaget's thinking about the origins of World War I was close to that of moderate turn-of-the-century socialists. For example, the assassinated French Socialist Jean Jaurès (1859–1914), whom Piaget (1916c, §§25–26) characterized as the heroic victim of narrow patriotism, had declared twenty years earlier that "there is only one means of abolishing war among peoples: to abolish war among individuals . . . to replace the universal struggle for life—which leads to universal struggle in the battle-fields—by a system of concord and unity" (Jaurès, 1895, 77).

For all its virulence, *Mission* advocates reform rather than revolution, remains highly individualistic, and pays no attention to the concrete relations between the war and social and economic structures. The "conservative spirit" certainly is a force of oppression and reaction, but it is far from that imperialism, "the highest stage of capitalism," to which Lenin, in a famous 1916 booklet, attributed the origin of wars. Piaget sides with the people: they are "tomorrow's force," the "anonymous but beautiful" mass that will rise under the shock of the war (60, 61) to participate in social reform.

In *Mission,* the notion of the people implies all the socializing commitments opposite to the church as agent of the conservative spirit. The last section of the poem, titled "The Idea and the People," contains a vigorous indictment of the church in relation to social questions.

"The church has betrayed the people" and transformed Christ's religion into a "bourgeois Christianity" (60). It has thus forced socialism to "vegetate" and stopped its "progress." It has preached a "vague morality" instead of helping to change "the order of the past."

Like many other Swiss-French Protestants, Piaget gives women a key role in the construction of the future world (Käppeli, 1990). He devotes an entire section of *Mission* to feminism (§XLI). "Feminism," he proclaims, "is a duty for the church, since all that touches upon social salvation must be its mission." Woman will regenerate society (62). The fact that men have maintained her "under tutelage" is a crime comparable to those of the bourgeoisie, conservatism, orthodoxy, and selfish nationalism (65).

> Peace, the death of interest-driven politics, patriotic idealism, humanitarian laws, social regeneration, the recovery of the proletariat, will all come out of woman's vote. Once she becomes conscious of her rights, woman will make impossible a crisis as gigantic as the one in which the past is perishing today.
>
> Such is the ideal, and a formulated ideal becomes a duty. Even if feminism jeopardized woman's grace and the family's tranquility, a duty would remain a duty, and feminism would have to remain a school of sacrifice to the idea, a painful struggle at the head of progress. (63)

Later, in *Recherche,* Piaget sees women's rights and universal suffrage as an indispensable step toward restoring social equilibrium (1918a, 209).

Piaget's social message is inseparable from his conception of the place of knowledge in the march of the idea. "Science and the people," he claims, "are always in solidarity"; "science becomes socialist, and socialism scientific" (63). Science, the people, and socialism have a common enemy, the church, which opposed "its dogma to science" and "its morality to social salvation" (63). Although the union of science and the people will take place "without the church," its goal is to "regenerate" the church and to "salute in Christ the eternal savior."

In pursuing the mission of the idea, Piaget tries to adhere to "present-day thought," which "tends toward the relief of suffering humanity" (63). Science is legitimate only if it promotes such relief. Since good may be achieved only "in harmony with the development of human reason," the progress of knowledge inevitably brings humanity closer to "the goal of morality" (51–52).

Mission in Its Local Context

The publication of *Mission* is the most important trace of Piaget's activity in the Swiss Christian Students' Association, but it is not the only one.

The exact date on which he joined the ACSE is not known, but it seems fairly certain that he did so no later than early 1914. In late 1913, after months of inactivity (M. Reymond, 1913), the ACSE's Neuchâtel high school group invited students in their last year at the gymnasium to join. Piaget began his last year at the gymnasium in September 1914, but he probably joined the ACSE before that. In February 1914 the group announced that "one of the members will present a paper on 'Sabatier's philosophy'" (Ecklin, 1914, 177); the chronological and thematic coincidence with "Bergson and Sabatier" (published in March) seems to point to Piaget as the paper's author.

Other evidence lends support to our hypothesis. Piaget's first text in the *Nouvelles* of the ACSE appeared in May 1915. It was a report of the colloquium of Swiss high school students that had just taken place at Evilard, close to Lake Bienne, not far from Neuchâtel. Piaget referred to the "sweet and well-known atmosphere of our annual colloquia"; commenting on a sermon, he noted that it evoked "Chanivaz," thus making the audience "relive last year's moments" (1915b, 198, 199). Chanivaz was a high school students' camp that was not officially part of the Association but was closely linked to it through its organizers and participants (see Rougemont, 1921, 27–28). It took place in August on a private estate on the shores of Lake Geneva, close to Allaman. Piaget was therefore recalling the summer of 1914, and the reference to the annual colloquia points to the previous spring. Since Piaget's activity in the Association may be traced to about May 1914, his membership in the high school group may be dated even earlier. Be that as it may, the traces of Piaget's participation in the ACSE show him as an active member who distinguished himself by his contributions to the life and the ideals widely shared by young Christian intellectuals.

The report of the Evilard meeting anticipates several major themes of *The*

Mission of the Idea and shows that by May 1915 Piaget was deeply imbued with the young-Christian sensibility. Thus, he points out "the nascent harmony" felt at the arrival of the Swiss-French and Swiss-German participants. The preacher of the first evening, he writes, "recounted today's religious disarray . . . and the immense task of a youth that does not yet know how to take life," and concluded on an optimistic note, "turned toward the future, toward the ideal for the realization of which we must work, even if in darkness" (1915b, 198–199).

The following day, a Swiss-German lecturer "stigmatized narrow patriotism, the God-Fatherland in the first place, while he hailed . . . a sane love for the fatherland, divine reality for which one might, and must, offer one's life." Both fatherland and Christianity seek to promote "the expansion of our good nature": "the good Christian is a patriot, just as the good patriot must remain Christian" (ibid.). The later exchange of reports among the French-speaking and the German-speaking group was for Piaget the most encouraging and "vital moment" of the colloquium, since it let everybody "perceive our unity of action" (ibid., 200).

The final lecture of the Evilard meeting, titled "What must tomorrow's generation be?" seems to have been typical of the discourse on youth within the Swiss Christian Students' Association. Piaget summarizes it thus:

> We are privileged in everything . . . privileged to be young, privileged to be able to meet among future intellectuals and to find outside the churches the strength that is lacking in official Christianity, privileged above all to be living today. Heroism surges everywhere, and under an appearance of universal destruction, our times, in their burning mold, cast a new world, an unknown and unforeseeable world that we, young people, will have to uphold. For that purpose . . . we need Christ, we need a living faith, purity, moral energy. (Ibid.)

The meeting at Evilard was a small-scale Sainte-Croix. The participants, Piaget reports, "returned to the plain stronger than before, and especially more united," "understanding each other better, and, above all else, better apprehending the ideal" (ibid.).

It was largely in meetings such as Evilard that Piaget and his contemporaries constructed their identity and became convinced of their redemptive mission. The local ACSE groups were imbued with the same exalted and melancholy atmosphere. In June 1915 the Neuchâtel group reported "little activity, many aspirations, a burning need of equilibrium. The most positive moment was the session in which Jean Piaget delivered his paper 'Essay on the empirical genesis of consciousness and its conciliation with religion' . . . We mean much to each other, we have apprehended each other, and we await dawn, the ideal that will come out of the present mêlée, and that tomorrow will establish" (Anon., 1915).

Piaget shared such a sense of communion. Thus, in 1915, when he took leave of the Friends of Nature, he declared that the moments that would remain most "alive" for him would be the "hours of friendship full of intimate and continuous comradeship," regretted not having "done enough for this friendship, since it is the only goal of the Club," and explained: "I do not despise your science, our science (for I am still one of yours); I say that this science results from friendship and not the other way around" (ms. 1915a).

That same year, in Sainte-Croix, Charly Clerc spoke of the "crisis" of the times and observed: "it seems that youth has shaken off its inertia." He saw in the war the occasion for a revival; he perceived the appearance of "sudden indignations," "new affections," "passionate sympathies," and surprisingly violent "new ideas" (Clerc, 1916, 14). *The Mission of the Idea* provides an example of the revival as perceived by Clerc.

The Mission of the Idea was enthusiastically received in the Christian youth environment, where it made Piaget appear as an original, cultivated, and courageous individual, half poet, half prophet, and one of the future leaders of his generation.

A review of *Mission* in *Jeunesse* (Youth), the journal of the Young Men's Christian Association, described the poem as bubbling with "youthful thought, lyricism, vitality, and revolt" and strongly recommended it "to cultivated readers, who joyfully welcome all thinking that is sincere, serious, original, and innovative, even if it opposes received ideas and established traditions" (Nicod, 1916). Piaget was described as an "idealist" who did not, however, "preach an abstract intellectualism. For him, the *Idea* is not simply an intellectual notion, but . . . a driving revolutionary force" (Nicod, 1916). The same issue of *Jeunesse* published an excerpt from *Mission* (§XV). The passage chosen—a quite contemporary scene, in which men in the trenches anxiously wonder about their place in the "superb impulse" toward the Whole—highlights the significance attributed to Piaget's poem.

Another review appeared in the newspaper *La Suisse libérale* on 9 February 1916 (Dardel, 1916). Its author was Otto de Dardel (1864–1927), the father of one of Piaget's friends at the Club of the Friends of Nature. Dardel was a leading figure of the Liberal Party, which defined itself not only politically, as federalist, supportive of private initiative and opposed to state control, but also religiously, as conservative Protestant. Dardel belonged to the synod of Neuchâtel's Independent church and had campaigned for the separation of church and state. His review of *Mission* reflects his political and religious convictions.

After observing that the young Piaget is going through a period of destruction and that he "advances through a demolition site," Dardel emphasizes that he "is on the right track," since he wants to reconstruct the church with and through Jesus. Dardel criticizes Piaget's overuse of anathema, his volubility, and his "somewhat breathless" invectives, but notes his "scientific and philosophical background" and praises the "youth rich with thought and hope that shines forth in each page of his little book." Yet Dardel thinks that Piaget "will end up discovering that the obstacle to the Idea's conquest of the world is less the forms [of faith, that is, dogmas], indeed often perishable, than the terrible fact of sin." In opposition to Piaget's extreme liberal and secular Christianity, he asserts the truths of evangelicalism. Moreover, Dardel is skeptical about Piaget's declared socialism. His review opens with the following comment: "It has been said that Jean Piaget is a future socialist. I am not so sure. He is starting his own evolution in a world in which everything evolves. We know nothing of where it will lead him."

A third review of *Mission* appeared on 29 January 1916 in the weekly *L'Essor moral, social, religieux*. Its author was the pastor Paul Pettavel (1861–1934), editor of the publication. The goals of the journal, founded in 1905 by two ministers of the Free Church of the canton of Vaud, was to promote solidarity, peace, cooperation, and justice and to awaken a religious feeling founded on the teachings of Christ, teachings that should govern religious, moral, and social life, including its most concrete economic dimensions (Schmitt, 1980). From the beginning, *L'Essor* enlisted prominent Christian intellectuals, such as the educator Adolphe Ferrière, who was close to the Rousseau Institute and one of the main figures of the progressive school movement; the engineer Auguste de Morsier, a kinsman of Edouard Claparède and advocate of social Christianity and women's vote; and Pierre Bovet, first director of the Rousseau Institute, who remained loyal to the journal throughout his long life.

During the war *L'Essor* actively joined two major debates. In 1915 and 1916 there was an exchange of articles on the hot topic of conscientious objectors. In 1917, an apology of the just war by Ferrière gave rise to passionate discussions; Romain Rolland observed that the "slaughterhouse Christianity" advocated by some was expressed "in a Protestant journal, perhaps the most liberal of all in French-speaking Switzerland" (Rolland, 1952, 1077; see also 1083–85, 1417–18). Toward the end of the war *L'Essor* defended Rolland and announced its support of a socialist type of Christianity. The journal's collaborators often took part in the activities of the Young Men's Christian Association and the Swiss Christian Students' Associations; and *L'Essor*'s precepts and values are all to be found, in a radicalized form, in *The Mission of the Idea*.

Paul Pettavel himself was active in the YMCA, and often attended the Sainte-Croix conferences. During his twenty-five years as a minister of the Independent Church in the industrial, leftist, and conflictive Jura city of La Chaux-de-Fonds, he championed all sorts of progressive causes, such as conscientious objectors' rights, consumer protection, the separation of church and state, and pacifism. Pettavel's political stance is consistent with a comment he made about his weekly *Feuille du Dimanche*: "It calls itself liberal; others call it socialist . . . in fact, it leans toward socialism out of liberalism" (quoted in Perrenoud, 1936, 35–36). Pettavel had chosen socialism because its program seemed to him to follow the teachings of the Gospel (ibid., 37). One of his former catechumens wrote that "he had the passion of making [others] love Jesus Christ" (quoted ibid., 29). It was also said that he had the "vocation and natural gifts" of a prophet (ibid., 27).

Paul Pettavel (1916a) saw in *The Mission of the Idea* "a sort of declaration of Youth for the new times." He was enthusiastic about this "prose poem (in good prose) made vibrant by pure sympathies and sacred wraths." Piaget sang "like an ancient bard and a young prophet . . . the promised coming of the Idea," and in so doing he "revealed himself, thus opening the heart of idealist youth." Young people, Pettavel said, should read *Mission* "so that their souls may vibrate"; older people should read it "to learn again the new life and anticipate the future times." Piaget's poem seemed to him "fresh," "vigorous," "extraordinarily alive," "moving," "stirring," and "a delicious comfort"—even if a certain amount of culture was necessary to read it with pleasure.

Pettavel thought that the poem expressed a "male and marked sensibility" that "perhaps" originated in suffering. He perceived in the text a "well-read" individual, born in a "cultivated milieu," "developed beyond his age," "strong in science, psychology, and life experience," who had devoted himself "to contact with nature, philosophical studies, and the passion of feeling and scrutinizing life," who had "taken the time to dream and meditate" and was endowed with a "penetrating mind" and an "enthusiastic soul." For Pettavel, Piaget had "glimpsed the great human ideal that reaches God because it descends from Him. Seized by the idea . . . he started to write to apprehend the idea, and to make it the substance of his life." Piaget (ms. 1916) later thanked Pettavel "for the way in which you understood my brochure's intent rather than its content, for I feel that you disagree [with it] on quite a few issues; I am therefore all the more touched by the sympathetic judgment you granted it in *L'Essor*."

Finally, a full appreciation of the reception of *Mission* must take into account the lengthy critical letter of a major figure of contemporary French-speaking Protestantism, already mentioned as the author of an exemplary progressive catechism and as an advocate of Christian socialism: the French minister Wilfred Monod. Monod was raised in a pietistic and Methodist milieu and was educated in orthodox evangelical theology. Though antiauthoritarian, he felt that the subjectivist attitude of nineteenth-century liberalism undermined the foundations of shared faith, and thus of the church itself. Above all, he championed the application of the Gospel to social issues. (On Monod, see Monod, 1938; Poujol, 1965; L. Gagnebin, 1987.) Early on during World War I, Monod protested against the manifesto of German intellectuals that asserted the superiority of their nation's *Kultur;* after the war, he celebrated the victory of "democratic nations" and proclaimed the end of "Bismarckian civilization" (Monod, 1915a, 1919). His attitude, however, is best expressed in weekly "meditations" aimed at the renewal of Christianity in a spirit of tolerance and forgiveness (Monod, 1915b).

There are unfortunately no traces of Piaget's contact with Monod.[2] From the minister's letter, however, we may deduce a certain closeness: he addresses Piaget as "My dear young friend," and at the end he writes, "I embrace you fraternally, as an old friend of your parents whose worthy son you are" (Monod, ms. 1915, 1, 12). *Recherche* reports that, after losing faith in a revealed and omnipotent God, Sebastian found consolation in Monod's *To Believers and Atheists* (see Chapter 12).

In his commentary on *The Mission of the Idea,* Monod is both encouraging and severe. For him, Piaget is "an authentic youth, and," he tells him, "I love you for the generous enthusiasm of your soul. There is much inspiration in your pages, and beautiful things. You have received from God more than *'one talent'*—a great joy and a great responsibility" (Monod, ms. 1915, 1). Yet Monod does not think that the text is ready for publication. He advises Piaget to condense, to correct grammatical mistakes and suppress improprieties of language, to rewrite obscure passages, and to eliminate absurd or comical images and metaphors. But he particularly dislikes certain excesses of language.

Piaget's expressions of virulence remind Monod of free-thinking and anticlerical writings. These, he notes, are devoid of *Mission*'s "generous mountain breath, the wind of white summits . . . the higher you aim, the better you must choose your arrows" (ibid., 6).

> Your ambition is to be the champion, the knight of Life against the powers of conservatism that paralyze it. You sound against Jericho the trumpets of the

Idea . . . Nevertheless, you may believe my experience, the work of life is silent
. . . In the long run, nothing resists a perseverant softness rendered unyielding
by a truth animated by indignation and love.   (Ibid., 3–4)

Monod then furnishes Piaget with a list of aggressive passages—on orthodoxy,
pragmatism, the bourgeoisie, patriotism, Christian good works, prayer and lit-
urgy, the church, pastors—that would needlessly antagonize favorably inclined readers (ibid., 4–6).

Monod is also attentive to theological, historical, and textual accuracy and
to what he considers distortions of the Gospel. For example, when Piaget asserts that charity and forgiveness constitute the essence of Christian morality,
Monod retorts that he forgets saintliness (ibid., 9). Most important, when
Piaget claims that Jesus was never concerned with the interests of the individual, Monod replies that "perhaps the greatest originality of the Gospel is the
concern for the single person," and explains:

> Social Christianity, just like socialism, wishes "to control things to liberate
> man." And if it has been possible to say, truthfully, "Perfect society is the goal
> of the soul," it is even truer to affirm: The goal of perfect society is the soul—
> the blossoming of the person made possible, the birth of the whole man. It is
> in this sense that Christian socialism always emphasizes, among the Rights of
> man, the "Right to salvation," which epitomizes them all.   (Ibid., 10)

Monod's comments are consistently inspired by his theological and religious orientation and by an extreme sensitivity to the distinction between
metaphysics and religion. When Piaget writes of the "sins of the brain,"
Monod cautions that "sin does not belong to the intellectual level of reality";
the phrase "metaphysics will pull religion out of its present torpor" sounds to
him like "orthodox language," and leads him to exhort Piaget to distinguish,
"always, [between] *religion* and *theology*" (ibid., 13); the idea that the "soul of
Humanity will one day be independent of personal souls" makes him wonder,
"This is metaphysics; but is it still religion?" (ibid., 14).

Monod thus clearly perceives that *Mission* is more philosophical than religious—and he is not satisfied with its philosophy. He considers that many of
the ideas are unclear and that Piaget himself is not entirely certain about the
"substance of his thinking." "You have written a *poem*," he tells him, "and I
like it as such; but it is not a philosophical study" (ibid., 6). He finds the very
concept of Idea enigmatic, and the poem's whole doctrine seems to him not
only obscure but perhaps even dangerous. According to Piaget, orthodoxy is
able to hinder and weaken the idea. For Monod, whose aversion of intolerance
surfaces here, the conservatives may hinder the Idea only by means of an idea,

doubtless their idea, but finally an idea to which men sacrifice their preferences, and even their lives, an idea they adore and which is their Divinity . . .

Without a doubt, the doctrinaires of *reaction* . . . are the enemies of humanity; but anticlericalism, irreligion, materialism, and monism also have their
doctrinaires; and it has not been proven, as you write . . . that "error serves
conservatism" . . . Do not give the impression of identifying "transformation" with "progress"; when it became the papal church, the Christian church
"marched"—but backward.   (Ibid., 8)

Piaget's identification of evolution and the good makes Monod wonder why, if
nature is indeed solidaristic, it is a "natural inclination" that leads the individual toward selfishness (ibid., 9).

Monod does not seem to have held the intellectual content of *The Mission of
the Idea* in high regard. Yet the very seriousness of his reading underlines the
sincerity of his encouragements and of his calling Piaget a talented "authentic
youth." As he told Piaget, "you are experiencing the truth of the saying, 'The
best thing that can happen to a young man is to devote himself, early on, to a
just and unpopular cause'" (ibid., 3). Monod's reaction to *Mission* thus coincides with Dardel's and Pettavel's, who did not agree with Piaget on every
point but admired his courage and his sincerity and praised him as a model
young Christian.

It is difficult to determine a larger public's reaction to *The Mission of the
Idea*. According to Mme. Marthe Piaget-Burger, the poem made Arthur Piaget
proud of his son and had a more profound effect on his immediate environment than would *Recherche* in 1918. The poem was obviously seen as an important product of the Christian students' milieu, and both the prepublication
announcement and the reviews show the place Piaget created for himself in a
context that approved of his intense sense of mission.

Conclusion: The Young Man's Mission

For Piaget, Jesus is the perfect model of youth. He is "the idea made flesh" (8);
he "fully understood the immensity of the heroism he would embrace," and
that is why "the clash between this young and humble man's exquisite soul and
the unyielding obstinacy of stupid traditions would be tragic" (9). Each young
man is a potential Jesus whose mission is to realize the idea (§IV, 7–8). Youth
is inherently in harmony with the idea and all it stands for; it is the "truly
moral period" of life, during which man is "in communion" with life and with
God. When a young man feels the idea springing in him, he revolts against the
world that surrounds him; he apprehends "the sacred value of the emerging

idea" and "experiences the ineffable state" of the individual who has become aware of his mission; "because he has not compromised, he feels the power, that is, the duty, of undertaking this immense struggle: to clear the way for the idea." During youth, "the self affirms itself and draws up its conceptions," the idea "raises itself to the metaphysical sphere [and] accumulates and coordinates all the potentialities, all the beauties of true theory, all the poetry of the soul."

The action of the conservative spirit begins only after the period of youth, in the form of compromises and the "ugliest of sins, fear when confronted with the idea" (8). The idea itself is young (11); and youth is like the idea: "When he enters life, the young man has a force nobody can oppose, a power of virtualities which, if realized, would stir life and nourish the idea" (27).

Youth is the recapitulative microcosm of the universal march toward salvation. Piaget describes the birth of humanity as the dawn of a collective youth, as the moment when man has left childhood and feels an "indefinite malaise" and an "anxiety" that are nothing other than the signs of an "august labor" (30). The young man is thus immanently linked to Jesus and must try to realize Jesus' teachings and to become the idea's incarnation. The obligatory character of youth's mission is a consequence of Piaget's postulate that "a stated ideal becomes a duty" (63). That is, at bottom, why *The Mission of the Idea* also communicates the idea of a mission.

Piaget's poems contain his first global "system," as well as certain fundamental assumptions or attitudes, at once stable and diffuse, that persist throughout his oeuvre, although they are neither reducible to nor based on observation or reasoning. In *Mission,* such leitmotifs are: the feeling or perception of a universal movement that it would be artificial to segment or stop, but that must be nevertheless understood; the identification of this movement with historical, evolutionary, and developmental change, and of change with progress and the good; the existence of an ideal destination, characterized by synthesis, harmony, and equilibrium, from which the movement draws its principles and laws; and the insertion of the individual in the movement as a microcosm in the macrocosm.

The images used in *Mission* to denote the idea and life (and including the good, the true, and the beautiful) demonstrate that all these entities are equivalent. Words such as "march," "impulse," "thrust," "motor," and "flux" evoke all that is good and worthy of being pursued. Creative movement is the common denominator of the poem's positive figures. This movement expresses a cognitive and aesthetic value that Piaget never relinquished. Starting with *Mission,* the themes of life as tendency and progress, and of the ultimate identity of all vital processes underlie the different aspects and periods of his work.

At the time of *Mission,* Piaget's specific originality was to establish an inherent link between an image of youth and a metaphysical system that involved doctrines about science, morality, and social action, as well as a project concerning his personal identity and future life. In a word, the "mission of the idea" was nothing other than the young Piaget's own mission.

According to Piaget, the "mission of the idea" is "the new birth of Christianity" (68)—and that is also his generation's mission: "When you understand that the idea leads the world, and when you see today that Christianity surrenders, you apprehend the urgent mission that is incumbent upon postwar men: to embark on the pursuit of a truth purer than the one that makes us live" (55). *The Mission of the Idea* itself is the personal expression of a man already committed to the pursuit of such a purer truth.

Piaget follows his own doctrines and injunctions. His attack on the conservative spirit is authorized by the Idea (27). *Mission* aims at "seizing" the idea and at the same time exposes the limits of the poetic sentiment (10). Piaget does not hesitate to assert the superiority of the thinker, himself having stayed "in the silence of the study" before launching "the young idea in the open" (10–11). He elaborates a metaphysical system and then attributes to metaphysics the power to save religion (55). He turns conversion into the basis of the "true life" before narrating conversion experiences in the first person. He describes the young man as the one who must "clear the way for the idea" (7) while himself clearing the way for the idea. In sum, it is in a youthful text inspired by the idea that Jesus, "the idea made flesh" (8), appears as the archetypal young man. Jesus is the model; *Mission*'s author, his apostle.

The Mission of the Idea has two epigraphs. The first one is Jesus' words: "Think not that I am come to send peace on earth: I came not to send peace, but a sword . . . And he that taketh not his cross and followeth me is not worthy of me" (Matthew 10:34–38). The second one, quoted in Greek, is the prayer of the blind men of Jericho: "Lord, that our eyes may be opened" (Matthew 20:33). The blind men's call may be read as that of all Christians or of all men, including Piaget himself; but it may also be read as a symbol of *Mission*'s goals: to open the reader's eyes. *Mission*'s author is willing to "take the cross," follow Jesus, and be, like Him, "an idealist, an innovator, a rebel" (44). In his quest to realize the idea, he upsets the established order and sets "a man at variance against his father" (Matthew 10:35). He must destroy before recreating. He advocates an awakening of conscience, but such a revival "takes place through gun and sword" (54). From the formal point of view, the identification of the narrator with Jesus and, a fortiori, with an apostle is manifest in a style that could be called evangelical.

A whole section of *Mission* (§XXI) is a prosopopoeia in which Jesus, "seized by a sacred wrath," anathematizes conservatives. Elsewhere (§§III, VII) the narrator himself utters maledictions, always in the style of Jesus' seven maledictions to the scribes and the Pharisees (Matthew 23:13–32). At least once Piaget uses Jesus' typical formula for addressing the masses or his followers: "Verily, I say unto you . . ." (33). Christ or Jesus appears variously, directly and indirectly, both as speaker and as quoted authority.

Piaget likes to teach by means of parables. The lonely traveler symbolizes the "life for the idea"; the stormy night illustrates the process of being born again; the children lost in the forest represent faith and doubt. Piaget's use of the didactic allegorical tale highlights his role as prophet on the model of Christ: "All these things spake Jesus unto the multitude with parables; and without a parable spake he not unto them" (Matthew 13:34); "but without a parable he spake not unto them: and when they were alone, he expounded all things to his disciples" (Mark 4:34), since, as he told them, "it is given unto you to know the mysteries of the kingdom of heaven" (Matthew 13:11; compare Luke 8:9–10). Piaget always explicates his parables, and in so doing, he enlightens the disciples who will propagate the Idea, whose gospel is *Mission*.

The Mission of the Idea as a whole may be related to the synoptic Gospels, and to Matthew's in particular. Matthew's Gospel provides the poem's epigraphs and most of the biblical quotations and paraphrases. Some of the poem's central features correspond to Matthew's spirit and rhetoric: the basically didactic goal, the emphasis on the communication of doctrine, the unification of themes by "discourses," and the use of exemplary narratives. Moreover, *Mission* contains several instances of "inclusion," a common Old Testament procedure found more frequently in Matthew's Gospel than in the others, which consists in beginning and finishing a section with similar words. More generally, *Mission*'s sections are short and relatively independent from each other, so that they can be readily used as pericopes (as was done in the YMCA journal *Jeunesse* in the issue that reviewed the poem).

In sum, an ensemble of conceptual and stylistic elements shows that Piaget designated himself as an apostle of Jesus and the Idea, and considered that his mission was to work for the realization of their doctrine on earth. "Yet," he added, "everybody's help is necessary for the rebirth of the idea." "Metaphysics is not an aristocratic art. The savant, who finds hypotheses, must place above them the grand edifice capable of enclosing them; the Christian, who has felt a life deep in his heart, must assimilate it by means of an interpretation provided by reason; the moral man, who wants a rule of life for his action, has to construct an idea to justify it [the rule]" (68). Metaphysics implies building a system, giving a rational formulation to the feeling of faith, and establishing life on an idea. Piaget's nascent life enterprise in December 1915 is precisely to elaborate such a metaphysics.

Three major projects intertwine: a project for personal identity (to integrate the thinker, the Christian, and the moral man); a moral, social, and political project directed at the new birth of Christianity and postwar reconstruction; and the more theoretical project of giving a philosophical and scientific foundation to the moral project, and thus to the new world and to "tomorrow's ideal." The young man feels the inner advent of the idea, asserts himself, and states his "conceptions"; he sees life as an "immense struggle" to "clear the way for the idea" (7): "And this thrust will by itself nourish [his] future existence. Such is the young man's metaphysics, such is the value of his whole life" (8).

In *Mission,* poetry and mysticism are essential components of metaphysics. Yet they open onto a "void" and cast the individual from excessive elation into sadness and melancholy (14). Such oscillation between extreme moods is one of the main sources of suffering of *Recherche*'s autobiographical Sebastian. Like his hero, Piaget aims at surmounting such instability and at the same time remaining loyal to Christ and Christian faith. By August 1917 he asserted the vanity of all intellectual metaphysics, claimed to have got rid of metaphysics and theology, and characterized the problem that made up his life as that of basing morality on science (1917a). It is through a reform of the self and a revolt against his milieu that Piaget gave to the projects formulated in *Mission* the increasingly precise and rational formulation that eventually became scientific work.

12

The Making of a New Identity

From 1915 to 1917 Piaget seems absorbed with his own personality, and particularly with the forging of a new identity, free of metaphysics and theology. In his efforts to understand evil and to believe in a humane God, he arrived at the idea that human beings themselves create God. This was a painful process, punctuated by doubts and crises. Yet, when asked if he had had a religious crisis in adolescence, Piaget replied, "No, because I promptly began to believe in immanence" (1977, 51). This was simply not the case, and Piaget's denial must be seen as a powerful repression of the deepest joys and sufferings of his youth.

The Magic Mountain

Much of Piaget's development during the middle years of World War I took place on the mountain. There he examined himself and the world, expressed in writing his doubts and his anguish, and worked out a new identity. Whether entirely fictional or autobiographically realistic, the mountain is the setting of his characters' illuminations, the retreat from which they contemplate the world.

Piaget's mountain was not that of the naturalist or the sportsman, but that of the sick. He was one of many young people during that period who were sent to mountain health resorts for treatment of tuberculosis or other lung ailments, and his psychology during the war years corresponds largely to the one ascribed at the time to the lung patient.

Piaget's cures took place in Leysin, the main Swiss-French mountain health resort. There is unfortunately little documentation of his stays there.[1] The town's records on residents go back only to 1920, and there are no traces of Piaget in *La petite revue*, a local "literary, artistic, and medical" magazine published from December 1916 to December 1917. Piaget's letter of resignation from the Friends of Nature, written in Leysin, is dated 25 September 1915 (ms. 1915a). His stay at that time may have lasted half a year. In February 1916, Piaget's letters are still dated from Leysin, and a May letter to Paul Pettavel states that he has been back in Neuchâtel for a month but must return to Leysin for the entire summer (ms. 1916b). His absence from Neuchâtel is confirmed by the fact that he was not enrolled at the university during the summer term of 1916 (mid-April to mid-July). Later he tells Arnold Reymond (ms. 1918c) that *Recherche* was written at Leysin, and the preface to the book specifies "September 1916 to January 1917." That Piaget spent Christmas 1916 in Leysin is confirmed by a passing remark in his mother's correspondence.[2] Writing on 20 March 1917 from Neuchâtel, Piaget informs Maurice Bedot that he returned from Leysin "three or four" weeks earlier (ms. [1917]). The letter to Rolland, dated 4 August 1917, is written from Leysin. In his autobiography (1952, 241), Piaget states that he had "to spend more than a year in the mountains."

On the basis of Piaget's letters and a few comments, we may presume that he sojourned in Leysin from at least September 1915 to April 1916, perhaps with interruptions, then from June or July 1916 to February 1917, and finally (most hypothetically, suggested only by the letter to Rolland) during the summer of 1917. Despite such long stays in Leysin, Piaget remained enrolled at the University of Neuchâtel from October 1915 to July 1918, with the exception of the summer term of 1916.

Nothing is known about the condition that took Piaget to Leysin. In his September 1915 letter to the Friends of Nature, he claims that "illness" forces him to resign from the club (ms. 1915a). In a May 1916 letter he mentions a case of measles as a threat to his lung (ms. 1916b). A March 1917 note by Piaget's mother states that he has returned to Leysin "with a bad flu."[3] *Recherche* (1918a, 147) is consummately oblique: "I was hurt, and retired to a nearby hill." In his autobiography, Piaget (1952, 241) recalls that, around 1914–15, in addition to his schoolwork and his research on mollusks, he read a lot and "began to write down" his ideas "in numerous notebooks." "Soon," he adds, "these efforts affected my health." This is all. From the address in Piaget's letters, we know that he did not reside in a sanatorium, but in at least two different pensions, "Les Buits" and "Beau Soleil." Although no traces of the latter survive today, an advertisement for "Les Buits" from *La petite revue* describes it as a "family pension open to consumptives [*pulmonaires*], convalescents, visitors." It therefore seems that Piaget's lung condition was not a declared tuberculosis. In the vocabulary current at the time, he may have been characterized as "fragile," "vulnerable," or "predisposed," apt to relapse (as suggested by the remarks on flu and measles). Although he did not have to follow the regimen of the sanatorium, he remained under medical supervision, at least in part by the physician Louis Vauthier (1887–1963). Vauthier (who later married Piaget's sister Madeleine) practiced in Leysin from 1914 to 1916; at that time he established the "Libres Entretiens de Leysin," "free conversations" that brought together patients from different countries with the goal of encouraging international understanding.

This scarcity of medical evidence is not a serious obstacle to understanding the psychological role illness played in Piaget's life, his perceptions of himself as a Leysin patient, and the personal and public use he made of his condition.

From the establishment of mountain sanatoriums in the late nineteenth century until the 1950s, when antibiotics began to be widely used, being affected by a lung disease and sent to the mountain for treatment were not only associated with suffering and hopelessness, but also frequently enveloped in an aura of spiritual grandeur. Novels and medical reports depict mountain-cure patients as individuals who, though cut off from active life and subject to a rigorous medical regimen, might embark upon uncommon voyages of self-discovery and self-renewal. The young Piaget's case fits such a description.

Leysin is a village some 1,450 meters above sea level in the Swiss-French canton of Vaud. Its development as a health resort began in the early 1890s, following the model of another Swiss town, Davos. Mountain cure combined aerotherapy (exposure to air deemed pure) and heliotherapy (controlled exposure to sunlight) with a strict hygiene and with meticulously defined daily periods of total rest and silence. Despite its necessarily restful ambiance, Leysin had a rich cultural life, made up essentially of lectures and concerts given by residents or guests. Piaget himself contributed to it: a letter to his future mentor Edouard Claparède shows him, as a member of an unspecified committee, arranging for a lecture by the Genevan psychologist (ms. 1916c).

Around 1910, tuberculosis was responsible for about half of the deaths of eighteen-to-forty-year-olds. Mountain cure was only modestly effective: according to one study, 47 percent of the 1,200 patients treated at Leysin's Sanatorium Populaire from 1912 to 1916 were dead by 1920 (cited in Heller, 1990, 338). The tuberculosis patient was seen as a model of courage and confidence, whose "wounded soul" provided "mysterious gifts . . . to the frivolous world" (Burnand, 1936, 210).

The basic regimen of the sanatorium cut patients off from their customary environment and activities. The idleness and silence it imposed could acquire a haunting quality, distort the sense of time, lead to potentially creative introspection, but also (and more frequently) to boredom and depression. In any case, it created a microcosm composed of sick individuals, each absorbed by his or her own condition, yet extraordinarily sensitive to signs from their narrow social world. For some of the more intellectual or religious patients, organic disease would become a creative illness.

The closing of national boundaries during the war modified the composition of Leysin's population. The internment of soldiers in Switzerland started in January 1916 (the procedure was later extended to civilians from refugee camps). Moderately ill or wounded prisoners of war were transferred from the belligerent countries to Swiss health stations (German-speaking for soldiers from the Central powers, French-speaking for soldiers from the Allied armies); Switzerland received a small fee from the soldiers' native country, and the interns themselves had to perform services in such areas as agriculture, forestry, and road maintenance. Leysin accommodated a total of about 6,000 interns for the duration of the war. Their presence affected the atmosphere of the town and the life of its residents (for collections of photographs, see *Album* and Jaccottet et al., 1918, both propagandistic). Piaget's concerns may have been nourished by his contact with Leysin interns. Their presence certainly made a difference for him: a letter to Arnold Reymond hints at lively conversations and the establishment of close relations with French patients, some of whom commented on the manuscript of *Recherche* (ms. 1918f).

Fiction coincides with the reports of doctors and other witnesses about the psychology of the ill and the atmosphere of the *cité douloureuse* (Vallette, 1929). Such convergence highlights the strength of the image of the mountain-cure patient and suggests its potentially formative role.

The most famous novel in this domain is *The Magic Mountain* (1924), by Thomas Mann, inspired in part by a two-month visit to Davos, where his wife spent half a year in 1912. Mann narrates the story of Hans Castorp, a young man who goes to a sanatorium for a short visit, is drawn into the role of the sick, relishes it, and stays seven years in the clinic, until the outbreak of World War I sends him to the battlefields with the German army. Like all *Bildungsroman* heroes, Castorp starts as a relatively simple and naive individual. Through personal encounters, reflection, observation, and the experience of unfulfilled love, he reaches a literally timeless kind of knowledge about himself and the world, before being prevented by the war from reaching the summit of that superior state of health that is attained through illness and proximity to death.

Some of the psychological themes of Mann's complex and often ironic masterpiece are found in lesser writings. One of them, *The "Hours of Silence,"* by the Genevan novelist and essayist Robert de Traz, is a depiction of the mountain-cure patient reportedly based on the author's visits to Leysin. The title borrows from a clause in a clinic's regulation: "The elevator stops during the hours of silence" (Traz, 1934, 176). For the writer, the "silence therapy" widely practiced as part of the cure implied that the disease was fought not only by medical means but also by "a slow decantation of the mind, by withdrawal into oneself and inner concentration" (ibid., 177). The book's epigraph, a quotation from Alexandre Vinet, encapsulates its main theme and highlights the religious dimension of the experience of illness: "Suffering is perhaps nothing other than deeper living" (see also Seippel, 1912).

Traz (1934, 7) observes that the real distance between Leysin and the plain is small, but that the psychological distance is infinite; others write of the "insurmountable psychological barrier" that separates cure towns from the "world of the living" (Burnand, 1936, 163). Stuck in an environment that encouraged them to focus on themselves, patients tended to meditate about their case and elaborate a "general idea" into which to incorporate it (Traz, 1934, 10). In this self-oriented process, patients pondered their identity, oscillating considerably about their own "inner truth." "Psychologically, the disease is a trembling hesitation to identify oneself; it is a painful and necessary deepening, a sometimes unbearable encounter with oneself, a passionate acceptance of one's own person, and also a refusal, a denial, a repudiation of oneself, a frantic flight that brings one back to oneself" (ibid., 40).

Recherche is Piaget's own description of his painful and hesitating journey from self-denial to self-rediscovery and redefinition, an inner quest largely carried out upon the magic mountain. Although he was neither an extremely serious medical case nor one of those lingering sick on whom novels tend to focus, he was aware that he belonged in the *cité douloureuse*. In a letter to Reymond, Piaget wondered if, in writing *Recherche*, he had not been "a victim of the harshness one contracts in Leysin" (ms. 1918c). *Recherche* itself confirms the town's significance. Introducing his disagreement with the "young socialists," Piaget explains:

> I was with you in the midst of the mêlée, but you suddenly lost sight of me, and you will not see me again. For I was hurt, and retired to a nearby hill. And from there, as I healed my illness, I saw a terrible sight. I saw that the battle we had joined was very little compared to the future struggle . . .
>
> I then decided to stay up there, not because I am particularly qualified to be in the limelight, but because I happened to be there and my injury immobilized me.
>
> And now I come to reveal to you what I saw. (1918a, 147)

As for the hero of the mountain-cure *Bildungsroman*, Leysin was for Piaget the place of crucial inner experiences, the importance of which extended far beyond the results of medical treatment.

In *Recherche*, written in Leysin, and precisely in the middle section, based on a diary kept during one of his stays there, Piaget asserts that illness is indispensable for "the thinker" (1918a, 115). Illness facilitates the interchanges between consciousness and the unconscious (Piaget here speaks of *tréfonds,* or "innermost depths"). The intensity of physical suffering, he claims, is proportional to the disequilibrium of the *tréfonds;* the more the latter is disequilibrated, the more it surfaces and "dominate[s] everything"; consciousness reacts proportionally and "concentrates" increasing amounts of intelligence and will aimed at understanding oneself, taming the bustle from the unconscious, and separating good from evil (ibid., 116). It is this process that led Piaget to write, while in Leysin in 1915, "The Mysteries of Divine Suffering."

"The Mysteries of Divine Suffering"

A "prayer for the coming year": that is how, in December 1915, Jean Piaget characterized "The Mystery of Divine Suffering" as he submitted it to Paul Pettavel and asked him to publish it in *L'Essor* as early as possible in January (ms. 1915b). Pettavel (ms. 1915, 2) responded enthusiastically: Piaget's text seemed to him revealing of the "mood of present-day youth," and its author "more modern than *L'Essor* has ever been." The text appeared in February 1916 under the slightly different title "The Mysteries of Divine Suffering." In seven long columns printed on both sides of a large sheet, it made up the whole first issue of "Youth's Corner," a monthly supplement Pettavel (1916b) offered to young people so that they could freely voice their psychological, moral, social, or religious preoccupations.

Piaget (ms. 1916a) later thanked Pettavel for the place he gave to his "meditation, and for the happy initiative to open *L'Essor* to youth," accepted (ms. 1916b) the pastor's offer to join what was probably an editorial committee related to the "Youth's Corner," and promised to advertise the supplement.

Like *The Mission of the Idea,* "The Mysteries of Divine Suffering" both illustrates the main themes and the style of socially concerned intellectual Christian youth, and embodies Piaget's spiritual life during the first half of World War I. On the one hand, it declares the revolt against the political and religious "orthodoxies" deemed responsible for the war; on the other hand, it manifests the anxious quest for a more humane God, and the exalted acceptance of a redeeming mission to regenerate humanity and Christianity. As in *Mission,* Piaget's message in "The Mysteries" is punctuated with quasi-mystical experiences and formulated within a Bergsonian framework. But the 1916 "prayer" anticipates Piaget's renunciation of metaphysics and theology.

When Piaget (1916c) claims in "The Mysteries" that "metaphysical suffering" is "eternal and perhaps definitive," when he underlines the "radical helplessness of the Creator and his creature" as they "try to enter into each other in a glorious and final absolute" (§51),[4] he foreshadows the evolution described to Romain Rolland in August 1917:

> Everyone is a metaphysician at eighteen, and in addition a theologian, if one is Swiss-French. But I believe I have got rid of all that; I have been trying for two years. I believe more than ever in Christ, but he teaches me to be human [*être homme*], and all religious belief would prevent me from doing so. Only faith is great, and faith is the decision to live in spite of the mystery that is at the bottom of everything. This is all my metaphysics, a metaphysics that is not at all intellectual, and that is merely the metaphysics implicit in all life. We cannot live without asserting an absolute value that gives sense to life. I assert it without proof: that is what faith is. Hence the great problem is to base morality on science, since faith is independent of metaphysics, and since metaphysics is vain, and that is the problem that makes up my life. (ms. 1917)[5]

"The Mysteries" does not present a mental universe stripped of metaphysics and theology and animated by the project of basing morality on science. But it points toward it.

Like *The Mission of the Idea*, "The Mysteries of Divine Suffering" wishes to inspire confidence in the future "reconstruction" (§59). Yet this optimism is made possible only because pain and evil are perceived as "the very breath of the creative impulse" (§52), and because war is accepted as an image "of the eternal turmoil in which God still moves" (§54). Such a view of evil enables Piaget to accept the existence of a transcendent God—but this is precisely the "religious belief" that, a year and a half later, in the letter to Rolland, he identified as the obstacle to his being fully human.

The Problem of Evil and the Discovery of Self-Creation

"The Mysteries of Divine Suffering" is a dialogue between a man and God. Starting with the man's despair before evil, it culminates in his discovery that humanity and God collaborate and suffer together; this discovery is presented as an illumination.

An anguished man climbs to the mountain and speaks to the "Father" at length (§§4–33). He first expresses desperation and sadness. Like the author of *Mission*, he curses "narrowness, reaction, orthodoxy, all those conservative inertias . . . that threw us headlong into today's chaos" and implores God to destroy all such "principles of death" (§21). But his message is above all the supplication of a creature who feels abandoned: "Oh, Father, where are you? What are you doing? What a formidable mystery is your silence . . . How can we believe in the goodness of man when you, the Just, do not even have the kindness to thrust us into an eternal void?" (§§8–9).

The man's desperate cry is heralded by three epigraphs: 1 Kings 19:4, Job 3, and Jeremiah 20:14–18. The first one corresponds to the moment of discouragement felt by Elijah, the only surviving prophet of Jehovah left in the land of Israel, during his long flight to the Horeb, "God's mountain": "'It is enough,' he said, 'now, Lord, take my life, for I am not better than my fathers before me.'" In the other texts, Job and Jeremiah curse the day of their birth. Although these Old Testament epigraphs sound a more pessimistic note than the New Testament ones of *The Mission of the Idea,* the quotation from Kings combines the theme of despair with that of the sacred mountain where one meets God and is endowed with a redeeming mission (Elijah will anoint kings and prophets). It thus prefigures the hopeful message delivered at the end of the "prayer."

The man's revolt against God's indifference is followed by an incensed attack on evil and cowardice, culminating thus:

What are you doing, my God, where are you? . . .
   Why is the cry of Jesus, isolated on his cross, his most human word . . . the hiccough of an agony that is the eternal agony of the good and justice? (§§28–29)

Father, why? why? why? Such is the complaint that summarizes my entire suffering . . . It would be a thousand times better to know and then die, than to be tortured by ignorance. When will you judge me sufficiently strong to bear the weight of truth? When will you reveal yourself, hidden God?
   My God, my God, why hast thou forsaken me? (§§32–33)

The use of Christ's cry on the cross (Matthew 27:46; Mark 15:34) pathetically underlines the man's predicament and the ultimate sources of his pain, and suggests the communion between human and divine suffering that will indeed turn out to be the object of the man's illumination.

When the man reopens his eyes after this tragic questioning of God, he finds himself surrounded by night and the calm of nature; then, "in the ecstasy of a distant and vague music, he recognize[s] the voice of the God of love. Overwhelmed by joy, he let[s] himself be penetrated by an infinite peace" (§34). At this point, God reveals to him that He is consubstantial with the perpetual creation of the universe (§38); that, similarly, man creates himself through his action in the world (§42); and that, through his struggle, man becomes not simply a "true image of divinity" and God's "collaborator" (§51), but God's own creator (§49). As He says, "trying in a perpetual becoming to reach the

absolute, to reach a real and full existence where I will not need to create incessantly in order to assert myself, I gradually generate the universe out of my
own substance, becoming conscious of myself exactly to the same extent that I
produce the world. To create the world is to create myself" (§38). "Like you,"
God tells the man, "I do not know everything" (§39). He creates "to assert"
Himself, but the "exterior" so produced becomes an obstacle to His full realization: "I eternally bump into that which I thrust in front of me" (§39). Hence
His question, analogous to humanity's, "Will I ever arrive at the absolute I
search for? Will I absorb in myself the world I created? Will I be 'God' one
day?" (§39).

The answer, God reveals, depends on humanity's capacity to participate in
the Plotinian cycle already postulated in *The Mission of the Idea,* and here made
explicit by the use of the terms *conversion* and *procession* in quotation marks:
"Life is a return to my being through the matter I thrust out of myself. This is
the 'conversion' of my creation, succeeding the initial 'procession'" (§40). God
emerges out of the creative opposition between matter and the vital impulse,
now energized by human action. The entire power of salvation thus resides in
humanity: "In the same way I create myself in creating the universe, you create
yourself in your painful labors" (§42). This is the reason why redemption had
to come through Jesus, the only *man* who knew "how to elevate himself to the
individual absolute, to the perfect independence of his soul" (§44). Since
Christ himself did not know that God could not prevent his tragic death, the
passion appears as an "eternal moment that concentrates in itself the history of
the universe" (§45). As the man tells God, "You created a battlefield in order
to create yourself" (§59).

After the revelation God exhorts the man to "continue the struggle: it is not
you alone, it is me you will create" (§49). The man realizes that God resides
nowhere else but in his own active participation in the agonies of the world.
Through the identity of divine and human suffering, man becomes "a true
image of the deity" (§51). To penetrate the mystery of divine suffering is therefore to understand the essence of humanity. Such is the man's illumination:
"By placing himself in the divine becoming, he understood the necessity of
each phase . . . And in a superb impulse he elevated himself to God's own suffering and experienced the ineffable existence whereby only what was best in
him apprehended in one instant a bit of eternity" (§50). This mystical experience dispels the "formidable mystery" (§8) of God's silence before His
creature's torments, and justifies humanity's anguishes and toils by turning
them into life's inherent condition.

Taking up the Bergsonian idea of self-creation (Jouhaud, 1992), Piaget next
postulates that human individuals are the autonomous and responsible au-

thors of their own lives, and identifies God with their inherent capacity to create themselves and the world. From *The Mission of the Idea* to "The Mysteries of Divine Suffering," God has replaced the Idea, and man has replaced God.

In *Recherche*, Piaget places the development presented in "The Mysteries" in the context of an encounter with the idea of destiny. Sebastian's anger was "man's sacred revolt against destiny, a revolt that is the source of all true religion . . . He repudiated the despotic God who gives Grace to some and denies it to others . . . for he recognized in that God the old enemy, the Moira," the mythological personification of fate (1918a, 27). Thus, Sebastian no longer believed in a revealed omnipotent God. "A God that leaves man in ignorance is a God that can do nothing against evil. If evil was useful or had a sense, we would at least know it" (ibid., 29). But that was not the case, and Sebastian suffered from his ignorance. "The Mysteries" formulates the knowledge he eventually gained.

Sebastian found the idea of a suffering God in Wilfred Monod's collection of prewar essays *To Believers and Atheists,* and shared in the comfort it had brought to "the anxious minds of Protestantism" (1918a, 29). Two essays in particular ("An Atheist" and "The Problem of God," about half of the volume) discuss the question of evil and argue in favor of a God who must struggle for the salvation of humanity. For Monod, such a conception of God was "not only in agreement with the essential postulates of Christian conscience, but also in harmony with several fundamental principles of the modern mind," including the social ideals of democracy, the identification of evolution and progress, the tendency to think of science and life in terms of becoming, the hope of vast economic and political reforms, and the readiness to accept a God who is no longer a support of the status quo (Monod, 1914b, 280–281).

Action and the Grasp of Consciousness

In *The Mission of the Idea,* Piaget found a solution to the problem of evil in the belief that God is powerless before circumstances for which only the conservative spirit is responsible. The war is not a God-sent ordeal, but a tragic event that makes God suffer together with humanity. In "The Mysteries" suffering becomes "the very breath of the creative impulse" (§52), and war "a cynically realistic image of the eternal turmoil in which God still moves" (§54). In his final address to the Father (§§56–61), the man of Piaget's "prayer" asks for the capacity "to remember the Creator's infinite suffering, a Creator whose agony constructs, day after day, in us and through us, his eternal divinity." Suffering is consubstantial with self-creation, and it is the price the man pays for knowledge acquired in a moment of illumination. This knowledge "is not good for everyone": "Only matured by his own suffering can man arrive at the acceptance of metaphysical suffering . . . This truth is only for the strong, for those who are not frightened by responsibility, by the true freedom that places in man himself his own support" (§51).

In conformity with the theology elaborated in *The Mission of the Idea* and "Bergson and Sabatier," Piaget holds that truth assumes transient forms: "What my reason understood is merely a symbol and a venturesome construction, but what my heart understood is eternally true" (§57). Yet truth is always for the privileged few who think rather than act. As he said in *Recherche*, progress is accomplished by those who are "strong enough to ignore action, and aim, in spite of facts, at the ideal" (1918a, 117) and let others remedy its miseries. "The Mysteries of Divine Suffering" highlights the metaphysical significance of this elitism.

In Piaget's "prayer" God observes that "life was obliged to adapt to action rather than to contemplation, and action deformed reality" (§47). God's assertion is consistent with the Bergsonian distinction between active and passive adaptation on which Piaget based his discussion of mimicry. Throughout his later career Piaget (for example, 1936, 1976b) asserted that the *activity* of the living organism is the condition of possibility and the "motor" of both psychological development and organic evolution. Such an assertion does not contradict his youthful critique of action. The "action" that, according to *Mission,* "The Mysteries," and *Recherche*, destroys the whole and deforms reality is not creative activity. Piaget criticizes the passive modes of natural selection or mass activism but fully accepts the active modes involved in creative evolution or in the psychological apprehension of *durée* and the *élan vital.* Bergson (1889, 114, 143) himself called "free every act that emanates from the self, and the self alone," and defined freedom as "the relation of the self to the act it accomplishes."

"The Mysteries of Divine Suffering" points toward a psychology according to which the thinking self is the creative agent of itself and the universe, and the grasp of consciousness is the key act of self-creation. As God explains, "my consciousness has followed degrees—the degrees of my creation—and it is only gradually that I understood my life" (§39). God creates Himself by "becoming conscious" of Himself as he "produces" the world (§38). Similarly, in Piaget's psychology and epistemology, human individuals construct themselves and the universe of objective relations largely by becoming conscious of their own actions and mental operations.

Piaget devoted one of his last books to the grasp of consciousness. There, he explained that "cognizance (or the act of becoming conscious) of an action scheme transforms it into a concept" (1974a, 332). The subject "looks at his actions and these are assimilated . . . by his consciousness as if they were ordinary material links situated in the objects—hence the necessity of a new conceptual construction to account for them" (ibid., 339). This conceptualization is genuinely creative, since it consists in "reconstructing, then going beyond . . . what was acquired on the plane of the action schemes" (ibid., 342). In accordance with the postulates of Piagetian constructivism, the subject "learns to know himself [only] when acting on the object, and the latter can become known only as a result of progress of the actions carried out on it"; for Piaget, this "explains the harmony between thought and reality, since action springs from the laws of an organism that is simultaneously one physical object among many and the source of the acting, then thinking, subject" (ibid., 353). Thus, more than half a century after "The Mysteries of Divine Suffering," Piaget "reconstructed" as psychological discourse the ideas about the constructive and creative role of the grasp of consciousness first formulated as religious insight in that youthful "prayer." The latter thus gives biographical substance to the idea that Piaget's constructivist epistemology results in part from the decline in the authority of religion; since the world is no longer revealed, we are left to construct it ourselves, particularly through science (Vandenberg, 1991, 37–38).

Only after subjecting the notion of self-creation asserted in "The Mysteries" to a strict purification of subjectivity could Piaget claim that "God is thought" (since He is "the condition of existence, and the condition of existence is thought"), and that "immanentism implies the identification of God, not to the psychological self, but to the norms of thought itself" (1928a, 34, 36). This conception of God is of great gnoseological and epistemological import. To the extent that man creates himself and the universe through his own action and grasp of consciousness, self-knowledge must be the royal way toward all knowledge, including that of the absolute. As Bergson (1907, 248) had put it when discussing the idea of divine creation, if creation is conceived as "unceasing life, action, freedom," then it "is not a *mystery;* we experience it in ourselves when we act freely."

Piaget in His Generation

Numerous indices in Piaget's youthful writings show that a sense of shared mission and common generational destiny was one of the defining aspects of his life. Beyond their rootedness in the Swiss Christian students' milieu, all his wartime texts partake in a movement characterized by a notably pathetic style, sympathy for Christian socialism, belief in the universality and freedom of the spirit as opposed to the base interests of politics, constant calls for peace, and the enthusiastic hope that humanity would be regenerated after the war.

Romain Rolland

The soul of this movement was Romain Rolland (1866–1944).[6] Many young people had been attracted to Rolland's political humanism through his *Jean-Christophe,* a ten-volume *Bildungsroman* published between 1903 and 1912. The name of the hero, Jean-Christophe Krafft, incorporates both "bearing Christ" and "strength." As the Child makes the bearer cross dangerous water, faith gives the individual the strength to advance against social currents. Krafft's development includes intense moments of revolt against the world; inspired by the forces of art, love, and friendship, he denounces individualism and nationalism. Born in Germany, Jean-Christophe settles in Paris; the Rhine is for him the symbol of a civilization based on common values, and on faith in an unknown God whom everybody can adore.

Rolland's impact on youth at the time of World War I is best encapsulated in the words God speaks to Jean-Christophe during his adolescent crisis: "Suffer. Die. But be what you must be: A Man" (Rolland, 1903–12, II:231). "Being a Man" implied never giving up the quest for truth, never ceasing to be sincere, living according to one's conscience, and being prepared for the solitude and lack of understanding that such attitudes are bound to incite. "Being a Man" was widely adopted as a sort of password among Rolland's admirers. Piaget's use of the expression in his letter to Rolland and elsewhere is typical.

Rolland's influence on youth was immense. Numerous testimonies reveal his prestige and moral authority. Not only celebrated personalities of European culture, but also young men, many of them at the front, wrote to him expressing their admiration for his oeuvre; for Piaget, who sent Rolland *The Mission of the Idea,*[7] the French writer was best understood by those soldiers who defended their country without feeling hatred or losing their love for humanity (1918a, 75–76). Although Rolland's stand during the Great War led many to call him the "conscience of humanity" and helped earn him the Nobel Prize for Literature in 1916, it also gave rise to violent slanders, to accusations of treason and defeatism, and to the banning of his publications in his native France, a situation to which Piaget alludes in "The Mysteries of Divine Suffering" (1916c, §27).

Rolland was in Switzerland at the outbreak of the war and decided to stay there. Until 1937 he lived mostly in the small town of Villeneuve, close to Vevey, on Lake Geneva. At the end of August 1914 he began writing against the war and nationalism in several Swiss newspapers and magazines; his most famous article, "Au-dessus de la mêlée" (Above the Battle), appeared in the prestigious *Journal de Genève* in September 1914.

The title "Above the Battle" became a symbol of Rolland's position. Giving up national allegiances, the thinker perceives the failure of all governments, of socialist parties and official Christianity, and asks intellectual elites to build "the enclosure of the city where the fraternal and free souls from all over the world will gather" (Rolland, 1914, 82). Being above the battle did not entail moral neutrality but a rejection of nationalistic passions and the will to look for the facts behind political propaganda. As for Rolland, fighting nationalism was for Sebastian the most urgent task (1918a, 73).

Rolland's attitude was largely inspired by Tolstoy's political and religious thought. Leon Tolstoy (1828–1910) sought to purify Christianity of mysteries and dogmas; he interpreted injustice and social inequality as a betrayal of Christian commandments, for which he blamed the established churches (he was excommunicated by the Russian Orthodox church in 1901); he advocated a nonviolent pacifism. In his biography of Tolstoy, Rolland (1913, 203, 4) called the Russian writer "our conscience," and wrote that Tolstoy's books were for many of his contemporaries "what [Goethe's] *Werther* had been for his [Tolstoy's] generation: the magnificent mirror of our potential for love, weakness, hope, fear, and despair." Rolland, in turn, became for Piaget's generation what Tolstoy had been for his, and the names of the two apostles of human fraternity and freedom of conscience often appeared together in the progressive Swiss-French press during the war. Piaget's 1917 letter to Rolland was prompted by an article on Tolstoy as a model of free humanity, and his major wartime texts are permeated by Rolland's ideology and style.

Socialism

The quest for a renewal of social and economic structures through socialism was a central component of the Rollandist movement. Piaget first disclosed his socialist sympathies in *The Mission of the Idea*. Bourgeois Christianity, he asserted, hindered socialism; in the new era, science would become socialist, and socialism scientific. In "The Mysteries of Divine Suffering," the French socialist and antiwar leader Jean Jaurès, assassinated by a young nationalist in 1914, is characterized as the man "who incarnated an ideal of humanity that could have saved the world, a saint, a prophet" (1916c, §25). *Recherche* would confirm Piaget's socialist allegiance. And in December 1918, after witnessing the November general strike in Zurich, Piaget wrote, "Recent events could do nothing other than reinforce my socialism" (ms. 1918f). This general allegiance to socialism appears to have evolved.

In September 1915 a group of antiwar socialists met secretly in the Swiss village of Zimmerwald (Lademacher, 1967). A majority sought to end the war by means of peace treaties that excluded land annexations; a minority (including Lenin) wanted the war to lead to revolution. Thus began the rupture between the revolutionary and the reformist currents of the socialist movement. In French-speaking Switzerland, "Zimmerwald's left," as it was called, was vocally supported by the magazine *Demain*, published by a young French socialist-revolutionary who was at the time a close friend of Romain Rolland's.

The Zimmerwald meeting encouraged the radicalization of a portion of the Christian socialist movement. The best-known and most spectacular case is that of Jules Humbert-Droz (1891–1971), a native of La Chaux-de-Fonds. According to his own memoirs (1969), Humbert-Droz studied theology only because he saw in Christianity a moral and social ideal, and in Jesus a prophet of human fraternity. He became a pastor and continued to defend his unorthodox ideas. In 1914 he organized the Neuchâtel group of the Christian Socialist Federation. During the war, inspired by a Tolstoian form of Christian pacifism, he became a conscientious objector and was imprisoned and deprived of civil rights. He gradually moved toward revolutionary antimilitarism, quit diverse socialist organizations, entered the Communist Party in 1920, resigned in 1921 from the Christian Socialist Federation, and became secretary of the Communist International. He returned to Switzerland in 1931 after clashing with Stalin, who in 1942 had him excluded from the party; he then rejoined the Socialists.

At the time of *Mission*, Piaget seems to have adhered to the most idealist, messianic, and lyrical forms of Christian socialism. A letter from January 1918, however, shows him (ms. [1918]) active in the Swiss-French Christian Socialist Federation: he calls it "our group," appears intimate with its leaders, and recounts his participation in the most recent meeting (May 1917), where the creation of *Voies nouvelles* had been decided. (In establishing this journal, the Swiss-French group broke with the Paris-based Union of Christian Socialists, which they regarded as too nationalistic.) In a brochure cited by Pettavel (1918a, 2), Piaget is listed as one of the Neuchâtel writers for the new journal; the list included Humbert-Droz and several future leaders of Swiss socialism.

Jenny Humbert-Droz, Jules's widow, did not remember Piaget's taking part in the *Voies nouvelles* or in the Christian Socialist Federation. But she recalled that her husband "greatly appreciated his conversations with Piaget" at the Swiss Christian Students' Association (to which they both belonged); Piaget, she also related, "was not a member of the Socialist Party, but was clearly left-wing, and very open about antimilitarism."[8] Humbert-Droz was imprisoned in Neuchâtel from July 1916 until January 1917, and Piaget's mother was among his numerous supporters. She told him, for example: "I have a deep contempt for those who have sentenced you, and above all so harshly, and who certainly are way below you." By the time she received from Humbert-Droz an unspecified brochure, undoubtedly his blazing defense speech *War to War:*

Down with the Army (1916), she had "already read it with great interest, lent by her son Jean."[9]

The foundation of *Voies nouvelles* throws light on the relations between Christian-socialists and social-Christians in a way directly relevant to an understanding of Piaget's position. Paul Pettavel, whose journal *L'Essor* advocated an evangelical form of social Christianity, knew the young members of the Christian Socialist Federation well. Indeed, he initially mentioned their new journal because he was upset that they had not told him anything about it.

Already in March 1916 a group of "young people who leave their corner and burst into their parents' bedroom" (that is how they signed) manifested their unhappiness about *L'Essor*'s moderation (Anon., 1916b). Socialism appeared to them "to have a general life project, a plan for a new world"; it seemed to be "the great counterpower against the war," the only movement that advocated "justice, fraternity, peace, international reconciliation, and an ideal and humanitarian democracy." But if Christ is the Savior, if the Gospel is indeed a "project for universal life and the plan for a new world," and if Christianity can be "the human and divine ideal of tomorrow's humanity," then, they urged Pettavel, proclaim it loudly in *L'Essor*. The youths ended their appeal by asking the pastor to help them surmount their "moral idleness" and "live." Pettavel (1916c and 1916d) responded sympathetically but called for restraint and exhorted them to read the Gospel and follow Christ.

In 1916 the young socialists were going through a period of self-conscious morosity. An account published in May summarizing reports from the different Swiss-French local groups described the situation as "sad and humiliating"; "the new phase," it commented hopefully, "must be more beautiful and fertile than the present one" (Monastier, 1916, 44, 47). When in July 1916, after nine months of interruption, *La voix des jeunes* (The Voice of Youth), journal of the Swiss-French Federation of Socialist Youth, was relaunched under the editorship of twenty-five-year-old Jules Humbert-Droz, the first editorial spoke of the "new vitality that animates" young people: "Our ambitions are huge. We wish to tell our young contemporaries how critical the times are for our generation . . . We would like to stimulate reflection and thought, to create personalities, strong and independent temperaments, which the world needs so much . . . We are perhaps mad with optimism. But we . . . are at an age when generous and disinterested impulses are still possible, when self-sacrifice for the good of humanity is still capable of filling the heart with enthusiasm" (Anon., 1916c). Such were the hopes and self-image of the young socialists whose expectations Pettavel was unable to meet.

L'Essor, however, welcomed Christian-socialist articles, and it was apparently not Pettavel's attitude that led the Federation to create *Voies nouvelles*. In a January 1918 message to his "Christian socialist friends," Pettavel (1918a) stated that he understood youth's feeling that *L'Essor* might be outdated, but he emphasized that social Christianity and Christian socialism pursued the same ideal. Piaget (ms. [1918]) responded immediately. He told Pettavel that he had participated in the discussion leading to the creation of *Voies nouvelles*, and explained:

> we discussed at length whether we needed an organ, and whether *L'Essor* would not satisfy the demands of any Christian socialist. I can assure you that you would have attended the discussion without the slightest displeasure: we all rapidly agreed that if *L'Essor* = P[aul] P[ettavel], we did not need anything new. But to us, who defended this equation, the Genevans and others objected that *L'Essor*'s committee and a portion of its readership would be unhappy to see the socialists take over the [journal's] columns.

The latter position won the day; Pettavel was supposed to be officially informed, but everybody forgot about it.

The same explanation was given by Hélène Monastier (1918), who was then president of the Federation and remained a lifelong militant pacifist and Christian socialist. She added, though, that Christian socialism would not profit from adopting *L'Essor* as its official organ: "We wish to make a pacifist and Zimmerwaldian propaganda . . . Since we want to proclaim our faith as Christians, our social faith, and our faith in the International, we must do it at our own risk, under our own flag." Pettavel (1918b) seemed content with the explanation, although he again advocated collaboration.

As the *Voies nouvelles* episode suggests, Piaget tried to steer a middle course between the center and the left of Christian socialism. In any case, it is difficult to assess just how active he was in the organized movement. Documentation is scarce.[10] Piaget's "retreat" to Leysin played a role in distancing him from youth organizations. He himself realized that having to spend the summer of 1916 in the mountains would make him "lose all direct contact with the student and high school groups" (ms. 1916b). Leysin clearly played a deeper role, consistent with its image as a place where individuals gain a better understanding of themselves and the world.

Piaget's narrative in *Recherche* confirms and completes the documentary evidence: "From the early years of his intellectual development, he [Sebastian] had been attracted to socialism, where he found . . . a life and an idealism that no longer nourished the churches and politics. But these concerns rapidly gave way to the moral and religious problems that almost by themselves govern all social questions. The war made him come back to the socialist idea" (1918a,

77). For Piaget, however, socialism had evolved in two opposing directions. One was pursued by the "orthodox" official parties, which approved each nation's war credits and became nationalistic. The other was pursued by certain progressive though somewhat incoherent minorities (Zimmerwald, which Piaget does not mention, is the obvious example) that represented a "new ideal" and were free (ibid., 79–80). In this lyrical phase, Sebastian identifies socialism with Christ's message and dreams of a "Christ-people" recommencing the mystery of the cross (ibid., 80–81).

The subsequent story corroborates Piaget's choice of a middle path and suggests that the radicalization of the socialist movement was not to his liking. *Recherche* includes two letters to "young socialists." The first one (ibid., 82–87) is placed at the end of the book's first part, before the narrative of Sebastian's great crisis. Sebastian writes that socialism is primarily "a faith" and "must be a science, an art, and a morality." Its duty is to create a "specifically new synthesis" that unites social and individual forces and reconciles science and faith. This first letter represents the period up to *The Mission of the Idea*. The crisis hinted at in "The Mysteries of Divine Suffering" has not yet occurred.

The second letter, in contrast, is placed after the crisis and opens the third part of *Recherche*. This third part, titled "The Reconstruction," is a theoretical essay, not Sebastian's story. The "Letter to Young Socialists" (1918a, 147–148) is therefore Piaget's, not his hero's. In it Piaget says that he will report the "result of the European war" perceived from the "nearby hill" where illness had forced him to retire. A portion of youth, he claims, moves toward nationalism, catholicism, and pragmatism; its more progressive faction favors an immature socialism. For him, however, it is necessary to find an intermediate point "between a reactionary right and a left without culture" (ibid., 172). This middle point would be a "liberal socialism" grounded on "human principles" and consistent with Piaget's belief that "socialism and human sentiment are one" (ibid., 204). For him, federalism is the best system, since it maintains the equilibrium between parts and wholes (ibid., 209). A bourgeois regime is "abnormal and iniquitous" because it does not assure the equilibrium between the individual and society; collectivism is based on the suppression of private property and is therefore nothing other than its opposite extreme; only "socialist cooperation" preserves "individual autonomy" while guaranteeing a just distribution of wealth (ibid., 210). For Piaget, the superiority of cooperative federalism is not specifically moral or political, but a result of "scientific principles" (ibid.).

The culmination of Piaget's theoretical edifice was therefore a "socialist" political system aimed at "social salvation." Nevertheless, as has been rightly observed, from the viewpoint of organized politics, the radicalization of socialism after 1915 "resulted in defections, even among the young, as shown by the example of Jean Piaget" (Liniger, 1980, 60).

In April 1918 Piaget's enthusiastic comment on a brochure about the contradiction between being a Christian and being a patriot highlights the religious and metaphysical dimension of his political choices. In her brochure, Renée Warnery (1917), a woman physician who was active in the Christian Students' Association, argued that the demands of the state during wartime were incompatible with those of individual conscience, and that conscientious objection should remain an individual choice. She thus implicitly rejected the revolutionary socialists' call for objection as a form of mass action. Piaget agreed with her, and, after acknowledging that "national defense is a compromise" (1918d, 120), he suggested that living itself entails compromises, yet should be inspired by the goal of "reconciling the two potentialities of life, fatherland and humanity" (ibid., 122).

Individualism, Science, and Self-Criticism

Piaget was imbued with the sense, which Romain Rolland exemplified in the highest degree, that the intellectual's universalistic outlook precluded partisan activism, and that the best way to accomplish his mission was to remain a totally "free conscience," above the battles that might lead to absorption into collective bodies. In spite of Piaget's aspiration to belong to the great "soul" of Humanity, no collectivity, including organized Christianity and socialism, could satisfy him. Piaget's sense of being apart was reinforced by the feeling that, contrary to his generation, he succeeded in abandoning mystical subjectivism.

This feeling is apparent in Piaget's review of a thirty-page brochure titled *The Christ*, by the pastor Pierre Jeannet, a leading figure in the Swiss Christian Students' Association. (On Jeannet, see *Cahiers de "Jeunesse,"* 4, 1920.) Jeannet's text (1917) is a direct and somewhat lyrical message on behalf of Christ. In it Piaget finds an "amazing concentration of humanity and humanities around a single figure. But, alas! one wonders whether that is logically possible and coherent, whether an intellectual who has experienced the true struggle of the brain and the heart, [and] has seen his own life risk being dislocated . . . may still believe in the possible plenitude of such a Christ" (1917b, 124). After the great emotions of *The Mission of the Idea* and "The Mysteries of Divine Suffering," Piaget wants logic and coherence: Christ's "plenitude" is possible, but it must result from a "synthesis" of heart and brain. Finding such a synthesis was for him a matter of survival.

The experiences Piaget depicted as violent mystical episodes were signs that his personality was severely dislocated. His self-criticism and his renewed commitment to rationality turn out to be part of a reconstruction of the self. Piaget's quest for a personal equilibrium shapes the story he tells in *Recherche* about his own life and underlies his theoretical thinking; his autobiographical novel thus illustrates the insights about self-creation and the grasp of consciousness formulated for the first time in "The Mysteries of Divine Suffering."

13

Recherche

R*echerche* (1918a) was for Piaget an extended self-criticism and a way of expressly inaugurating and justifying a personally and intellectually new phase of his own life. The book is divided into three parts. The first two narrate the development of Sebastian; the third is a theoretical essay. (Unless otherwise indicated, all numbers in parentheses in this chapter and the next refer to *Recherche*.)

The first part, titled "The Preparation" (11–87), is the longest. It deals with Sebastian's background and present situation. His contacts with religious groups, philosophy, science, and literature are all disappointing. None relates science and faith harmoniously; all display a state of "disequilibrium." Sebastian no longer believes in revelation; he has not yet found a universal human faith, but he thinks that socialism may provide the desired synthesis. He also starts thinking of a "science of genera."

The second part, titled "The Crisis" (91–143), is the shortest. It deals with Sebastian's fall toward atheism, his mystical recovery of faith and sense of mission, and his struggle against the sensual and egotistical passions he discovers in himself. Oscillating violently from doubt and depression to certainty and enthusiasm, Sebastian desires to restore his equilibrium. This personal goal matches his projects for humankind at large, which are also conceptualized in terms of disequilibrium and equilibrium.

The third part of *Recherche*, titled "The Reconstruction" (147–210), is no longer the story of Sebastian, but a theoretical essay. It consists of a "Letter to Young Socialists" (147–148) and three sections: "Science" (149–198), "Faith" (199–201), and "Social Salvation" (202–210). In this essay Piaget proposes a "research program" based on "scientific principles" and aimed at solving the problems that tormented Sebastian; he builds on Sebastian's science of genera and develops a theory focused on the equilibrium and disequilibrium between wholes and parts.

Piaget's treatment of *Recherche* in his autobiography is extremely limited. He says: "during the year I spent in the mountains I was haunted by the desire to create, and I yielded to the temptation. Not to compromise myself on scientific grounds, however, I avoided the difficulty by writing—for the general public, not for specialists—a kind of philosophic novel the last part of which contained my ideas. My strategy proved to be correct: No one spoke of it except one or two indignant philosophers" (1952, 243). *Insights and Illusions of Philosophy* offers a similar version: "I did not wish to present this as a 'serious' text, and I incorporated it in a kind of philosophical novel" (1965, 9). Piaget also told Jean-Claude Bringuier (1977, 9) that he knew the ideas presented in *Recherche* "were debatable, a bit bizarre; if I wanted them to be tolerated," he added, "I would have to put them in fictional form." Finally, the quotations from *Recherche* provided in Piaget's autobiography (1952, 243) are concerned exclusively with the equilibrium and disequilibrium between wholes and parts.

Scholars have focused on *Recherche* as an anticipation of Piaget's later thought (see Chapman, 1988, 19–30; and Kaye, 1980, for particularly nuanced readings). Piaget's explicit goal in publishing *Recherche*, however, was not to camouflage doubtful speculations in a fictional narrative but, on the contrary, to provide the indispensable background for an adequate understanding of his theoretical ideas and to launch a career in professional philosophy. Restoring the original linkage between Sebastian's spiritual development and Piaget's equilibrium theory helps uncover the original scope of the theory. Sebastian aspired to work for the postwar reconstruction of society; Piaget's theory aimed specifically at furnishing a scientific basis for such a task. The reactions to *Recherche* focused on its author's goal and criticized (or praised) the book mainly in connection with its moral and political dimensions.

The Swiss-French *Bildungsroman*

Recherche exemplifies a particular sort of autobiographical *Bildungsroman*. In the Swiss-French Protestant milieu, formation novels appeared as the ideal means of communicating the results of introspective self-examination, especially in relation to the processes of conversion deemed to be the foundation of faith. Personal testimonies or psychological reports of crisis and conversion were indistinguishable from comparable narratives in fiction, and all may be seen as contributions to the "experiential" and "inductive" theology favored by Swiss-French liberals.

The typical formation novel narrates the development of a personality through interaction and confrontation with an environment. The formative principle is the experience of the world through spiritual trials. The process of *Bildung* takes place primarily during adolescence and youth; it is a quest for identity and certainty, at the end of which the hero is prepared for a new life. In general, a *Bildungsroman* is a hidden autobiography and a work of didactic intent. Thus it also often turns out to be a *roman à thèse,* or "thesis novel," aimed at proving the superiority, legitimacy, or correctness of a certain doctrine (Suleiman, 1979; on the *Bildungsroman* in general, see Berman, 1983; Hirsch, 1979; Jost, 1969).

Recherche fits the pattern of the formation-thesis novel, in the style characteristic of the Swiss-French nineteenth century. It narrates a process of preparation, crisis, and reconstruction. The disequilibrium Sebastian perceives in himself and in the world is both the leading theme of his developmental story and the problem Piaget sets out to resolve. But the distinctive features of the novel proceed from its connection to Protestantism. Sebastian evolves largely through an encounter with his own conscience rather than with external events; the trials he undergoes take the form of a religious crisis; his discovery of truth is a grasp of consciousness of the self and the adoption of the "personal faith" that will sustain his life.

Piaget did not lack models. One of the reviewers of *Recherche* saw in it the influence of Romain Rolland's *Jean-Christophe.* For Piaget himself, "The admirable *Jean-Christophe* depicted the anguish of the times more than it provided a solution for it" (70); the comment underlines the difference between his novel and Rolland's, and between *Jean-Christophe* and deliberately Protestant formation-novels. Closest to Piaget, Samuel Cornut, his godfather, published in 1903 a *Bildungsroman* titled *The Testament of My Youth,* which narrates in the first person an individual's quest for faith. Through crises and revelations, Cornut's hero discovers for himself a religion without priests or churches, based on his conscience, and animated by love. The same developmental pattern shapes *The Two Houses,* a 1914 novel by Pierre Jeannet, intended as the first volume of a Protestant *Jean-Christophe.* This novel, as a reviewer put it, is "not a literary, but a religious work" (A. J., 1916, 203). Its title, an allusion to Matthew 7:24–27, which most readers surely recognized, summarizes the story: after adopting a weak faith "built on sand," the hero goes through a spiritual crisis out of which emerges a genuine faith, erected on the solid rock of his own conscience. Jeannet's novel was regarded as depicting the real experiences of young Christians. According to one reviewer, a member of the Swiss Christian Students' Association, the hero "is clearly one of us, a Swiss-French like those we encounter in our meetings and associations" (G., 1915). For another reviewer, the loss and recovery of faith through inner suffering was a topic "of great current interest" (Nicod, 1915).

From the perspective of Swiss-French Protestants, the novels by Cornut and Jeannet end happily. They therefore contrast with a novel such as Roger Martin du Gard's 1913 *Jean Barois*, the story of a Catholic man who fails to overcome the "disequilibrium" (as he calls it) between science and religion. For a contemporary observer, there was no Swiss-French Jean Barois thanks to Flournoy's religious and epistemological doctrines (Picot, 1920, 582–583). And for Piaget in *Recherche* (70), Jean Barois is an antihero, the opposite of everything Sebastian pursues.

The Motivation for *Recherche*

For the young Piaget himself, the primary significance of his *Bildungsroman* derived from its autobiographical dimension. Late in life he readily admitted that Sebastian was himself (1977, 10). That must have been clear to the contemporary public. Indeed, in his preface to *Recherche* Piaget reports that the novel was written from September 1916 to January 1917—"I had just turned twenty, and that is its explanation and justification." He adds that since then he has evolved "in a direction that can be easily determined"—but that is necessarily inferred from Sebastian's development.

In a letter not yet found, Arnold Reymond scolded Piaget for the insolence and pretentiousness of *Recherche* and criticized its mixture of personal and intellectual discourse. Piaget's reply is his most extensive comment on the autobiographical meaning of his novel:

> You must first know that the second part [of *Recherche*, "The Crisis"] is based on a diary I kept in Leysin, without knowing I would use it later. It is simplified, but entirely true. The essence of Sebastian's character is a rather violent pride, sustained by a continuous lack of adaptation.
>
> This being so . . . does he have the right to make judgments that he knows are the result of a particular moment of his character? . . .
>
> You think he does not . . . I, on the contrary, feel free to do so. In that case, what are the conditions necessary for avoiding insolence and pretentiousness? 1. Be sincere. 2. Tell the reader what you are doing.
>
> As far as sincerity is concerned, there is nothing I have written that I did not experience . . .
>
> As far as the second point is concerned, my judgments would be absurd in

an essay or a memoir. But I write a confession. I take care to devote a third of the book to describing the character's personality.

Here we get to the heart of the question. You find this confession pretentious . . . [But] in my book, the philosopher does not appear. It is a study of
the self. I need it to make the philosopher understood when he speaks (which
will be, for the first time, in my dissertation).   (ms. 1918d, 1–2r)

Recherche, then, was for Piaget a truthful portrait of his spiritual experiences, a
confession, a study of the self supposed to throw light on philosophical ideas
to be formulated later.

Yet Piaget's reduction of *Recherche* to a "confession" is largely tactical. He
claims that his book is not an essay—but that is precisely what he calls it in the
preface. Similarly, the absence of "the philosopher" is spurious. The third part
of *Recherche* elaborates a philosophy, and Piaget himself (ms. 1918a) initially
asked Reymond to review his book in a major philosophical journal. *Recherche*
is as much a philosophical statement as a confession.

Piaget told Reymond that he felt "morally obliged" to reveal the self before
letting the philosopher speak (ms. 1918d, 2r). Was it necessary to give *Recherche* to the public? "I am convinced [it was]," he wrote; "everything I saw in
my generation pressed me to do so" (1918e, 1r). The reading of *Recherche* that
follows below therefore approaches the work not only as an autobiographical
self-description but also as a self-definition and a self-transformation, as the
means whereby Piaget surmounts and supersedes his own present self and
offers a generational model. Indeed, in close analysis *Recherche* appears
as Piaget's conceptualization and revision of his own identity—less an accurate self-portrait than an existential choice constitutive of an evolving consciousness.

"The Preparation"

The first chapter of "The Preparation" sketches Sebastian's personality and
sets the stage for the rest of the narrative. The first sentence reads: "As the war
sustained in every mind the greatest disequilibrium ever endured by thought,
Sebastian concentrated in himself the pains of a world in labor" (11). This initial statement presents all the basic elements of *Recherche:* the war exacerbates
an already existing disequilibrium of ideas, which is responsible for the world's
suffering; Sebastian is a sort of microcosm whose center is thought; his (and
Piaget's) project will be to restore personal and universal equilibrium through
a reform of knowledge.

Before the war, Sebastian gets involved with the great currents of thought;

he sees science penetrate everywhere and is enthusiastic about "popular revivals." The war brings to light the failure of "intelligence" before the "passions" (12). The rare figures who stay free seem paralyzed by their need of faith and science simultaneously. A dedication to faith leads to compromises that drown reason in a "cloudy mysticism"; a commitment to science demands submission to a crippling "scholasticism" (12).

Sebastian's revolt against such a situation betrays his "passion to dominate" and an "apostle's pride" (13). These are sometimes moderated by love and pity; he then implores God's help, and offers in return "to fulfill the divine mission of lessening evil" (13). Sebastian cannot rest until his ideas are organized as a "coherent whole" (13); he "doubts too little" and "does not analyze himself" (13–14). He seeks the absolute and disdains practice; he distinguishes between moral truth and reality and considers that "devotion to truth is life's only beauty" (14). His quest for an ideal absolute makes him explain the war as a special case of universal processes. Reassured by this "vision of things," Sebastian undertakes the "quest for a faith" that would be "human, . . . accessible to all, and capable of nourishing by itself the postwar renewal" (14).

Sebastian first turns to Catholicism. The encounter with young modernists, who disregard both philosophy and science to cultivate mysticism, shows him the inadequacy of symbolism. Yet Sebastian respects their "assertion of the value of life," which seems to him to be a "true faith" (20). He then becomes aware of "the social significance" of the problem of reconciling science and faith. This problem is responsible "for the entire present-day disequilibrium" (21). Sebastian understands that life, as a value, is distinct from life as known through science. The latter mingles good and evil, order and disorder, values and nonvalues (22). Sebastian sometimes wonders why faith should not limit itself to the realm of values and leave to science the knowledge of reality. His "thirst for absolute truth," however, makes him trust metaphysics as a means of uniting being and value, science and faith: "If we attain the Absolute, we will know why values are values, and Sebastian had not given up [the idea] of reaching the Absolute" (23).

Having rejected the Catholic notions of revelation and of an omnipotent God, Sebastian looks to Protestantism. He is initially struck by its "intellectual anarchy" (31). He castigates orthodox Protestants for their quest for rational certainty and for their individualism; "to be alive," he writes, religion "must unite the social and the individual" (35). The more progressive young people, with their "Bergsonian Protestantism" and their "Latin pragmatism," seem to Sebastian weakened by "incoherence": "Nothing was comparable to the disequilibrium of this youth" (37). Sebastian joins the Christian students, and the intense experience of a common "*élan* toward God" (39) enables him to forgive them their incoherence (40). Still, the students' movement lacks "a doctrinal basis" capable of providing the equilibrium between symbolism and dogmatism, science and faith, the quest for truth and the quest for value (41). The question is, what will provide such a doctrine—science, faith, philosophy?

Sebastian first looks to philosophy. This was natural, for he had always philosophized, and had been led to Protestantism by a "philosophical hope" (42). All philosophical schools seem to Sebastian concerned with the problem of science and faith (44). All take science into account, though in different ways between the two extremes of conventionalism and materialistic realism. As for faith, some admit it in a traditional sense; others deny it. Some are in between, such as those who have a mystical faith in science, yet wish to suppress all religion; "this contradiction is not uncommon in this century of intense disequilibrium" (44). All misunderstand faith (43–44). Sebastian is temporarily attracted to Fouillée, reformulates his concept of *idée-force* in terms of equilibrium, and wishes to turn his philosophy into a biological and psychological science of life (45–46).[1] This science, however, cannot provide a basis for asserting values: faith is still necessary.

The longest section of Sebastian's encounter with philosophy is devoted to Bergson. Even though critical of some aspects of Bergsonism, Sebastian adheres to what he perceives as its "logic," and realizes that a "science of genera" must start with biology. Before committing himself to such a project, he makes "a last effort within philosophy" by looking to pragmatism, "the most interesting of contemporary movements" (54). To the extent that pragmatism accepts mystery and advocates action and faith, Sebastian is a pragmatist; but he ends up rejecting pragmatism's identification of the good, the useful, and the true (56).

Sebastian then turns to science. He is full of hope, since he already has a "sort of mystical confidence" in evolutionism (57). He is, however, disheartened by science's dogmatism and ignorance of philosophical questions. The sciences, Sebastian observes, can be arranged along a continuous circle; the maximum of dogmatism is located in biology, the minimum in mathematics (59). He is particularly irate at the "scholasticism" of biologists. Psychologists seem to him less naive than biologists. Yet the weakness of James and Flournoy, who helped create such new sciences as religious psychology, "the experimental theory of knowledge," and psychical research was that they remained within philosophy and close to pragmatism, "bankruptcy of all knowledge" (64).

Literature does not fare much better than the sciences. Sebastian dreams of a "literature of ideas" (66), but he is disappointed by the conservative Catholicism of such authors as Maurice Barrès and Paul Bourget. He admires Charles Péguy's goodness and sincerity but considers Romain Rolland a better observer of the times. *Jean-Christophe* is for him the last product of an "impulse toward social salvation" characterized more by its "convulsions" than by its "equilibrium" (70). It describes the end of an era but does not offer solutions for the future.

After his tour of European culture, Sebastian ponders the causes of its deplorable state. Since the beginning of the war he has devoted himself to the reconstruction and "looked in present-day thought for the origins of today's evils" (71). The war appears to him as the expression of a disequilibrium of the "social organism." This "universal disequilibrium," which causes him intense personal suffering, is that between science and faith (72). While waiting for an answer from "his God," Sebastian is possessed by "the desire to act immediately" and realize his ideas even before they are coherently organized (73). He thus turns to socialism. He was attracted to it at the beginning of his intellectual life; after an interlude of moral and religious preoccupations, the war brings him back to "the socialist idea" (76–77). "If the social cause of the current disequilibrium is the opposition of science and faith, the solution to the problem will be found only if a new faith satisfies collectivities and individuals alike" (77). Socialism could furnish the solution, if it was more coherent; still, it is the only movement that searches for a "new ideal" (79–80).

"The Preparation" concludes with a letter from Sebastian to his young socialist friends who understand that socialism is neither an economic school nor a political party, but a faith. Socialism, he says, "must be a science, an art, and a morality. It must be a Life, strong and equilibrated" (82). It must pursue the "synthesis" of science and faith (83). Sebastian proclaims the need to find a new ideal in order to overcome the social and intellectual disequilibrium, and asks youth to get down to work and "be men" (87).

"The Preparation" portrays Sebastian's reactions to his environment and introduces the book's central theme, disequilibrium. Sebastian sees himself and the world in terms of disequilibrium; his sense of self may be dictated by external circumstances, but it is also that which he projects onto the world in order to understand it. Which comes first is impossible to tell. Whatever Sebastian says about the world applies to himself, and vice versa.

Disequilibrium is "universal"; it pertains to the entire "social organism," including individual minds and "thought" as an abstract entity; nowhere is it more intense than among the young Christians with whom Sebastian sympathizes. The war "sustains" it, but its cause lies in the opposition of science and faith as it evolved during the nineteenth century. This opposition turns out to be a sort of ideal type of disequilibrium, an epitome of the antitheses that characterize for Sebastian the present moment of history as well as his own personality: passion versus intelligence, certainty versus doubt, practice versus the ideal, symbolism versus Revelation, conventionalism versus realism, metaphysical speculation versus analytical reasoning, individuals versus collectivities.

The opposition between life as value and life as empirical reality (embracing good versus evil, order versus disorder, and value versus nonvalue) is the key to Sebastian's intellectual ambition. His thirst for the absolute drives him to pursue a unitary conception of life, capable of explaining why values are values yet taking into account the nonvalues present in reality. Such a theory of life would realize his aspiration to reconcile the quest for truth and the quest for value while providing the "doctrinal basis" and the "new faith" needed to restore equilibrium. Sebastian's crisis does not fundamentally alter the projects thus "prepared," but it gives them a fuller existential dimension, invigorates them through a conversion experience, and thereby provides them with the qualities of "life" so avidly pursued by the young Christians.

"The Crisis"

"The Crisis," based on a diary Piaget kept at Leysin, is the nucleus of *Recherche*. It is conceived as a pivotal moment between "The Preparation" and "The Reconstruction," between the past and the future, between Sebastian's somewhat conceited criticism of his whole era and Piaget's apparently clearheaded blueprint for a new world. It is a present time made up of tormented self-examination, desperate doubt, mystical raptures, and metaphysical gloom; and it derives from a self-analysis that leads Sebastian to discover the sinful roots of his creative energy. "The Crisis" furnishes the self-portrait that Piaget considered (ms. 1918d) an indispensable introduction to his future philosophical writings.

"The Crisis" is the rite of passage that every *Bildungsroman* hero must undergo on his way to authenticity and truth and takes the form of a confrontation between the hero and his own conscience. "The Crisis" is perfectly clear on this point: a "voice" tells Sebastian that he does not yet know the "combat" and the "purifying fire" that, like every "constructor of ideas," he will have to face (91). He feels the crisis coming, but prefers to keep "arguing and constructing" and to ignore the mounting doubt.

Sebastian's doubts concern the very essence of his desire: "he wants truth to coincide with the good, with his faith," but the "voice" reminds him that he is not "sincere." Piaget speaks of "the eternal doubt" as Sebastian's "inner foe," as a "demon" that springs suddenly into his consciousness, particularly at night, "when the subconscious overcomes the mind"; he also mentions the "silent struggle" that forces the "demon" back "into the unconscious without even leaving a clear memory" (92). Sebastian suffers from anxiety and insomnia; he has "chaotic dreams" that blend "the madness of reason and the anguishes of faith with the howling of unbridled lustful animals" (93). He tries to escape through work but must again and again face doubt and atheism; unable to accept his failure, he goes to the mountain in search of faith and serenity and, "like an old anchorite, he exhaust[s] his physical strength in order to vanquish his demon" (ibid.).

In Sebastian's crisis, doubt and loss of faith are connected with a surging of unconscious carnal desires, a discovery of the self through dreams and introspection, and theoretical reflections. Once, for example, Sebastian has a partly allegorical dream revealing that all system-builders are liars. Upon awakening he feels a great peace; his identity is reduced to a small "hub of consciousness" that observes the disintegration of the self, as well as Sebastian's development. Sebastian sees himself receiving from God the "sacred mission to reconcile through his life science and religion" (96), developing a theory of equilibrium, discovering that the "problem of values" stays outside science, and therefore doubting. Thus, a dream is followed by an introspective self-examination, which in turn leads to a theoretical discourse that brings the reader back to Sebastian's present.

After his dream, Sebastian in effect reviews the years of "The Preparation." During that time, remarks the narrator, "Sebastian's life was purely intellectual" (96). The crisis changes that. Doubt becomes the most important component of his identity and "henceforth poisons his whole life" (101). As in the earlier hypnagogic self-perceptions, Sebastian feels his ego disintegrate and melt into a "gray universe" (102), into an "immeasurable night, eternal and silent" (103), a "total grayness" and an "immense fog" (101) devoid of feeling and values (102) and permeated by "agony and despair" (101).

A "revelation" takes Sebastian out of his depression. While walking in the shade of huge dark pines, he feels the attraction of "the whole, the abyss of passions and sensations"; but the contrast with a luminous view of the plains and the Alps reveals to him "[t]wo attitudes between which one must choose, passion or the good" (105). As a "voice" tells Sebastian, passion is not an "increase of life" (105). On the contrary, it destroys "all equilibrium" and "denatures" the "forces of love and sacrifice" (106).

Sebastian is now certain that his *recherche* will be successful. The very existence of a quest proves to him that there is an absolute "source of all the values of truth and the good." There would be no quest without a hierarchy of values; truth is moral, because when we decide to maintain only the truth, we make a "moral decision." "The person who searches therefore asserts a moral value, he is a believer" (107).

Realizing the connection between truth, faith, and value effects a "transfiguration" in Sebastian (109). Science, he now thinks, gives knowledge of good and evil but does not explain the root of things; it is incapable of knowing the "absolute value"; the good and the beautiful are for it no better or worse than the bad and the ugly. Faith, in contrast, gives life meaning, described as the "supreme reality" and as partaking in the "ultimate order of the universe" (109). The practice of science and the "annihilation of metaphysics" do not suppress faith but are its allies (110–111). Faith must assert values, never pretend to be knowledge (111). Sebastian thus regains his "equilibrium" and experiences a mystical joy, sometimes anguished and ecstatic, sometimes "sweet" (as when he spends a whole night praying and talking "with God about science and faith"; 112).

The recovery of faith strengthens Sebastian's trust in his own "mission" and in "theoretical research" and makes him dream of "fantastic projects, an entire scientific summa, a course synthesizing the sciences of life, a broadened equivalent of [Auguste] Comte's course of positive philosophy and claiming, like him, to bring about social salvation" (113). All this effects a "revolution" in his personality (114). Sebastian "lived only through his brain" (114). But now, the project for a "scientific synthesis" overwhelms not his brain but his heart, for it makes him realize that his life will be "the tragic life of the thinker, a life of struggle and abnegation," dominated by the "sacrifice" of his "entire being to his thought" (ibid.).

The life of the thinker is the existential personal concomitant of the equilibrium theory: truth "is an ideal"; life is composed of "two realities," real disequilibria and an ideal equilibrium to which the disequilibria "tend" (114–115). The thinker must "submit to truth, never to reality"; he must "realize the ideal equilibrium," and to do this requires total self-sacrifice (115). He must know illness, for illness favors the manifestation of the individual's "inmost depths" and leads to a heightened state of consciousness, self-understanding, intelligence, and will (116). He must refuse action as a deformation of the ideal; he must revolt and learn to be alone (116, 117).

The thinker's self-sacrifice must include celibacy. Instead of accepting himself and others as they are, the thinker must try to incarnate "an unreal and perhaps unrealizable ideal" (118). He must therefore refuse human love and marriage. Like every other passion, love includes an element of selfishness and is therefore contrary to the thinker's absolute self-sacrifice to the ideal. Piaget quotes Tolstoy's famous *Kreutzer Sonata* to emphasize that sexual love belongs to reality, whereas the thinker must live according to the ideal (118, 119).[2] Sebastian, however, realizes that he is motivated by pride and selfishness rather than by true love of humankind, and that he is animated by the passions to know with certainty, to feel, and to dominate, all contrary to true love (120–125).

Sebastian's life oscillates between periods of disequilibrium during which he is dominated by anguish, desire, and mystical enthusiasm, and moments of equilibrium during which he is animated by grace and God's love. Sebastian examines himself and finds a sinful pride in each of his thoughts and feelings: "There is only pride in my apostolate" (125). His mystical episodes, always in the mountains, bring him the "atrocious" suffering distinctive of the "constructive mind" that has not yet attained the "ideal equilibrium" (128).

One night Sebastian climbs to a mountain pasture; there he "experiences" salvation through Christ instead of grasping it intellectually; he feels in "communion with God in the consciousness of Christ" and returns from the "sacred mountain" confident in his vocation (132, 133). He now understands that equilibrium, which is an ideal, "can be found only by means of disequilibrium—such is the great law of real life" (135). The individual and the species tend toward a "physical" sort of equilibrium, whose "inner version" is "moral equilibrium" (ibid.). The most disequilibrated individuals, such as Tolstoy or Pascal, are those who live the fullest lives and are also the most equilibrated: Christ is simultaneously the most disequilibrated and "the most equilibrated son of man who ever existed" (136).

Sebastian realizes that he must follow his ideas to the very end, and he feels an intense joy (139–140). He has "become aware of himself" and "vanquished his passion" (141–143). "The Crisis" closes with Sebastian claiming "Victory! I have recovered my God, my true God. Am I good, am I bad? I no longer know; I live, I suffer and cry of joy, that is all I know. I know I will do something great, and I do not care whether it is God or myself who does it" (143).

This is the kind of happy ending one could expect. Sebastian is now ready to pursue the "divine mission" of furnishing, as a thinker, the basis for social salvation—which is what Piaget proceeds to do in the third part of his novel.

After Sebastian's crisis, equilibrium and disequilibrium, the ideal and the real, are no longer opposites; rather, as science and faith, they require each other. Equilibrium is to be pursued by means of disequilibrium, the ideal through reality, ataraxia through activity. Passion destroys equilibrium, but the search for equilibrium cannot be conducted without passion. The surging of elements from the unconscious is a sign of disequilibrium, but it also drives consciousness to levels of knowledge and self-awareness that bring the individual closer to personal equilibrium and to the apprehension of the ideal. The Absolute is not an immutable transcendent entity, but an unceasing immanent process of equilibration (the word is not in *Recherche*). Christ becomes the thinker's supreme model, and the theory of equilibrium emerges as a constitutive part of its author's identity.

14

The Theory of Equilibrium: From Personal Crisis to Universal Salvation

The third part of *Recherche*, "The Reconstruction," is the discursive elaboration of the insights and revelations that ushered Sebastian out of his spiritual crisis. The theory of equilibrium developed in "The Reconstruction" has a clear personal significance. Piaget published his novel with the explicit purpose of disclosing the intimate personal roots of his theorizing. Sebastian suffers from disequilibrium, and he finds a personal equilibrium when he discovers that disequilibrium and equilibrium are indissolubly connected in the progress of the real toward the ideal. The reconstruction of his identity is a first step toward the accomplishment of the social, moral, and intellectual reconstruction that is Piaget's ultimate goal.

In his autobiography, Piaget (1952, 241–242) explains the origins of the theory presented in *Recherche* in the following way: A lesson by Reymond on realism and nominalism sometime during the academic year 1914–15 gave him a "sudden insight," dispelling the "state of uncertainty" in which he was plunged concerning the status of zoological species and the "reality or non-reality of society as an organized whole."[1] Piaget discovered that the two problems were basically the same. He "suddenly understood that at all levels (viz. that of the living cell, organism, species, society, etc., but also with reference to states of conscience, to concepts, to logical principles, etc.) one finds the same problem of relationship between the parts and the whole" (see also 1959a, 9). The question of species and totalities was logical; thanks to Reymond, Piaget grasped "the fundamental unity of the biological and the logical" (1959b, 45).

This realization was the starting point of his "system." The theoretical part of *Recherche* elaborates the thesis that "[i]n all fields of life (organic, mental, social) there exist 'totalities' qualitatively distinct from their parts and imposing on them an organization," that the whole and the parts are in relations of reciprocal preservation or predominance over the other, and that only "reciprocal preservation" constitutes a "stable" form of equilibrium.

Although Piaget's explanation of his basic idea is perfectly adequate, only a more detailed examination of the entire "system" will allow us to unearth the larger meaning it had for him at the time he wrote it, and which is summed up in the title he gave it, "The Reconstruction."

Piaget's Research Program

"The Reconstruction" opens with a "Letter to Young Socialists" in which Piaget announces the need to constitute a force between a "reactionary right" and a "left without culture" (148). The essay itself begins with a section on science. For Piaget, science should turn from the study of quantity to the study of quality; he proposes to build "upon the ruins of metaphysics" a science of life concerned exclusively with the relations of equilibrium and disequilibrium among qualities (150). The "postulate" of Piaget's theory is that "to every material movement definable by its physical properties . . . corresponds an original quality"; for example, two rhythms combined into one give rise to a new quality that cannot be described merely as "the result" of the two others (ibid.).

All the phenomena of life may be understood as quantitative or qualitative equilibria, that is, respectively, in mathematical and physical terms or in psychological terms (151). The adjective "biological" applied to the opposition between the ideal equilibrium and the "unstable equilibria of the real" (63) denotes the scope of a theory aimed at embracing all living phenomena. Yet, more than strictly biological, Piaget's science of quality is also psychological. As he explains, individual qualities must be related within a "total quality" for us to be aware of them, and they do not exist unless we are aware of them. Thus, I would not be conscious of the whiteness of the paper and blackness of the ink if the two "were not fused in my consciousness in a certain whole, and if, despite this whole, they did not remain, respectively, white and black" (151–152).

Equilibrium therefore exists not only between "discrete parts" but also between the whole and the parts. Mechanical and psychological equilibria differ in that, for example, three mechanical forces combined into one disappear as discrete forces, whereas three qualities combined into one persist together with the fourth one resulting from their combination. The distinction of the mechanical and the psychological corresponds to two modes of scientific activity, the mode of "laws" and the mode of "genera," the former proceeding from the parts to the whole, the latter from the whole to the parts (152–153).

For Piaget, the qualitative science of genera requires that consciousness be considered not as a "force" but as a "sui generis equilibrium" (152–153). He thus realizes Sebastian's wish to transform Fouillée's philosophy of the *idée-force* into a science: the "idea" is no longer a state of consciousness, but a "group of forces"; the ideal becomes a "limit" in the mathematical sense, "the full equilibrium toward which tend the unstable or false equilibria of reality"; thus is established a "science of life" that studies "mechanical equilibria" as well as the "inner light" through which we grasp them (46).

Piaget believes that understanding genera in terms of equilibrium (something, he points out, Bergson did not do) renders their study compatible with "mechanistic science" (153). He never mentions, however, the source of his concept of equilibrium or why it became the core of his theory. As we shall see, he elaborated the notion of "assimilation" explicitly against Le Dantec's, and it is likely that the notion of equilibrium also derived from the French biologist.

Indeed, Le Dantec believed that a view of life (in its widest sense, from organic functions to social phenomena) based on the idea of equilibrium would replace all previous philosophies. The language of equilibrium, which he claimed to have borrowed from physics, and in particular from the principle of conservation of energy, seemed to him capable of providing a "mechanical" explanation of everything. All organic and inorganic bodies would no longer be considered as entities or as individuals but as "parts of a whole, of an equilibrium" (Le Dantec, 1908, 2). Nothing exists by itself, since everything belongs in a balanced system (Le Dantec, 1907, 141). According to Le Dantec, this way of seeing things leads to a denial of individuality, the immortality of the soul, and free will, thus turning scientific biology into a "negative religion" (1908, 270).

Here, as in the case of "assimilation," Piaget borrows his vocabulary from Le Dantec, yet he never becomes a true disciple. Sebastian admires the biologist's genius and his "powerful synthesis" but deplores his materialistic simplemindedness (60); Piaget considers Le Dantec's psychology "naive" (160) and firmly denies that his own theory of equilibrium is a "vain repetition of Le Dantec's biology in the language of quality" (155).

Piaget's early science of genera was based on the contrast between the vital order (genera) and the geometric order (laws). *Recherche* reconciles the two, for Piaget now uses *genus* in its general logical sense of a class containing smaller classes (in his words, a whole composed of parts) and claims that the equilibria of genera are just as "mechanical" as that of physical equilibria. Piaget calls "mechanical" the processes of equilibrium and disequilibrium between the whole and its parts. Yet his science remains, as he claims, Bergsonian, because it deals with processes, not with fixed states, and because the paradigm for these processes is psychological.

Piaget speaks of equilibria among "qualities" and calls his science of genera "qualitative." "Quality" refers to the features that make something what it is, and thus differs from quantity and relation; it is inherent in the subject and irreducible to other categories. Basically, Piaget's choice of "quality" as a central concept again reveals his Bergsonian and psychological orientation.

In *Creative Evolution* Bergson (1907, 300) wrote that qualities (color, sound, and so forth) are the first things we distinguish in the world. These qualities consist in numerous "elementary movements"; their permanence, therefore, is only apparent: however we represent it, "every quality is change" (ibid., 301). It is perception that solidifies "into discontinuous images the fluid continuity of the real"; thus, "What is real is the continual change of form: form is only a snapshot view of a transition" (ibid., 302). Piaget's characterization of his project as a qualitative science or a science of quality emphasizes the "tendency" of qualities toward equilibrium, and such a focus on tendencies is an expression of his Bergsonism.

The equilibrium of the genus is an equilibrium between parts and wholes, of which there are two "elementary forms": when the "partial qualities" are compatible with the "qualities of the whole," there is "reciprocal action and conservation"; when they are incompatible, the whole "maintains its unity at the expense of the parts, and vice versa" (153–154). Life, Piaget explains, is defined by assimilation. The living being "assimilates, that is, reproduces substance identical with itself" (155). It therefore remains "stable" as a totality. The influence of the environment implied by assimilation modifies the qualities of the parts without destroying the quality of the whole: "The better I assimilate, the more I remain identical with myself" (ibid.).

Assimilation designates the action of making or becoming alike; in physiology, it denotes the process involved in digestion and nutrition, whereby an organism converts extraneous material into a substance identical with its own. Although, as we shall see, Piaget differed on important points with Le Dantec, the place the concept of assimilation occupies in his system—as the defining operation of life in all its forms—originates with the French biologist, and in particular with his "law of functional assimilation." According to this law, the functioning of an organism is not simply sustained by assimilation: it is an external manifestation of the internal processes that produce the substance of the organism (Le Dantec, 1896, 251).

Piaget emphasizes that organic equilibrium takes the first of the two "elementary forms" of equilibrium, in which the parts are compatible with the whole. Consequently, there is a "parallelism" between "the equilibrium of qualities presupposed by consciousness, and the reactions of the organism" (156). By means of this "parallelism," Piaget fuses the organic and the psychological in a way (the theory of equilibrium) he deems compatible with "mechanistic science."

From the postulate of a "parallelism," Piaget draws the four laws that "govern all of biology" (ibid.). The first law states that every "organization" tends to preserve itself as an equilibrium between a whole and its parts. According to the second law, the second elementary type of equilibrium (incompatibility of parts and the whole) is a compromise between the first form and the action of the environment. As declared in the third law, all possible equilibria are a combination of the first two; and (the fourth law specifies) all tend toward the first form (157). Life is therefore "an organization in unstable equilibrium" that tends toward stability. Piaget designates the "stable equilibrium" (first type) as the "law" toward which unstable equilibria "tend"; he calls the former "ideal" and the latter "real" (158).

Piaget follows the standard vocabulary of dynamics: a body is said to be in stable equilibrium when it returns to its original position after being disturbed, and in unstable equilibrium when it continues to move in the direction given to it by the disturbing force. His application of such language to all processes, be they biological, psychological, or social, helps him overcome the Bergsonian opposition of the vital and the geometric orders he maintained in 1912–1914 (and, in "The Crisis," attributed to Sebastian; 53). The definition of evolution as the march of real equilibria toward stable equilibrium is for him neither teleological nor metaphysical, since stability is a result, not a goal, and since the "interplay" of qualitative equilibria is no less "mechanical" than that of physical equilibria (158–159).

Since equilibria are simultaneously qualitative and mechanical, Piaget believes that his theory makes possible a psychology that is experimental yet allows for consciousness. He explains that "only the conception of a real, individual organization controlled by an ideal organization permits the understanding of consciousness as a pure internal translation of physico-chemical phenomena" (160). This rather cryptic statement (and they are numerous in "The Reconstruction") does not imply materialistic reductionism. Piaget's comments on James's "stream of consciousness" and Bergson's "intuition of duration" as a "march" toward stability and equilibrium clarify his psychology (160–161). Consciousness is the whole; sensations, perceptions, and memory are parts (or "partial qualities"). The first two are "not yet equil-

ibrated with the whole," while the third has become integrated into the equilibrium of the whole (161). Piaget describes this conception as an "advanced
Bergsonism," in which "duration" is replaced by the "tendency" of qualities to
equilibrate each other (ibid.), and the notion of an "unconscious psychological
force" by that of "the biological equilibrium itself" (162).

Thought must also be understood in terms of equilibrium. The understanding is thought operating on quantity. Autistic thinking, in contrast, is purely
qualitative, and proceeds by means of the kind of "symbolism" of dreams,
imagination, art, mysticism, and metaphysics. Reason is a synthesis of understanding and autistic thinking; it therefore combines genera and laws, qualitative and quantitative knowledge (165). Value is the quality of that which can
inspire human activity. Science limits itself to saying that *if* life is considered
as a value, then the "norm" of all values is given, both socially and individually,
by the ideal equilibrium of the first type (compatibility of parts and whole,
with interaction and reciprocal conservation; 166). As for the rest, Piaget
claims, "One must believe or not believe, that is, live or not live" (ibid.). Insofar as the realm of values is independent of science, it is purely "metaphysical"
and requires faith, not knowledge (166–168).

Piaget's theory applies also to sociology and political thought: the whole is
society, the part is the individual; morality is the equilibrium between the two.
The "ideal social equilibrium" is an equilibrium between the conservation of
society and its effect on individuals, and the action of individuals on themselves and on society (171–172). Internationally, patriotism must be made to
serve humanity as a "guiding ideal," while nationally, a "broadened socialism"
must secure the equilibrium between the whole and the parts (172). Having
thus explained that the "biological equilibrium of qualities" is the basis of both
psychology and sociology, Piaget claims that his "scientific conception" based
on the distinction between real and ideal may elucidate the fundamental problems of morality, aesthetics, and religion (173).

Morality is the subject of the very long fifth chapter of "The Reconstruction." Piaget first claims that "evolutionary moralities have proved that the
good is life itself" (173). This adds nothing to what he declared in *The Mission
of the Idea*. Piaget realizes that "such a vague point of view" gives rise to different, even contradictory moralities, and he therefore wishes to clarify (172).
The following line of thought emerges from a rather obscure discussion: the
good is life; "absolute altruism" represents the "blooming" of life (175); altruism embodies the ideal equilibrium among individuals, and between the person and society; disequilibrium is evil; the maxim of morality is "act in such a
way as to realize the absolute equilibrium of the organization of life, both collective and individual" (177).

For Piaget, morality necessarily involves the individual and society; the "laws of sociology" concern "moral" equilibrium (169). Although the equilibrium of an individual's qualities is "purely psychological but not moral" (177), "moral equilibrium coincides with the ideal psychological equilibrium" (178). Egoism, pride, and passion are disequilibria. Thus, what follows from the theory of equilibrium is "Christian morality" itself. This discovery fills Piaget with satisfaction: "Scientific morality does nothing other than confirm the views adopted by individual conscience . . . and in the same way that we know how to reason before we know Aristotle's logic, or how to digest before knowing physiology, we know how to practice the good before learning to know biological equilibria" (182). The problem of freedom, Piaget states, is irrelevant to morality, since all that counts is the personal responsibility that results from an individual's belief in an absolute value (183).

Morality belongs to the realm of the will, but the real and the ideal are also related in aesthetic feeling. Beauty is "the love the individual feels for the ideal equilibrium"; art must therefore "construct an ideal equilibrium" (185–186). Like the thinker's effort to reach truth, the artist's attempt to realize beauty is a "moral impulsion" (185). Finally, insofar as the ideal and the real may be related through a combination of will and feeling, they furnish "the experimental basis for a psychology of religion" (173).

Indeed, religion can also be explained in terms of equilibrium. The real strives after an ideal equilibrium that is approachable but unreachable. The suffering entailed by such a situation is accompanied by the "feeling of absolute value the individual attributes to his moral ideal." The "sacrifice" of the person to values is for Piaget a specifically religious way of approaching the ideal equilibrium (190). A true religion must realize the equilibrium between fanaticism (predominance of the collective over the individual) and mysticism, which is the opposite; it thus includes sacrifice and commitment to the ideal social organization (191). Such a religion, which Piaget sees as based on science, includes no creed, requires no metaphysics, and boils down to a personal yet nonmystical assertion of faith.

For Piaget, mysticism and metaphysics are forms of "autistic thinking." Both proceed by "concentrating" in symbols the qualities of the objects we are interested in, and by "displacing" onto the symbols the "affective contents" of those qualities. The symbolic outcomes of mysticism are analogous to artistic creations; those of metaphysics are the intellectual exterior each person gives to his or her faith in an absolute value (194–195). All metaphysics "individualize" absolute value as some kind of entity (reality, the ideal, God). In contrast, for science, such values remain a "mystery" (198). Thus Piaget achieves the reconciliation of science and religion and is ready to elaborate his conception of faith.

Piaget believes that his religious attitude embraces the best of all religions, including Christianity. God, he says, is the absolute value. Thus conceived, He "engenders" all possible values, and therefore deserves the name "Father" (199). Such a God is transcendent, since absolute value transcends reality, and immanent, since absolute value is within everything, everywhere (199–200). By virtue of the "continuous opposition" between the ideal and the real, the individual feels miserable before the absolute value and cries for help (200). The reply is Jesus' sacrifice: by letting himself be crucified, Christ attested the absolute value forever. True Christianity, the one whose rebirth Piaget has sought since *The Mission of the Idea,* is contained entirely in the "[n]ecessary trilogy of God source of all value, man prostrated before holiness, and the Cross that saves" (201). The reconciliation of faith and science in turn provides the clue to social salvation.

For Piaget, the most important contribution of science to social salvation is that it shows the interdependence of morality, religion, aesthetics, and education. Each discipline establishes a different sort of link between the individual and society, the parts and the whole. Morality defines the "three cardinal duties: to realize the ideal equilibrium in oneself, in others, and in society itself" (205). Politics must apply the same rule. In aesthetics, an equilibrium must be found between art for art's sake, and a more substantial "literature of ideas" (206). As for religion, the "church of tomorrow" (or the "ideal church") must be a "synthesis" of the Catholic and the Protestant, an equilibrium between the collective and the individual (206–207). Education must enlighten. For example, the "psychological difficulties" of harmonizing individual autonomy with social community in the religious realm originate "more in the believer's lack of culture than in an intrinsic cause" (207). Culture presumably implies knowledge of Piaget's theory of equilibrium.

Education leads to the establishment of social reforms aimed at the equilibrium of society within itself, with other societies, and in general. For Piaget, only cooperation "conforms to the ideal equilibrium," and only "a confederation provides the equilibrium between the whole and the parts" (210). Internally, the best political system is a federalist and cooperative socialism, while internationally, patriotism is made compatible with the idea of humanity (209–210). Thus is resolved "the most pressing problem among those posed by the war, that of the moral personality of societies. For it is in Humanity alone that we can commune with each other in our various undertakings: It alone will reconcile science and faith" (210).

The reference to the "moral personality of societies" in the next-to-last sentence of *Recherche* is no mere metaphor. Michael Chapman (1988, 5) has acutely suggested that the young Piaget's system gave him "a solution to his immediate problems of identity in the form of a life project that satisfied the conflicting sides of his personality." This statement is accurate, as far as it goes. But I wish to go further. Piaget's thinking, nourished by a vast culture and encompassing a large number of topics, is obviously irreducible to introspective self-examination. His system, however, was not just a "solution." Rather, Piaget's conceptualization of his personality provided the paradigm for his other speculations, and his self-analysis was the generative act of the theory of equilibrium.

Piaget's Self-Analysis

As a quasi-technical term, *self-analysis* designates the relatively systematic study of oneself by oneself using the tools and vocabulary of psychoanalysis. There is no evidence that, at the time of *Recherche,* Piaget resorted methodically to such techniques as free association and the analysis of dreams, as he did later on (Vidal, 1986a). Nevertheless, even though he did not, for example, interpret Sebastian's nightmares (93, 96) psychoanalytically, he examined the constitution and dynamics of human personality with a predominantly psychoanalytic vocabulary.

The theoretical problem of the relation between the individual and society claimed Piaget's attention just at a time when he anguished over the authenticity of his own personality. Maybe this was natural in a voracious reader whose thinking bore the mark of many authors, and who was aware of his numerous intellectual debts; it was perhaps to be expected in an individual who saw his own passions as contradictory with the ideal purity he professed; it illustrates, at any rate, the simultaneous assertion, so common among the young Christians, of the most extreme individualism and the most ardent desire for community with others. *The Mission of the Idea* proclaimed the quest of an "absolute Humanity" that would harmoniously integrate all individual souls and would, like a "symphony," transcend its components into a "superior whole." *Recherche* translates this mystical quest into the language of equilibrium without, however, eliminating the personal dimension highlighted by Piaget's letter to Romain Rolland.

The Letter to Romain Rolland

For Piaget, an equilibrated personality provides the model for the most desirable form of equilibrium, in which the parts and the whole are compatible and "conserve" each other. "My personality," Piaget writes, "tends to conserve its partial qualities (the believer, the philosopher, and so on) in the same way as these qualities tend to conserve the personality" (154). The relations between an individual and his environment involve the same type of equilibrium: the more a person is able to assimilate, understand, and be influenced by the external world (these terms are for Piaget equivalent), the more he is himself and has "more individuality" (156).

Individual equilibrium is both internal and external, "psychological" and "moral." "An individual," Piaget writes, "is an equilibrium between his own individual tendencies and his fulfillment of the social equilibrium" (177). There is, moreover, a special link between individuality and absolute value, since the latter is the "source" of everything that "has or could have worth" in the former, and even of "all the values the ideal personality could know" (199). The "moral personality of societies" (210) that Piaget wishes to regenerate is "moral" in that it involves the relation between the individual and the collective, and is a "personality" in that its equilibrium entails the agreement and the mutual conservation of the whole and the parts.

Recherche thus conducts the reader from Sebastian's private difficulties to the question of the personality of societies, that is, from intimate psychological self-examination to the contemplation of the broadest problems of humanity. Since the theory of equilibrium applies to everything, individuality necessarily appears as a microcosm. But the reason why it emerges as a microcosm of universal processes is that, as demonstrated by Piaget's letter to Rolland, it is itself the pattern for the description of those processes.

In June 1917 the Genevan literary magazine *Les Tablettes,* outspokenly anti-militarist and "Rollandist," published a special issue on Tolstoy. Rolland contributed a short essay titled "Tolstoy: The Free Spirit," in which he sees the Russian writer as the perfect model of his own ideals and attitudes.

Rolland (1917, 3) opens by recounting how, in his personal diary, Tolstoy imagines himself as "an ensemble of loved beings." In general, he then says, "a great personality contains in itself more than one soul." Tolstoy was a great artist, a great Christian, and a creature of "unbounded instincts and passions." He was, however, governed by "free reason." Now, for Rolland, it is precisely this "free reason" that was most lacking during the war. Tolstoy was the supreme exemplar of free man. This is best revealed in his religious attitude. As Rolland explains, Tolstoy never considered something true simply because the Gospel said it; on the contrary, for him, the Gospel contained the truth only because it was in harmony with his own moral conscience (ibid.). Giving up the capacity to think by oneself is for Rolland "the core of all evil." "The freedom of the spirit is the supreme treasure." There have never been many free men, says the writer; but that small number must preserve the "flame of liberty" for the masses, who follow only "collective passions" (ibid., 4).

In a letter written from Leysin on 4 August 1917, Piaget (1917a) reacts to Rolland's text. He starts by telling Rolland the "impression" made on him by the article on Tolstoy, which he calls a "hymn to free reason": "How right you are ... to call for free souls! ... I thank you sincerely for this plea that each time touches me in a peculiar manner." He then comments on the connection between free reason and the collective makeup of the self.

Every person, he writes, carries within himself a large number of other individuals who keep on living their own lives, and who influence, direct, and even coerce the soul in its most intense moments. The word *image*, Piaget holds, does not adequately denote such inner individuals, "for each of these images is a true living being whose roots reach into the deepest areas of the self; only some aspects of them emerge into consciousness." The great difficulty is to take others' images without turning them into an internal "despot." The existence of a "society" within each individual may lead to the loss of individuality; such is for Piaget the "[b]eauty and misery of solidarity."

Tolstoy, Piaget continues, is one of the few individuals who succeeded in dominating his inner crowd. "In a moment of freedom, one manages to discern the 'selves' who are in oneself, and to transform them from masters into true friends." In such a moment, which Piaget characterizes as rapturous, the individual is "simultaneously one and many." Freedom and free reason reside in this experience of being "oneself, and at the same time in communion with great and beautiful beings." The "true self" emerges as a "small wave" pushed from behind by other waves in the rising tide. *The Mission of the Idea* celebrated this mystical absorption into the "great soul of Humanity," which is in *Recherche* constitutive of a personality's equilibrium.

After these reflections, which he characterizes as a commentary on Rolland's essay, Piaget acknowledges that there is something "comically sad in looking for free reason without showing what one does with it." The problem is for him personal: "I would like to tell you my dreams and my certainties, and to implant more deeply in my innermost self the image that represents you ... while at the same time protecting myself from your influence." Piaget then tells Rolland that "ten times" he restrained his desire to go see him, motivated "perhaps by independence, certainly by pride"; and adds, "I am disgusted by this strange mixture of pride and self-satisfaction, and I appear just as I am: a good young man who takes himself seriously."

Piaget's letter to Rolland shows him most concerned by the idea of the self as a dynamic unity of several "souls" or inner personalities. *Recherche* reformulates the question in psychoanalytic terms.

The Context of Piaget's Psychoanalytic Discourse

Piaget uses the notions of "complex" and "sublimation" to examine, respectively, the collective makeup of the self and the problem of the passions. In both cases, he makes room for the "unconscious." Moreover, he describes metaphysics and mysticism as forms of "autistic thinking." Finally, Piaget's analysis belongs to the realm of morality. In his own vocabulary, the analysis of the self is "moral" (rather than just psychological) because it involves the relations between the individual and society. It is "moral" also in the more conventional sense of qualifying conduct according to principles of right and wrong.

The psychoanalytically oriented discourse of *Recherche* is dependent on a definite context. In his autobiography, Piaget indicates that he discovered psychoanalysis in Zurich, where he spent a semester in 1918–19. There, he recalls, he read Sigmund Freud (1856–1939) and the journal *Imago*, occasionally attended lectures by Carl Gustav Jung (1875–1961) and Oskar Pfister (1873–1956), and followed the courses of Eugen Bleuler (1857–1939). Piaget also observes that the initiation to psychoanalysis and psychiatry "made me sense the dangers of solitary meditation; I decided to forget my system [that is, *Recherche*] lest I should fall a victim of 'autism'" (1952, 244).

By means of a pathological label, Piaget succinctly condemns the grandiose speculations of his youth. In *Recherche* itself, however, he had already done the same with respect to his mystical and metaphysical tendencies. Psychoanalysis had already helped him analyze himself. Contrary to what Piaget claims in his autobiography, he did not discover psychoanalysis in Zurich. It is even likely that Zurich attracted him *because* it was the Protestant capital of psychoanalysis. By the time Piaget went to Zurich, Jung had already fallen out with Freud and was evolving his own brand of analytical psychology. The Protestant minister Pfister, in contrast, remained devoted to the Freudian cause and was a personal friend of Freud's. He was convinced of the value of psychoanalysis for the education and cure of souls, and in 1913 he published a comprehensive book titled *The Psychoanalytic Method*. Bleuler, a psychiatrist renowned for his elaboration of the concept of schizophrenia (of which autism was considered a symptom), directed the Burghölzli, which was the first official mental institution to incorporate psychoanalysis and where Jung had worked from 1900 to 1908. In his paper "On the History of the Psychoanalytic Movement" (1914) Freud acknowledged the importance of Zurich in the international diffusion of his doctrine. In the circle of the young Christians, if Zurich meant anything related to psychology, it was psychoanalysis.

In an homage to Jung, Piaget (1945b) hints at the circumstances of his first contact with psychoanalysis: a talk given by Théodore Flournoy, supposedly on Freud and Jung. This was in fact a talk titled "Religion and Psychoanalysis," delivered in 1916 at Sainte-Croix at the annual meeting of the Swiss Christian Students' Association. Flournoy was a pioneer explorer of the unconscious and a main figure in the introduction of psychoanalysis in French-speaking circles (Cifali, 1983). As a pragmatist and a liberal Protestant, Flournoy shared with his friend William James the idea that "whatever it may be on its 'farther' side, the 'more' with which in religious experience we feel ourselves connected is on its 'hither' side the subconscious continuation of our unconscious life" (James, 1902, 386). Freud, on the contrary, did not even contemplate the idea of a "farther side"; as he explained in *The Future of an Illusion* (1927), religious ideas were for him the delusive fulfillments of the oldest, strongest, and most urgent wishes of humankind.

Jung (1963, 162) considered Flournoy a "revered and fatherly friend"; his 1902 medical doctoral dissertation, *On the Psychology and Pathology of So-Called Occult Phenomena,* bears the mark of Flournoy's work on mediums. In 1913 Flournoy helped Jung break with Freud. His talk highlights the role played by religious questions not only in the Jung-Freud rupture but also in Piaget's first encounter with psychoanalysis. Flournoy unhesitatingly allied himself with the Zurich psychoanalytic school, which he identified with Jung, Pfister, and Bleuler. He remarked, for example, that "the general spirit of the Zurich school must be much more attractive to the religious people of our land than that of the Vienna school, since it attaches more importance to the points of contact and the relations of mutual support that exist between psychoanalysis and religion (Christianity in particular)" (Flournoy, 1915, 220, n. 1).

In the notes on which he based his talk, Flournoy (1916) opposed the Freudians' "Judaic notion of religion" to the Zurich school's "Christian ideal" and asserted: "we have to get used to the equivalence of a double vocabulary: mystical [and] psychoanalytic." Elsewhere he pointed out "the contrast between the purely psychobiological and narrowly positivistic tendency of the Viennese school, and the Zurich school. Without giving up scientific rigor," he added, "the latter exhibits a much greater open-mindedness, a more delicate sensitivity, a much more lively concern for moral, religious, social, [and] pedagogical questions" (Flournoy, 1913b, 203).

Flournoy's reflections illustrate the Swiss reception of psychoanalysis. In Switzerland, psychoanalysis was first welcomed by liberal Protestant intellectuals, including educators and pastors, for whom religion had to be discussed in terms other than Freud's rationalistic materialism (Cifali, 1984). Piaget's initial apprehension of psychoanalysis bears the mark of the Zurich school (with an emphasis on the notion of "complex" and criticism of Freud's alleged "pansexualism"). Its orientation to self-examination was also consistent with the spirit of Sainte-Croix. The theme of the 1916 conference was "Christianity and Neopaganism"—"neopaganism" being the anti-intellectualist trend of youth. Flournoy's talk was thought to be a good introduction to the topic; claiming to adopt the stance of a "modern psychoanalyst," a Zurich minister attributed young people's moral crisis to an excessively strong repression of instincts (Cuendet, 1916).

The Interpretation of Mysticism and Metaphysics

In *Recherche,* psychoanalysis is initially mentioned in Sebastian's wholesale critique of contemporary culture. Within psychology he attacks the "parochialism of specialists," be they experimentalists, pathologists, introspectionists, or psychiatrists. The Americans' abuse of questionnaires, he comments, led them "to delicious puerilities . . . by means of a complicated mechanism of curves and calculations." As for psychoanalysis, "A Viennese doctor discovered the basis of the entire unconscious psyche in the sexual instinct, and immediately his school generalized his theories, which were at first correct, and gave rise to the same puerilities" (63).

The narrative of Sebastian's crisis anticipates the theoretical objections to psychoanalysis formulated in Piaget's "reconstruction." As we saw in the previous chapter, at the beginning of the "preparation," Sebastian becomes aware of his "passion to dominate" and his "apostle's pride" (13). Near the onset of the crisis, he doubts the sincerity and purity of his intentions. This doubt is the "demon" that leaps into the conscious mind from the *subconscious,* and is forced back into the *unconscious* after a struggle (92). "Subconscious" is a descriptive word designating that which is not conscious.[2] "Unconscious" is a theoretical concept of psychoanalysis naming one of the subsystems of the psychical apparatus; as implied in Piaget's usage, it is largely made up of the repressed (in Sebastian's case, anxiety-arousing ideas related to faith and sexuality; 93).

Later, in "The Crisis," Sebastian adheres to the ideals of chastity and love of humanity advocated in Tolstoy's *Kreutzer Sonata* (118–119), yet once again feels driven by egotistic passions. In spite of appearances, his life was not, as he thought, "purely intellectual" (96). His love was an abstraction, and "not the motor of his life"; his vocation was motivated by "pride and selfishness," by an "obscure desire to be great" (121). Sebastian feels in himself "the revolt of the beast recently muzzled," in three forms. One is the *cupido sciendi,* "a passionate thirst for intellectual certainty" combined with the desire "to explain scientifically the bottom of things" (121, 122). Another is the "mystic's *cupido excellendi,*" the passion to dominate (124). The third is the *cupido sentiendi,* Sebastian's sensual attraction to reality.

After each episode of creation and mystical communion, Sebastian wants "to plunge into the abyss of sensations and feelings, love and be loved, participate in the silence of souls embracing each other" (122). He knows that, to be pure, his "ecstasies" should exclude passion. Yet he goes as far as thinking that perhaps a woman could replace God as a companion to share his suffering (128). Incapable of vanquishing the "insatiable demon," however, he interprets it in such a way as to make it acceptable.

Sebastian is aware of "the close relation between mysticism and sensuality," but he turns around the theory according to which the "religious instinct" is a sublimation of sexuality (122). For him, "Mysticism was practically the normal state, in which man consecrates his powers of love, communion, and sacrifice to the close union with the ideal . . . Those powers appear in the ecstasy of love only because of an abuse of passion, because all passion is precisely a deviation from the normal state" (122–123).

Mystics are "capable of sensual passion" because they have been "endowed with a life that is stronger than the average" (123). Instead of mysticism's being a transformation of the sexual instinct, sexuality is a deviation from the normal powers of man, powers that the mystic possesses to a particularly strong degree. Such a deviation is a "disequilibrium"; equilibrium is restored as the individual strives after God in the course of mystical ecstasy; when it is attained, the individual feels "a great peace" and is touched by grace (123–124).

In "The Crisis," metaphysics is the core of Sebastian's vocation. Mysticism is one of the psychological processes leading to personal equilibrium, and is therefore a valuable component of Sebastian's personality. Less positively, "The Reconstruction" describes mysticism and metaphysics as forms of autistic thinking. Although Piaget used the same psychiatric label in *Recherche* and in his autobiography, it does not fulfill the same function in the two texts. In the autobiography, Piaget brushed aside youthful speculations; in *Recherche*, he combined self-criticism and self-understanding within the theory of equilibrium.

According to Bleuler in his 1911 psychiatric masterpiece on schizophrenia, autism was one of the fundamental symptoms of the disorder. He defined it as the "detachment from reality, together with the relative and absolute predominance of the inner life" (Bleuler, 1911, 63). Autistic thinking (Piaget's favored expression, very common in Bleuler) is made up of wishes and fears; instead of being bound by logical laws, it is directed by affective needs. Autistic patients are apathetic toward the external world, and hold their fantasies and illusions as more real and valid than reality; they think "in symbols, in analogies, in fragmentary concepts, in accidental connections," yet are also able to exhibit "normal," "realistic" thinking (ibid., 67).

In Piaget's description (165), autistic thinking is one of the main types of thinking (together with reason, understanding, and value judgment) and possesses two main features: it concerns quality rather than quantity, and it proceeds by a "symbolism" such as can be found in dreams, imagination, art, mysticism, and metaphysics. Since, he explains, qualities are unknowable in the pure state, autistic thinking "individualizes" them under the form of symbols, instead of "depersonalizing" them as do the other forms of thought. This it does by way of two mechanisms: the "concentration" in one symbol of qualities drawn from the diverse objects of our interest, and the "displacement" of the "affective contents" of those qualities onto a new object (194).[3] Thus originate religion and metaphysics.

The "core of the religious fact" is for Piaget "the feeling of absolute value the individual attributes to his moral ideal," and it is "naturally surrounded by accessory manifestations," which he describes as "eruptions of autistic thinking" (190). These manifestations "envelop the roots of faith already in the subconscious"; on the outside, they take the form of metaphysical systems and religious doctrines (ibid.). Thus, the beliefs that accompany conversion and prayer (which Piaget considers as religiously more essential events) are nothing other than "the autistic symbols that allow feelings to become attached to the concrete elements of the ego" (191). Piaget observes that, like historical religions, secondary religious phenomena allow religion to be studied scientifically (190).

Metaphysics works in the same way, but "embrac[es] rational knowledge under autistic symbols on a much larger scale" than mysticism (195). Its virtually unique symbol, Piaget declares, is the "intellectual surface" the individual gives to his faith in an absolute value (195). Beyond pure faith or the will to act, the empirical phenomena of religion and metaphysics are inherently pathological, symptoms of disequilibrium. Autistic thinking represents an unstable equilibrium; only reason synthesizes in an equilibrated fashion both qualitative and quantitative knowledge. As Piaget says, the thinker is "a madman" because he forces himself to "follow his thought completely," confronting paradox and ignoring external action (117).

By conceptualizing Sebastian's inclinations in psychiatric terms, Piaget repudiates his own metaphysical and mystical phase, while at the same time he understands it and gives himself the means for moving in the direction of the "ideal equilibrium."

Pride, Egoism, and Complexes

In his letter to Romain Rolland, Piaget conceived of the individual personality as a sort of inner "society" made up of autonomous persons dwelling in the deepest areas of the self and only partially emerging into consciousness. Far from being merely theoretical, this notion of personality conveyed Piaget's self-perception—his ambivalence about communion and solidarity with others, his desire and reluctance to let the individual be absorbed into humanity, and his quest to reconcile uniqueness and originality with insertion in a social and intellectual universe of which he was highly aware.

Sebastian encounters his inner society intensely during the crisis. Once, upon his return from the "sacred mountain," he feels a "crowd" emerge from his "unconscious." Each one of the "personalit[ies]" composing the crowd is "part of his being"; the crowd itself is "concentrated in [his] single small self" (132). Sebastian apprehends "the necessity of duty, sacrifice, life, [and] his vocation" as the "pressure" of the real soul of humanity crystallizing in his own unique person and endowing it "with a new life" (133). When he "amalgamates" his experiences "with his own substance," Sebastian feels in himself "his friends, sharing his personality, each one occupying a particular area," and he gains strength and consolation from his "continuous community" with this "beautiful and great ensemble" (141). Illness facilitates the individual's access to this unconscious inner society (115–116).

Having rejected (in his letter to Rolland) the word *image* to designate the elements that compose it, Piaget calls them "complexes," and reformulates the personality question that so agitated Sebastian in terms that fit his theory and bring him close to the Swiss vanguard of dynamic psychology.

In the theoretical part of *Recherche*, "complex" designates an ensemble of past ideas, emotions, and sensations, and of the interiorized "images of fellow creatures" (179). Our personality is the whole; complexes are "autonomous partial qualities" involved in the processes of equilibrium (ibid.). Like its conceptual companion "autistic thinking," "complex" clarifies the crucial personal, moral, and social problems Piaget wishes to resolve, and in particular the tormenting question of pride and egoism.

According to Piaget, interactions among individuals lead, within each person, to the development of "an infinitely complicated and nuanced image" of the others, which becomes an "inherent part of our own substance" (178). As he explains, this vocabulary is not metaphorical: "current research on the subconscious" has uncovered "the existence of such personal 'complexes' accounting by themselves for the entire mechanism of the deep activity of the self" (178).

The "complex" is not an invention of the Zurich school. The *Studies on Hysteria* (1895), coauthored by Sigmund Freud and Joseph Breuer, include the notion. Breuer spoke of the "ideational complexes" produced during Anna O.'s "absences," and disposed of by being given verbal expression under hypnosis. In the case of Emmy von N., Freud explained that when portions of unconscious complexes emerge into consciousness, what is usually perceived is the general feeling (of grief or anxiety, for example) attached to the complex. Yet "complex" is not a key Freudian notion.

The theory of complexes grew out of Jung's experimental studies in word association. The reaction to a stimulus-word was observed to be determined by emotionally charged "ideas" (thoughts, feelings, or memories) connected either directly or through intermediate links to the stimulus-word. Jung observed that these determinants of the reaction grouped themselves, and termed such a group a "complex" (see especially Jung, 1910, 1911). The association test thus became a method for discovering complexes; prolonged reaction times, faults, disturbances of memory, or failures to react were considered "complex indicators." In the healthy individual, the combination of complexes results in a relatively unified personality; in schizophrenia, both Jung (1907) and Bleuler (1911) noted, complexes behave like autonomous beings or subpersonalities that dominate a patient's entire personality at different times, and are responsible for his or her delusions and hallucinations.

In *Recherche,* Piaget employs *complex* in essentially the same way as Jung and Bleuler. In addition, he integrates it into the theory of equilibrium as a constitutive, fundamental concept, applicable to a vast array of phenomena from art to mental illness.

Piaget defines beauty as the love of the ideal equilibrium. Sensations "equilibrate themselves as a complex," and complexes may "crystallize around the image of a specific individual" (186). When, instead of simply reflecting reality, they conform to the first type of equilibrium (compatibility and mutual conservation of the whole and the parts), they "become aesthetic." An aesthetic complex is capable of integrating the worst physical and moral disorders, and it is all the more beautiful in that it "inundates the whole individual." Piaget therefore concludes that aesthetic realism is inadequate, since true art does not copy reality but "constructs an ideal equilibrium" (186).

Like art, religion entails complexes (194–195). Under the effect of autistic thinking, those complexes take on a sort of independent life, part conscious and part unconscious. The Catholics' saints provide one example. Another, furnished by cases of "nervous disorganization," consists of the "hallucinations and 'presences' well known to psychologists." Yet, as Piaget emphasizes, all religious life requires the individualization of complexes into symbols.

Most important, the notion of complexes sheds light on individual morality and on the problem of evil, and thus serves the goal of the theory of equilibrium, which is to help humanity advance toward religious, moral, intellectual, and political salvation. In *Recherche,* as we have seen, "moral equilibrium coincides with the ideal psychological equilibrium whereby the whole and the parts are in a state of harmony and reciprocal conservation"; the good is "ab-

solute altruism and abstinence from all passion" (178). "Moral disequilibrium" is defined by the incompatibility of the whole and the parts and gives
rise to two groups of evil: "egoism, pride, and derived vices," and the different
forms of passion (ibid.). The equilibria and disequilibria in question are those
of the human personality, and therefore those of complexes.

Indeed, for Piaget, the theory of complexes furnishes "the most psychological interpretation that may be given of the moral phenomenon" (178). It demonstrates in particular the immanent nature of morality. For although egoism
is censured by society, its "true condemnation" consists in the feeling of disequilibrium each person experiences when he or she acts selfishly (178–179).
Since we are essentially composed of complexes, which are images of other
persons, egoism is actually self-inflicted; to be generous and to love the other
implies enriching and loving one's own "qualities" (179). Piaget maintains
that he is not advocating a "disguised egoism," since "equilibrium does not
ensue" if you love others only for yourself; equilibrium requires an unreserved
altruism (179–180).

In sum, combining the theory of equilibrium with the theory of complexes
enables the young Piaget to advocate a morality of altruism while disposing of
Sebastian's pride and egoism. In the final analysis, morality is more a matter of
self-awareness than of moral conscience. For if we do not *feel* the disequilibrium that selfishness is supposed to generate in us, then there is no "true condemnation" of the selfish act. Complexes should function as a moral
homeostat, but the absence of a sense of disequilibrium goes together with that
of a guilty conscience, and nowhere does Piaget say that we necessarily feel
either when we act selfishly.

Sensuality, Sublimation, and Scientific Morality

The theory of complexes, thanks to which egoism is transfigured into altruism,
does not suffice to solve Sebastian's most intimate problem, the conflict between sensual drives and the ideal of purity. The more he strives after love and
humility, the stronger is the revolt of the "insatiable demon" of the passions.
Passions, the second main form of evil, are "a composite of altruism and egoism . . . a struggle between the divine and the diabolical in man" (181). Passion
is a disequilibrium because it entails the elimination of certain parts of each
partner's self, in such a way that each partner tends to identify entirely with the
other. It is, therefore, always selfish and contrary to "biological morality"
(ibid.).

Piaget here develops the theory, first formulated as a commentary to
Sebastian's crisis (122), according to which sensuality is a deviation of an
individual's mystical powers. He aims his theory against psychoanalysis (181–

182). Psychoanalysis, he explains, sees in "subconscious and sentimental life" a derivative of the sexual instinct. Sexuality is transformed by means of sublimation, which Piaget defines as the "transfer of psychical energy from an object of lesser value to an object of higher value." But since psychoanalysis "lacks a criterion for its value judgments," the difficulty lies in determining the value of the object. Thus, by implicitly turning passion into the source of the good, "classical psychoanalysis" gets into a teleological vicious circle: the good, which is an empirical result of sublimation, is also (by definition) the goal of sublimation. Piaget asserts that his theory avoids this mistake (182).

The theory of equilibrium characterizes values in terms of an "ideal organization," which is itself defined by the equilibrium between the whole and the parts. It therefore demonstrates that the "sublimated state" is the "ideal" or "normal" state. It is thus possible to accept that everything may be "tainted with sexuality," while avoiding the "somewhat grotesque assertion of pansexualism." Finally, and always in Piaget's own view, the theory of equilibrium encompasses the interplay of complexes in "subconscious" mental activity without employing the notion of "libido," which is metaphysical and spoils "such an interesting psychology" with a "verbose" biology.

Piaget's critique of psychoanalysis fits with a system he himself characterized as a Bergsonism that is "advanced," nonmetaphysical, "without duration" (161, 53). Observing that Bergson had been obliged to "put forward a psychological unconscious force," Piaget proposed to replace it by the notion of biological equilibrium (162). This rejection of Bergsonian "duration" also applies to Freudian "libido."

The most important consequence of Piaget's inversion of the theory of sublimation is moral and psychological: while it allows for passion and sexuality, it liberates individuals from guilt and releases them from making a conscious effort to untangle good and evil. According to Piaget, scientific morality confirms the views of conscience, but since "we know how to practice the good before learning to know biological equilibria" (182), we may rest assured that the processes of equilibrium will take us automatically toward the ideal.

The Logic of Life and the Logic of the Self

Recherche exposes Piaget's ambivalence regarding the relations between science and values. Piaget asserts that science does not dictate values; rather, if by an act of faith we define life as a value, then science shows that the ideal equilibrium of the first type is the "norm" of all value. In his view, however, science actually confirms the beliefs of individual conscience, and we practice the good without knowing anything about equilibria. Piaget's article "Biology and War," dated 20 January 1918, throws light on these and other issues touching on the relations among values, science, and the self.

"Biology and War" was solicited by the Zofingue student society (to which Piaget did not belong). Zofingue was founded in 1820 with the goal of promoting a Swiss national conscience through contact among academic youth. At the beginning of the twentieth century, under the influence of students who also belonged to the Swiss Christian Students' Association, Zofingue became animated by a more religious, especially social Christian spirit. During World War I the society opened its meetings and its magazine, the *Feuille centrale,* to discussions on the issues that gripped progressive youth (socialism versus imperialism, pacifism versus militarism, and so forth). Romain Rolland's favorable impression of Swiss youth derived for the most part from his contact with Zofingue.

"Biology and War" opens by posing the problem of the unity of personal identity: a naturalist, Piaget explains, will be unable to say anything on the subject "for a long time to come": "He can try literature, since it is alive and aims at human not scientific truth, but he cannot yet integrate his attitude as a human being with his science. He is too much a human being to adopt an a priori attitude which would go against his loyalty as a scientist" (1918c, 374–375). Since Piaget considers that scientific facts by themselves do not reveal whether "war is or is not a part of the internal logic of biological equilibrium," he tries to reason "on the basis of a sort of 'pure biology'" (ibid., 376).

"Pure biology" should disclose the "normal laws of evolution." We know from *Recherche* that "normal" means in fact "ideal." Piaget thus chooses not to worry "about the perpetual obstacle that reality presents to the free play of evolution." Since ethics "postulates that life and the good are identical," "pure evolution" coincides with humanity's "moral aspirations" (ibid.). Piaget's "demonstration" of this presupposes the theory of equilibration.

Once life and the good are defined as identical, there are for Piaget only two ways of "justifying war by biology": by showing that Darwinism explains evolution, or by reducing Lamarckism "to the narrow interpretation Le Dantec gave to 'functional assimilation'" (ibid., 376–377). Piaget is referring to Le Dantec's (1906, 1912b) idea that life, that is, functional assimilation itself, is a struggle between the individual and the environment. Assimilation is an organism's transformation of foreign substances into its own substance. "Imitation," in Le Dantec's terminology (for example, 1912a, 122–125), is the exact opposite. His model of equilibrium is the scale (Le Dantec, 1907, 138); equilibrium is therefore a mechanism of compensations and opposite actions.

Piaget's idea that assimilation and imitation are not antithetical shows that his notion of equilibrium is based not on the scale but, like assimilation, on the integration of parts into an increasingly rich and complex totality.

According to Le Dantec, a personality will be diminished if, instead of assimilating, the individual imitates or is assimilated. He acknowledges that there is no assimilation without imitation: "the victor retains the trace, the precise memory of the defeated" (Le Dantec, 1912c, 83). The French biologist applied this reasoning to all processes, from cellular growth and organic pathology to knowledge acquisition. Even affective relations among human beings illustrated the universal struggle: we are invaded by another's "image," and that is why love is like a chronic illness (Le Dantec, 1912c, 271–299).

In an autobiography, Piaget recalled his opposition to Le Dantec in relation to epistemology alone: knowledge, he says, is not simply imitation, "as Le Dantec believed," but assimilation to the organism's structures (1959a, 9). Yet Piaget's efforts to make assimilation and imitation coincide in a single constructive process applied to all levels of life, and in particular to interpersonal relations and the structure of the self. In a passage from *Recherche* disputing Le Dantec, he claimed: "The better I assimilate, the more I remain identical with myself. In contrast, the more I change, the less coherent I am, and the less assimilating power, personality, I have" (155).

Thus, for Piaget, any theory of life postulating that its basic processes are "struggle" or "competition" could only be misguided. August Weissmann's theory of heredity, he observes, could be interpreted as implying a "doctrine of harmony," since the coordination of the hereditary particles may influence the "relationships between individuals." But even in this case selection, that is, competition, remains the primary mechanism of evolution (1918c, 377).

Curiously, Piaget conflates Weismann's particles and Freud's "libido." One could see "in the transmitted germ plasm a psychological force, one could call it *libido,* and show how the 'sublimation' of such an unconscious energy leads to love, art, and religion" (ibid.). Yet, as also argued in *Recherche,* this doctrine implies "a rather unscientific teleology" (ibid.). In conclusion: "either particles and libido are mechanisms and, with selection alone being involved, only egoism and struggle can be deduced; or else they are entities, and we are off biological ground" (ibid.). Piaget here echoes Le Dantec's critique of "particles," familiar to the Friends of Nature, and presupposes the reversal of the theory of sublimation.

Science, Piaget claims, proves that "natural selection cannot explain evolution," and that the heredity of acquired traits is an undoubted "experimental fact" (ibid., 377–378). The Lamarckian preservation of acquired characteristics supposes "assimilation"; thus, when he based the whole of biology on assimilation, Le Dantec made the tenets of Lamarckism explicit (ibid., 378). Yet by making assimilation and "imitation" inversely proportional to each other, Le Dantec opposed the individual and the environment. Now, just as much as Darwinism, a Lamarckism based on the opposition between assimilation and imitation implies that "egoism is the basis of every society," that struggle is "the internal logic of life," and that therefore "war is necessary" (ibid., 379). But such a conclusion contradicts the theory of equilibrium.

While Le Dantec's idea that assimilation and imitation proceed in different directions may apply to digestion, "the opposite is true with regard to psychological phenomena" (ibid.). In conformity with what he explained in *Recherche,* Piaget asserts that "one is the more oneself the better one understands one's environment," that in every "conscious phenomenon" assimilation and imitation are directly proportional to each other, and that "this is the case for all phenomena essential to life" (ibid., 379–380). Thus, he concludes,

> the more one examines the mechanism of life, the more one discovers that love and altruism—that is, the negation of war—are inherent in the nature of living beings. Only later complications due to environmental inertia, and thus competition, force living creatures to a restricted assimilation, that is, egoism, stupidity, struggle, and, in the human species, war. To struggle against war is therefore to act according to the logic of life against the logic of things, and that is the whole of morality. (Ibid., 380)

As Gruber and Vonèche (1977, 38) suggest, "Biology and War" may be read as an opinion against the war and the doctrine of its biological inevitability, or as an early statement of Piaget's biological position between what he described as Darwinism and a certain form of Lamarckism. But "Biology and War" must be also seen as an expression of Piaget's resolution of his personal crisis, and its transmutation into the starting point for universal salvation. From the theoretical point of view, the article applies the principles of the theory of equilibrium. As in *Recherche,* the question of identity must be settled before any larger conclusion can be reached. Thus, the article starts with the announcement that "a naturalist," the implied author, is not yet able to integrate his attitudes as a scientist and a human being, and that consequently his argument must be ultimately grounded on an act of faith (the identification of life and the good). In Piaget's vocabulary, this act of faith enables the individual to maintain the integrity of the self, that is, to "conserve" its "partial qualities" (believer, philosopher, scientist, and so forth). It has an integrative value. Later on, the crucial part of Piaget's "demonstration" in "Biology and War" turns out to be a discussion of the makeup and functioning of the self. As in *Recherche,* the individual personality is the model for the equilibrium of the first type, both in its internal operation and in its relations to the environment (the more a person can assimilate, the more he or she possesses "individuality"). The "logic of life," in sum, is the logic of the self.

Epilogue

In his autobiography, Piaget claimed that he incorporated his theory of equilibrium into a philosophical novel to avoid compromising himself on scientific grounds. Such a claim, however, masks the existential and intellectual significance of *Recherche* to him. Piaget saw himself as a "militant philosopher" (ms. 1918a), considered *Recherche* his first truly philosophical statement, and planned to complete a doctorate under the direction of Arnold Reymond. He was still thinking about it in December 1924 (ms. 1924), and he later said that his only regret in succeeding Reymond in 1925 as professor of philosophy at the University of Neuchâtel was that he could no longer submit a thesis since he held the chair (1965, 10). He aimed *Recherche* not only at his peers or at young socialists but also at a professional philosophical public. He wanted his criticism and ideas to be heard and pondered; and the fact that he was unsuccessful changes nothing with regard to his initial hopes and desires.

The Reception of *Recherche*

Just after the publication of *Recherche*, Piaget wrote to Reymond asking him to review the book: "If you think that the ideas formulated have some value, either social or philosophical, would it be too much to ask you to write something for the *Revue de métaphysique* [*et de morale*]? If, on the contrary, you find my book banal, would you write for the *Revue de théologie et de philosophie?* . . ." (ms. 1918a). Although the *Revue de théologie et de philosophie* was well known in French-speaking Switzerland, the Parisian *Revue de métaphysique et de morale* (Journal of Metaphysics and Moral Philosophy), established in 1893, was the foremost French philosophical journal. As its title suggests, the *Revue* represented (to a certain extent) a reaction against positivism, and it was unquestionably the very best mirror of the movements and debates of turn-of-the-century French philosophy and social science. Piaget's attempt to get his name into that eminent journal gives the measure of his ambition and of the value he attributed to his ideas.

Reymond, who had not yet seen *Recherche,* proposed instead to write for the Genevan *Semaine littéraire,* the leading Swiss-French literary magazine. Piaget (ms. 1918b) said he was happy to accept. He obviously did not anticipate the severity of Reymond's criticism, who went so far as to declare that he commented on *Recherche* only because it revealed the perilous aspirations of a section of Swiss-French youth.

Reymond (1918b, 550) attributed the "curious mixture of passion and reason" that, for him, characterized *Recherche,* to what he took to be its model, Romain Rolland's *Jean-Christophe,* a book he openly disliked. He remarked on the summary and superficial character of Sebastian's critique, commented that it was all the more surprising that Sebastian constantly borrowed from the authors he disparaged, and pointed out its lack of originality. He then pursued two main critical points. The first was that Sebastian's religious attitude was incoherent, since it combined belief in a "living" personal God with the idea that God is a sort of abstract value. The second was that Sebastian, like other young Christians according to Reymond, lacked a conception of justice.

Alluding to Rolland, Reymond castigated those who placed themselves "above the battle" and refused to condemn Germany. For him, the almost complete absence of details about Sebastian's circumstances and national origins turned Piaget's hero into a *heimatlos,* a stateless person. The diffusion among Swiss intellectual youth of a "nebulous," "neutral," and "insipid" internationalism appeared to Reymond an extremely dangerous development for the country's identity. He hoped that Piaget, "whose philosophical and literary talent [was] so full of promise," would realize that his "solution" was inadequate and had to be modified (ibid., 551).

The *Revue de théologie et de philosophie* printed a review by Samuel Gagnebin (1882–1983), a professor of mathematics and physics at the University of Neuchâtel who had initially been trained in theology. Gagnebin's review was friendlier than Reymond's and reflected better the contents and spirit of *Recherche.* For example, he described Piaget's book as a "confession modeled after *Jean-Christophe,*" yet pointed out that Sebastian was a "Swiss Jean-Christophe, and more of a philosopher than an artist" (Gagnebin, 1919, 131). He also noted that Sebastian traced the roots of the war to the disequilibrium between science and faith, and he devoted almost half of the review to summarizing Piaget's ideas. His main criticism was the same as Reymond's: the absence from *Recherche* of the idea of justice, and especially the lack of explicit condemnation of "Germany's crimes" (ibid., 133).

Furthermore, Gagnebin thought that biology was "too narrow a basis on which to found a morality" (ibid.). He argued that if the essential features of human nature could be defined once and for all, then one could perhaps infer from them a moral ideal, and thus establish a scientific morality; humanity, however, is constantly evolving and changing, and therefore morality can be grounded only on personal moral experience. Gagnebin, who in 1912 had published an intelligent and sympathetic essay on Edouard Le Roy's Bergsonian and conventionalist "philosophy of intuition," remarked the insufficiency of Piaget's emphasis on scientific reason as the means to solve the question of science and faith (ibid., 134). He then commented on the vagueness of Piaget's program to reconcile individualism and socialism. Piaget, he wrote, seemed to know nothing of concrete social problems; his "solution" was purely verbal and "serenely ignore[d]" earlier attempts at establishing a "social equilibrium" (ibid., 134–135). Finally, the questions Gagnebin formulated on the theory of equilibrium highlight its obscurities and contradictions: How can one scientifically establish the ideal equilibrium if it is never realized? How can its immutability be proved? How can equilibrium be simultaneously qualitative and mechanical? (ibid., 135).

La Revue romande, a predominantly literary "journal of Swiss culture," published a lengthy review by the Neuchâtel writer and critic Wilfred Chopard (1895–1958). Chopard (1918, 7, 8) saw in Piaget "one of the most gifted minds of our generation," and in most of *Recherche* a "psychological autobiography" centered on the desire to reconcile the "impulses of faith and the positive data of science." For Chopard, the best part of the book (which he thought would be familiar to many readers) was the discussion of contemporary philosophy. Yet he found Piaget's critique of science arrogant, and said that only his youthfulness could excuse his immoderate ambition and self-confidence. For Chopard, ambition was Piaget's "illness," as Piaget realized when he accused himself (under Sebastian's guise) of *libido excellendi* (ibid., 9). After reviewing in detail the section on literature, Chopard concluded that Piaget was "incompetent" in the matter. While marveling at Piaget's ease among the "clouds of metaphysics," Chopard perceived in his ideas about the "reconstruction" a total lack of realism. Thus, he concluded, *Recherche* "can have no more than a documentary interest, and inform us about the psychological development of a young man who thinks" (ibid., 10). Such a comment could not have pleased the young Piaget, for whom *Recherche* was far from being exclusively an autobiography.

The only frankly positive review of *Recherche* appeared in *L'Essor* and was written by Adolphe Ferrière (1879–1960), Paul Pettavel's successor as the journal's editor. Ferrière liked *Recherche* so much that in 1920 he printed two excerpts from it in the journal.[1] Ferrière, a spirited polygraph, was a friend of Pierre Bovet's and one of the great prophets of the progressive education movement (see Gerber et al., 1981). He was deeply concerned about the relations between faith and science; in 1915 he had finished a substantial dissertation on the "law of progress" in biology and sociology. According to those who knew Piaget, however, Ferrière embodied exactly the turn of mind that he abhorred—that of a sincere and productive but hyperbolic and hazy cosmic visionary. Thus Piaget could scarcely have been satisfied with the reception of his book—or in particular with the fact that only Ferrière (1919, 2) unhesitatingly praised *Recherche* and saw in its publication the sign that "a philosopher is born."

Beyond *Recherche*

The accusation of pretentiousness and lack of contact with social and political realities may have humbled Piaget and helped induce a new crisis. In his later analysis of the dream of a "twenty-two-year-old student" who was clearly himself, Piaget (1920b, 21) reported the dreamer's "moral crisis" and desire to attain an "independent spiritual position" at a time when he was moving to another city. *Recherche* appeared at the time Piaget was moving to Zurich; and while the negative reviews might have distanced him from professional philosophy, they left his ideas almost intact. Even though the kind of work Piaget did after *Recherche* differs greatly from what he had done until then, it does not nullify the theory of equilibrium or its moral, political, and religious underpinnings.[2]

In *Recherche*, Piaget characterized the theory of equilibrium as an "advanced Bergsonism" (1918a, 161). Elsewhere he asserted that it boiled down to "Boutroux rethought through Bergson" (ms. 1918e). Emile Boutroux (1845–1921) was a leading figure in the reaction of French metaphysics and philosophy of science against mechanism and determinism; significant traces of his ideas can be found in the works of the main turn-of-the-century French thinkers, including the two most important for Piaget's development, Henri Bergson and Léon Brunschvicg.

Boutroux's most influential work was his 1874 doctoral thesis, a dense and swiftly argued little book on "the contingency of the laws of nature." Boutroux claimed that to the extent that all phenomena are characterized by change, natural laws can be predictive but are not necessary. He stated, for example, that "the true condition of man always is the passage from one state to another"; and he concluded that all laws are relative (Boutroux, 1874, 123). Laws do not exist before things; they presuppose their existence. They do not govern phenomena, but only express them (ibid., 135–136). As we move from matter to humanity, essence appears as less and less primordial, and we realize that it consists in the being's existence. What Boutroux called "the doctrine of contingent variations" did not deny science but, on the contrary, doomed all attempts at knowing the universe without taking experience into account (ibid.). As he later explained, natural laws are compromises that bring mathematics as close as possible to experience; they are methods whereby we assimilate things to our intelligence and subordinate them to the accomplishment of our will; as mental constructs, they "are the chain that links the exterior to the interior" (Boutroux, 1895, 142–143).

Boutroux's emphasis on transformation over permanence and on freedom over determinism appealed to Piaget. As he wrote in *Recherche* (1918a, 48), Boutroux looked for the "fissures" in the edifice of scientific determinism through which the "creative impulse" could surge. For Sebastian, however, Boutroux's premises "had a psychological rather than a metaphysical significance. They inform us on the work of the mind . . . The contingency of natural laws thus became entirely subjective" (ibid., 49). He believed that the "alleged fissures" were "illusory," and that the creative impulse of life could be understood in conformity with the "underlying logic" of Bergsonism (ibid., 49, 53). Thus, he necessarily moved in the direction of psychology.

Recherche does not explicitly present psychology as the central discipline for the realization of its objectives. Indeed, as Jacques Vonèche (1992, 27) points out, it does not even hint at the genetic psychology of intelligence that Piaget developed later. But it does contain most of Piaget's ideas about social, or rather, moral psychology. A few months before finishing *Recherche,* Piaget told Romain Rolland that his main problem was to base morality on science. At the end of the book he reminded his readers that the crucial problem raised by the war was that of the "moral personality" of society.

Implicitly, however, psychology was for Piaget the pivotal science. It was the starting point of the theory of equilibrium, and, through the psychological and psychopathological analysis of the individual personality, it furnished the paradigm for the conceptualization of all social and mental phenomena. Piaget's outlook was characteristic of the times. In 1908, for example, a French poll revealed that "the aversion to metaphysics, the interest in pathological psychology, and particularly in sociology, are the distinctive features of the present generation"; it also found that the favorite readings of students and teachers all dealt with psychology (Binet, 1908, 210, 212). Piaget's readiness to consider psychology as the key science was also consistent with a liberal Protestant perspective that regarded religion mainly as a psychological phenomenon, and theological discourse as largely grounded in psychological self-examination. Bergson fit right in, since his view of life as creative evolution rested on the postulate that "duration," or time as experienced in consciousness, was also the essence of life. With such background and interests as he had starting about 1912, Piaget seemed destined to become some kind of psychologist-philosopher.

Piaget's mature psychological thinking bears very deep traces of Bergsonism. The textbook image of Piaget as the creator of a developmental theory based on the succession of clearly demarcated age-related stages masks his emphasis on the continuity of development and his focus on processes rather than on states. As species were for the naturalist convenient but not fully natural divisions of continuous evolutionary tendencies, so would stages be for the psychologist. As the Bergsonian student of life stressed the role of active adaptation in speciation and evolution, so would the psychologist consider activity as the defining feature of psychological function and as the motor of development. Most fundamentally, the idea that psychology provides the nexus between the theory of life and the theory of knowledge is basic to Bergson's philosophy.

Nevertheless, it is not easy to see exactly how Piaget ended up studying children. About the time *Recherche* appeared, Piaget left for Zurich with the aim, he says in his autobiography (1952, 243), "of working in a psychological laboratory." He was enrolled at the University of Zurich, in the department called "Philosophy I," during the 1918–19 winter term (October to March; see *Verzeichnis*). The professors he mentions in connection with experimental psychology, Arthur Wreschner (1866–1932) and Gotthold-Friedrich Lipps (1865–1931), also taught courses in philosophy, pedagogy, and mental development. For Piaget in retrospect, their teachings seemed to have "little bearing on fundamental problems" (1952, 243).

Zurich was the Protestant capital of psychoanalysis, and it is very likely that Piaget was attracted to it precisely for that reason. For psychology alone, he could more profitably have gone to France, Germany, or even Geneva. But Zurich united intellectual and personal interest. Piaget's (1920b, 20–21) later analysis of a dream suggests that he moved to Zurich while in the midst of a spiritual crisis, analogous to earlier crises, and during which, not unlike Sebastian, he doubted the purity of his motives and feared to find "disreputable instincts" (ibid., 21) at the bottom of his intellectual quest. The little that is known of his activities in Zurich confirms his interest in psychoanalysis as a theory and as a self-analytic tool.

In October 1918 he wrote: "My impressions of Zurich are excellent. I am going to start working with Lipps. Up to now, I have mainly done psychiatry at the Burghölzli" (ms. 1918b). The director of the latter institution, Eugen Bleuler, taught a variety of psychiatric topics (which the *Verzeichnis* does not specify), as well as a clinical course including hypnosis and other "exercises." There were other courses, on diagnostics, child and adolescent psychopathology, and psychotherapy, as well as lessons on nervous diseases, "with demonstrations." Piaget also recalled hearing lectures by Jung and Pfister. We do not know anything specific about his curriculum in Zurich, yet it is clear that psychoanalysis occupied a prominent place: his first psychological article, based on a lecture given in Paris in 1919, deals with psychoanalysis and child psychology, at the time a Swiss specialty; the first meeting he attended as a psychologist was the Seventh International Congress of Psychoanalysis (Berlin, 1922); in the early 1920s he underwent analysis and was sometimes identified as a psychoanalyst; and Pfister (1920, 295) described him as a young scholar "from whom the psychoanalytic movement can certainly expect important contributions."

Piaget (1975, 106) claims that by the time he arrived in Paris in the fall of 1919, he already wished to study the development of knowledge by means of child psychology. At the end of his 1919 Paris lecture (1920b, 58) he mentioned that the "correlation" of unconscious and mental development had not yet been investigated. Such a statement, like others in Piaget's writings of the early 1920s, was the formulation of a project. Chance also seems to have played a considerable role. In Piaget's words (1952, 244), he "had an extraordinary piece of luck." Pierre Bovet, he recalls (1975, 107), had recommended him to Théodore Simon (1873–1961). Simon, a former collaborator with Alfred Binet (1857–1911), asked him to standardize Cyril Burt's intelligence tests with Parisian children. Piaget "started the work without much enthusiasm, just to try anything" (1952, 244). Yet soon his attitude changed, and his investigation of children's reasoning through intelligence tests turned into the beginning of a long and productive career.

In 1921, at age twenty-five, Piaget moved to Geneva to work at the Rousseau Institute. He submitted to the local university one of his researches (1921c), on comparison in the child, as the thesis that would allow him to teach as privatdocent. His first papers on child psychology reveal the influence of Pierre Janet (1859–1947), whom Piaget (1975, 107) considered his "true teacher in psychology at the time," and reflect his interest in psychoanalysis, as well as his earlier concern for the relations between parts and wholes, now approached from the angle of the logic of classes and relations. The idea of equilibrium resurfaces in the 1930s, in the definition of adaptation as an equilibrium between assimilation and accommodation, takes on an increasingly important role in Piaget's theorizing starting in the 1940s, and culminates in 1975 in *The Equilibration of Cognitive Structures.* It is from within psychology that Piaget rejects Bergson's idea that the analysis of time must be based on the intuition of inner duration, and argues "that nothing could be more erroneous than this Bergsonian interpretation of the psychological genesis of temporal relations" (1946, 215).

At the same time, Piaget did not abandon biology. After the discovery of *Creative Evolution* and the debate with Roszkowski, natural history became a theoretical and methodological dead end. In the preface to his dissertation (1921a, 1), dated September 1918, Piaget stated that malacology should become "biological" by means of biometrics, and in connection with the statistical work "carried out by botanists and psychologists." He contemplated two investigative approaches: genetics, or the experimental study of heredity; and "a sort of indirect genetics" based on correlating morphological and environmental characteristics. Finally, he described his dissertation as merely a catalogue built on past researches "done by someone who no longer understands anything, [and] who cannot go any further without changing methods" (ibid., 2–3).

Piaget's self-imposition of radical methodological and theoretical changes was a sequel to the debate with Roszkowski. Already before finishing his dissertation, he had tried unsuccessfully to use statistical methods (ms. 1918g); later he even claimed that he had moved to Zurich "to study statistical and biometrical methods applicable to mollusks" (ms. 1918h). Upon leaving Zurich, he used what is now known as Spearman's rank order correlation coefficient in an article on the relation between altitude and morphological variability. He thus pursued the "indirect genetics" mentioned in the dissertation, and took the initial step of a "long-term research" (1920a, 125) on the mechanisms of adaptation, the heritability of acquired characteristics, and the relations between the genotype and the phenotype (ibid., 126, 133). Piaget explored these questions throughout the 1920s; in 1928, he explained that he was trying to determine whether lake *Limnaea* were fashioned by their environment, or "preformed in the polymorphism" of pond populations (1928b, 17).

Piaget's major analysis of the question appeared in a monograph on the adaptation of *Limnaea* to lake environments (1929a; shorter version, 1929b). Piaget focused on the degree of shell contraction, a morphological feature dependent on the organism's motor activity. After studying more than 80,000 specimens, he concluded that, in order to explain such features, a *tertium quid* was necessary between mutation and the heredity of acquired characteristics. For him, morphological traits formed by the organism's activity become hereditary by means of "kinetogenesis." Kinetogenesis was the word used by the American neo-Lamarckian Edward Drinker Cope (1840–1897) in his 1896 *The Primary Factors of Organic Evolution* to name the inherited effects of motion; the mechanism accounted in particular for (apparently) linear evolutionary trends, such as the evolution of the modern horse from five-toed ancestors.

Piaget's 1929 publications on the adaptation of *Limnaea* hinted at the relation between his biological and his psychological work. His first explicit statement on the subject, however, was the introduction to *The Origins of Intelligence in Children* (1936), where he used the research on *Limnaea* to support his views on the continuity between biological adaptation and intelligence, and on the analogy of biological, psychological, and epistemological theories. In later writings, particularly *Biology and Knowledge* (1967), *Adaptation and Intelligence* (1974b), and *Behavior and Evolution* (1976b), he partly updated some notions and vocabulary. Nevertheless, he never contradicted the basic position he had adopted in his youth: the notion of life as a continuous creation of increasingly complex forms, the rejection of Darwinism and mutationism, the emphasis on the organism's activity and on a constructive concept of assimilation. Piaget's abandonment of natural history and his adoption of biological methods and language did not fundamentally alter his outlook on evolution, nor did they wipe out its distant Bergsonian roots.

The young Piaget, however, cannot be reduced to his enthusiastic but somewhat ambivalent penchant for the philosophy of creative evolution. At the time he entered the domain of psychology, his thinking was irrevocably marked by his Protestant background, and much of it involved reconciling the individualism and immanentism of his religious attitude with the universality and objectivity supposed to distinguish science.

In his autobiography, Piaget (1952, 246) wrote that when he arrived at the Rousseau Institute, he organized his research to gain "objectively and inductively knowledge about the elementary structures of intelligence" so that he could later "be in a position to attack the problem of thought in general and to construct a psychological and biological epistemology." The project of developing such an epistemology, however, was still inseparable from that of basing morality on science (as put in 1917 to Rolland) or solving the problem of the moral personality of society (as formulated in *Recherche*). In turn, basing morality on science was Piaget's way of establishing the equilibrium between the different parts of his personality that he had been pursuing since *The Mission of the Idea*.

The Rousseau Institute was very open to the psychology of religion and to questions of moral education, and rapidly accommodated Piaget's multidimensional projects. For example, while writing about the relations between religious feelings and child psychology, the Institute's director, Pierre Bovet (1925), used Piaget's findings to show that children's religious attitudes were consistent with their cosmogonies. Reciprocally, as we shall see, Piaget argued that children's ideas about the world evolve in the same way as the liberal tradition claimed religious attitudes had evolved—from transcendence to immanence.

After his arrival at the Institute, Piaget organized a group to investigate the psychology of religion. The group, he reported, asked: "From which point of view can we say that one religious experience is superior to another? Has this question a psychological meaning? And if it is an exclusively religious question, which criterion will faith have at its disposal to settle the matter and yet remain sheltered from any questioning from psychology?" (1923, 43). Piaget believed that the question had a psychological meaning, and that there was a way to demonstrate the superiority of certain religious attitudes. Indeed, a significant part of his work in the 1920s constituted a defense of the immanentist attitude characteristic of liberal Protestantism against contemporary efforts to restore transcendence as the foundation of religious faith and theological knowledge.

Early on, Piaget argued that the psychological and philosophical orientations of Swiss-French religious philosophy were convergent, "and that this convergence is indispensable for our intellectual equilibrium" (1921b, 410). He affirmed that the dissociation between psychology on the one hand, and faith and religious experience on the other, was a "temporary attitude, aimed at assuring the equilibrium of psychologists themselves as flesh-and-blood persons who want to keep believing while valuing the empirical method"; as one such psychologist, Piaget hoped to connect his religious quest "to the cult of classical logic, simultaneously rationalist and empirical" (ibid., 412, 410).

According to Piaget, the psychological tradition of Flournoy and Bovet was characterized by two features that he summed up as "empirical Kantism." One was the conviction that the foundations of the "values of faith" can be discovered empirically in the concrete mechanism of religious phenomena; the other was a systematic skepticism about the possibility of knowing anything beyond scientific data. As for the "logical" tradition, for Piaget it was represented by his teacher Arnold Reymond.

Piaget adopted the key ideas of Reymond's argument about the objective features of Protestantism—an argument he regarded as his own "moral and intellectual catechism" (1921b, 412). He claimed that the spiritual history of humankind was the process of objectification whereby "individual thought subjects itself to a simultaneously logical and moral norm that transcends it, and which is for the logician the true object of religious experience" (ibid.).

Piaget sought to continue within empirical psychology the Swiss-French tradition, and to provide an equilibrium between faith and science that would supersede the old system of totally separate domains of experience. He proposed to replace what he described as Kant's "faith" in the existence of a transcendental realm by a "rational faith" in "a God that increasingly forms one body with the world, that is, with reason and its cadres" (ibid., 410). All values, including God, thus appeared as immanent to the mind; the "norms" of reason were for Piaget simultaneously logical and moral.

Piaget's position was akin to that of the French philosopher Léon Brunschvicg (1869–1944), whose courses he had followed in Paris, and whom he considered one of his masters. In Brunschvicg's "historico-critical" perspective, progress in science and ethics are inherent in those domains and tend toward immanentism. History, which the philosopher describes as a progress of *conscience* (consciousness as well as conscience), proceeds from the acceptance of external reality to the primacy of the mind as constructive agency; the progress of science is also that of humanity's self-understanding; being is a function of thought; judgment, rather than concept or category, is fundamental because it synthesizes form and content in a unity; and mathematical judgment, simultaneously created by the mind and rooted in experience, is the highest expression of the *intériorité* (inwardness or internality) toward which science and morality tend. Religious truth results from a purification of human judgment, from a gradual elimination of egocentrism enabling the individual subject to become universal. For Brunschvicg, God is universal Reason.[3]

Studying the relation between Brunschvicg's neo-Kantian idealism and Piaget's work in the 1920s would take us far beyond the scope of this book. Piaget believed in the complementarity of genetic psychology and historico-critical epistemology, and in the parallelism between children's mental growth and the history of science (see especially 1924a and 1925a). Much of what he was trying to accomplish consisted in formulating and investigating Brunschvicg's philosophy empirically. This project did not exclude the domain of values and its religious foundation.

In 1922 Piaget spoke about psychology and religious values at the Sainte-Croix meeting of the Christian Students' Association. One participant described Piaget as a "master in psychoanalysis and general philosophy" (Abauzit, 1922, 550). Another reported that he was a success among the younger generation, who seemed "to distrust metaphysics and to have complete confidence in psychology" (P. F., 1923, 12). Explicitly following Flournoy's principles, Piaget postulated a strict separation between science and value judgments. Two conceptions of God would be for science equally true "as in-

dividual symbols of a unique ineffable reality" (1923, 49). Nevertheless, he argued, even if science cannot say that one value is more legitimate than another,
it can establish the "psychological or biological superiority" of one of them. It
is capable, for example, of tracing the evolution of transcendence and immanence as individual attitudes, and thus of showing that, "from the empirical
point of view, and only relative to individual psychological development, one
religious type is more evolved than another, and therefore superior" (ibid.).

For Piaget, science did not deal with values themselves, but it could help
explain value judgments. A scientific psychology of values would thus investigate, in a developmental perspective and assuming "a parallelism between
logic and the theory of values," the logical links between judgments whose
premises it does not discuss (1923, 56). Once a personal experience had been
formed, Piaget claimed, psychology could "control" it and check its logical
structure; for example, a militarist socialist would be led to examine whether
or not militarism and socialism are logically compatible, and would then have
to make a moral and practical choice. Logical and moral experience are closely
linked; contradiction in logic and contradiction in morals were for Piaget "the
two sides of the same phenomenon" (ibid., 69).

Thus could science establish, "from the immanent and biological viewpoint
of life and thought," a criterion based on the principle of noncontradiction,
interpreted as a "law of psychological equilibrium" (ibid., 77–78). In Piaget's
view, the principle of noncontradiction implied that the more a value has potential to generate other values, the higher it is; love is therefore the supreme
value (ibid., 80). After praising the "young psychologist's efforts to establish
the means of discovering the internal logic of religious experience and the hierarchy of values that governs it," a skeptical YMCA reviewer decided to "wait
for the confirmation that the study of facts will enable him to furnish" (Anon.,
1923).

A couple of years later, on the basis of his research and of contemporary
works in psychology and anthropology, Piaget asserted that the principle of
noncontradiction was a psychological and moral necessity, and a function as
biological as nutrition (1924b, 1925b). The books on the child's mental growth
that made him famous started appearing: *The Language and Thought of the
Child* (1923), *Judgment and Reasoning in the Child* (1924), *The Child's Conception of the World* (1926), and *The Child's Conception of Physical Causality*
(1927). Their common theme is that the main feature of the child's "mentality" is its "egocentrism," or the incapacity to adopt somebody else's point of
view, and that development is a movement away from it, toward objective
thinking and interpersonal cooperation.

The disappearance of egocentrism was for Piaget both moral and intellectual. It was linked to a grasp of consciousness of one's thought processes, a process that took place about the age of seven as a result of "contact with others and the practice of discussion" (1925c, 234). "Cooperation," he claimed, "is the empirical [moral] fact whose logical ideal is reciprocity" (1928c, 203). The most obvious example of the connections Piaget established between the development of judgment in morality and in other domains is his description of children's causal explanations as evolving from a supernatural and transcendent physics, where physical law is assimilated to a coercive social or moral law, to a truly mechanistic, implicative, and causal physics, immanent in the cosmos (see especially 1928d). "Every progress made in the different moral and social domains," claimed Piaget (1933, 483), "results from the fact that we have freed ourselves from egocentrism, and from intellectual and moral coercion."

In March 1928 the Swiss Christian Students' Association invited Piaget to discuss immanence and transcendence as religious attitudes. Speaking to an audience described as deeply influenced by the dogmatic revival, Piaget claimed that, by approaching values as empirical facts, psychology and sociology had discovered the law of evolution that governed them in the individual and in society. In his opinion, such a law showed the "psychological" superiority of immanentism, confirming, for example, the idea that the "gloomy mythology" of the passion of Christ exemplified "the inhuman nature of the moral and religious attitude of transcendence" (1928a, 29). Science thus substantiates what *The Mission of the Idea* proclaimed.

In accordance with Brunschvicg, Piaget asserted that the immanentist attitude was not subjective but, on the contrary, the most objective possible one. "Immanentism," he said, "implies the identification of God, not with the [subjective] psychological self, but with the [universal and impersonal] norms of thought" (1928a, 36). For Piaget, religion, morality, and science converged in a unique grasp of consciousness of the norms of reason that embodied, all at once, an immanent God, cooperation, justice, and every free and sincere intellectual search for truth. In sum, "From the viewpoint of morality, the ego is subjected to norms such as reciprocity or justice. These are the very norms of reason, which apply to action as much as to thought. Morality is a logic of action, as logic is a morality of thought. The activity of reason is one and the same" (ibid., 37). This statement would appear as one of the main findings of *The Moral Judgment of the Child* (1932).

The impassioned debate that followed Piaget's talk reflected the disagreements that were dividing Protestantism at the time. For example, although Reymond (1929) had no sympathy for the neo-orthodox position, he accused Piaget of being an extreme subjectivist. The debate culminated in June 1929, when the Group of Former Members of the Christian Students' Association invited Piaget to clarify his position. Piaget concluded that

> if, beyond men, one examines the currents of thought that propagate from generation to generation, immanentism appears as the continuation of the impulse of spiritualization that characterizes the history of the notion of divinity. The same progress is accomplished from the transcendent God endowed with supernatural causality to the purely spiritual God of immanent experience, as from the semi-material God of primitive religions to the metaphysical God. Now—and this is the essential point—to this progress in the realm of intelligence corresponds a moral and social progress, which is, ultimately, an emancipation of the inner life. (1930a, 54)

Thus Piaget's antiauthoritarian and antidogmatic immanentism appears as a global metaphysical attitude, encompassing not only religion but also the philosophy of science and the psychology of intelligence and morality.

The aim of *The Moral Judgment of the Child* was to demonstrate the direction in which moral judgment evolved, and to reconcile sociology and psychology by presenting development as socialization *and* as an immanent process. As far as the former project is concerned, *The Moral Judgment* described children's development as the progress from a heteronomous ("other-governed") morality, characterized by obedience to norms seen as eternal and unquestionable, to an autonomous morality, characterized by cooperation, reciprocity, and the creation of rules in a system of social contract. The advancement of morality thus paralleled the historical progress from transcendence to immanence in religion. In psychogenesis, morality paralleled the growth from egocentrism and attachment to concrete appearances, to the capacity to consider diverse points of view and think abstractly. Piaget's reasoning extended into politics: if moral progress is immanent, the factors that determine nationalism and the arms race are less economic or societal than psychological; they manifest a lack of universality of human reason and demonstrate that, from the international point of view, man is still a primitive or a child (1930b, 1931).

Examined as a whole up through the publication of *The Moral Judgment*, Piaget's oeuvre manifests a view of mental and historical development that is the same in different domains, including conceptions of physical causality, use of language, reasoning, epistemology, the history of science, and morality. Development in all these realms is a movement from egocentrism, concreteness, heteronomy, authority, and transcendence, to objectivity, abstractness, autonomy, contractual reciprocity, and immanence. This movement is progress: from the child and the primitive to the adult and the modern; from undemocratic theocracies to parliamentary democracies; from dogmatic religions to liberal Protestantism. In sum, Piaget's research led to a description of the development of the moral judgment that confirmed his earlier evolutionary ethics, reformulated and realized his youthful project of basing morality on science, granted scientific and philosophical superiority to liberal Protestant values, gave a seemingly objective foundation and justification to subjective experiences and beliefs, and restored the "equilibrium" of the psychologist who, as Piaget said in 1921, wished to believe and remain a scientist.

As a young man, Piaget took himself very seriously and was animated by an immense ambition. Nothing was more important for him than his own convictions; and his later development shows that even after his conversion away from mysticism and metaphysics, he would not relinquish them. He turned the antidogmatic passion of *The Mission of the Idea,* the mystical intuition of a constructivist perspective reported in "The Mysteries of Divine Suffering," and the grand speculations of *Recherche* into our century's most original, insightful, and influential depiction of child development, into an oeuvre that can be rationally discussed, and into observations open to replication and falsification. In the process, he remained loyal to himself—so loyal, indeed, that his empirical results often seem to illustrate his hypotheses rather than test them. Whatever this might entail for the future of psychology, it will not diminish Jean Piaget's stature within the history of science. For transforming one's existential situation into an intellectual legacy for all is, by any standard, a remarkable accomplishment.

Notes

Introduction

1. Many books aim at presenting Piaget. Some are very successful in communicating Piaget's psychology in a style more accessible than his. Few, however, offer an adequate balance between his psychology *and* his epistemology, not to mention other areas, such as religion, sociology, or perception, which are usually missing. In this respect, the anthology by Gruber and Vonèche (1977) and the presentations by Battro (1969), Boden (1980), and Kesselring (1988) are the best; Battro's (1966) dictionary is serviceable. See also Piaget's own summaries (1947, 1970a; Piaget and Inhelder, 1966) and collections of essays from the 1940s through the 1960s (1964, 1970b, 1972). The almost exhaustive *Bibliographie Jean Piaget* (Geneva, Fondation Archives Jean Piaget, 1989) supersedes previous bibliographies and constitutes an indispensable tool. The existence of a bibliography compiled outside Geneva deserves to be mentioned (McLaughlin, 1988).

2. "Swiss-French" and "French-speaking Swiss" translate *suisse romand.* French-speaking Switzerland, or *Suisse romande,* comprises the cantons of Geneva, Neuchâtel, and Vaud (the canton of Jura was created in 1978), and major portions of the cantons of Fribourg and Valais. I discuss questions of Swiss-French identity in Chapter 8.

3. I am especially indebted to the work of Lejeune (1971) and to the essays by Olney (1980a), Gusdorf (1956), and Starobinski (1970a), collected in Olney (1980b). See also Eakin (1985), Olney (1972), Pascal (1960), and Weintraub (1978).

4. References: Piaget (1952; 1959a; 1965, chap. 1; 1966; 1976a); for the conversations with Evans and Bringuier, see Piaget (1973) and (1977). See also Piaget and Beth (1961, 144–145, n. 1).

1. Neuchâtel, an Orderly Little Town

1. The title of this chapter is borrowed from *Neuchâtel, petite ville rangée* (North, 1960), a book of pencil drawings and some text that sympathetically celebrates, some-

times with gentle irony, the charms and constraints of Neuchâtel's orderliness. On Neuchâtel, see *Le pays de Neuchâtel*, Courvoisier (1963), and *Histoire du pays de Neuchâtel; Visages* includes an excellent anthology of travelers' descriptions; Froidevaux (1990) is the indispensable bibliography. A major source for a detailed chronicle of Neuchâtel during World War I is the annual *Messager boîteux de Neuchâtel*, a "historical almanac" in existence since 1708. See also Faessler (1969). On Switzerland in general see, most recently, *Nouvelle histoire;* on World War I in particular, see Ruffieux (1974, chap. 1), Kurz (1970), and Ruchti (1928–1930). Attinger et al. (1921–1934) remains the chief historical dictionary.

2. See A. Piaget (1935) for a selection of his work. On Arthur Piaget, see A. Du Pasquier (1923), *Musée neuchâtelois* 32 (1945), and Schnegg (1953).

3. There is no study focused on *nervosisme*. Useful elements can be found in Fischer-Homberger (1970, 81–106), López Piñero (1983), and Zeldin (1977, 828–844); Steiner (1964) deals with the German and Austrian situation, Oppenheim (1991) with the British, and Lutz (1991) with the American. There is a large body of publications addressed to the *nerveux* and their families; for a good example of such medical-popular literature, see Borel (1873). Concerning paranoia in the French-speaking domain, the discussions by Sérieux and Capgras (1909) and Binet and Simon (1910) give a good idea of how problematic were both the illness and the concept. Piaget's characterization of paranoia corresponds with the "classical" descriptions, such as those in the writings of Emil Kraepelin, Eugen Bleuler, or the French authors just mentioned.

4. See the final judgment (twenty-eight typewritten pages) by the Swiss supreme court, issued 25 November 1915. Tribunal Fédéral, Lausanne, Section de Droit Public, A.10446.

5. For Piaget's enrollment at the university, see *Autorités*. Information on his studies is drawn from "Procès-verbaux de la Faculté des Sciences de l'Université de Neuchâtel" (manuscript notebooks, Archives de l'Etat, Neuchâtel), sessions of 13 July 1917, 24 April and 12 July 1918 (all including reports on Piaget's *licence* examinations), and 7 February 1919 (on recent doctorates).

6. See *Histoire de l'instruction, Histoire de l'Université*, A. Piaget (1917), Tribolet (1905); for a comparison with other Swiss universities, see Marcacci (1986), table 2; *Schweizerische Hochschulstatistik*, tables 1 and 10; and Tribolet (1905), tables on p. 35.

3. Natural History

1. For the announcement of Piaget's admission to those societies, see *BSN* 39 (1911–12), 140; *Revue suisse de zoologie* 22 (1914), "Bulletin annexe" 1 (March), 13; *Actes de la Société Helvétique des Sciences Naturelles* 97 (1914), 216.

2. The first of the three letters from Fuhrmann to Piaget (AJP), dated 24 July 1912, alludes to an ongoing exchange on problems of determination.

3. Thirteen letters and postcards (1912–1918) from Piaget to Bedot are at the Museum of Natural History of Geneva; nineteen from Bedot to Piaget (1912–1915), plus the one to Fuhrmann, are at the Piaget Archives. One of the latter (Bedot, ms. 1913) confirms Piaget's (1952, 239) recollection of having a paper rejected because of his age (and Bedot's offer to publish it). The article was Piaget and Romy (1914). After meeting Piaget's friend Marcel Romy, the president of a local naturalists' society who had

initially accepted the paper for its journal (Zobrist, ms. 1913a), expressed surprise that they were high school students, claimed that his society published "only works by men who have proved their ability in the sciences or in letters," compared the article to "classroom recollections," and regretted that Piaget had not informed him about his status at the outset of their correspondence (Zobrist, ms. 1913b).

4. Piaget's interest in biometrics had started earlier. In September 1918 he told Bedot: "You were right to send me back my statistical study some time ago. It is indeed superficial, and since I do not think I can do any better for now, the best thing is to let the matter rest" (ms. 1918g). Neither Piaget's study nor a relevant letter from Bedot has been found.

5. Twelve letters from Yung to Piaget (1912–1915) are kept at the Piaget Archives. On 30 September 1912 Yung responds to Piaget's offer to determine the specimens from his draggings; on 9 November 1912 he tells Piaget that he will send him all the dragged specimens. The rest of their letters concern different aspects of their collaboration.

4. The Friends of Nature

1. Rossetti gave no clear indication of his sources. The Friends borrowed freely for their talks, hardly ever gave credit, and often did not even place borrowings in quotation marks. But the manuscripts quoted here were private lecture notes, and their authors were high school students whose personal thought was merely beginning. Communicating ideas was the important point; what might be condemned in another context was here seen as a source of instruction and, when discovered, of simple amusement (PV, 30 November 1911: Piaget discovers that the paper his friend Marcel Romy is reading comes straight out of a popular manual on mollusks; everybody laughs and enjoys the situation).

2. See Bowler (1983; 1984, 243–253); Buican (1984); *Revue de synthèse* 100 (1979), special issue, "Les néo-lamarckiens français."

5. Piaget Discovers Bergson

1. As illustrated in Gunter's (1986) bibliography, Bergson has generated a huge volume of writings. The best short recent introduction in English is Kolakowski (1985). Grogin (1988) surveys the "Bergsonian controversy" in France; Pilkington (1976) assesses aspects of Bergson's influence. Most of Bergson's writings are gathered in *Oeuvres* (1963) and *Mélanges* (1972). His courses are currently being published by Presses Universitaires de France under the editorship of Henri Hude. I am here particularly indebted to Kolakowski and Pilkington.

6. Natural History and Creative Evolution

1. The *Zoologischer Anzeiger,* where the quoted article appeared, used an enlarged spacing of the letters as a form of emphasis.

7. At the Threshold of Biology

1. A card from a Dr. Piguet to Piaget (Neuchâtel, 17 November 1912, AJP) shows that Piaget had already asked for the reference.

2. See *Journal de conchyliologie* 61 (1914), 373 (Roszkowski, 1912), 374 (Roszkowski, 1913), 406 (Piaget, 1913e), 407 (Piaget, 1913d); ibid., 62 (1916), 282 (Piaget 1914j).

3. From a July 1914 letter from Arnold Reymond to Piaget we know that Piaget wrote about "X chromosomes" in a paper (not found) on "moral conscience according to Cresson." Reymond, who was Piaget's teacher and mentor in philosophy, points out that the *moralistes philosophes* to whom the paper might be directed would not understand what is meant by "X chromosomes." It is perhaps in connection with such language that Reymond begs Piaget to "find a less barbaric terminology to designate the opposition between individual morality and collective morality" (Reymond, ms. 1914). The comment makes sense. On the one hand, by 1914 it was known that the accessory, unpaired X chromosome played a key role in sex determination. On the other hand, the French philosopher André Cresson (1869–1950) had been interested for several years in the question of "naturalism" in philosophy and ethics. In a 1913 book on the relation of the individual to the species, he argued that the individual's behavior always served the perpetuation of the species; but he did not mention chromosomes, and he stated that no consensus existed on the laws and mechanisms of heredity (Cresson, 1913). Piaget, increasingly concerned by the moral, social, and political aspects of the relation between the individual and society, might have discussed Cresson's thesis with the help of an updated vocabulary: the X chromosome, after all, helps determine the offspring's sex regardless of the individual parent's desires or interests. Piaget alludes to Cresson's book in the last part of *Recherche* (1918a, 175).

4. As for Wacław Roszkowski, after leaving Switzerland in 1914 he carried out scientific missions on behalf of the St. Petersburg Academy of Sciences. He settled in Warsaw in 1918, became full professor of comparative anatomy at the university in 1927, and was later administrator of the National Museum of Natural Science and editor of its periodicals. During the German occupation of Poland in World War II he helped organize clandestine teachings, and was murdered by the Nazis on 3 August 1944. His body disappeared, but a symbolic grave marker was erected at the Powazki cemetery (Feliksiak, 1987). I gratefully acknowledge the help of Professor Ryszard Stachowski, of Adam Mickiewicz University (Poznan, Poland), who located and translated for me Feliksiak's biographical article on Roszkowski.

8. The Protestant Context

1. On the history of liberal Protestantism, see in particular Barth (1947), based on a 1929–30 course, often insightful but necessarily partial (Barth was a major critic of liberalism), Reardon (1966, 1968), and Welch (1972, 1985). See Perriraz (1961, pt. 3) for a historical sketch of French-speaking Protestant theology in the nineteenth century. Baubérot (1985) and Encrevé (1985) are the two most important recent sources on all aspects of French Protestantism in the nineteenth and twentieth centuries; I am substantially indebted to both here. The critique of Swiss-French Protestantism by the

future cardinal Journet (1925) is polemical but enlightening. On Swiss-French philosophy (including its relation to the Protestant temperament), see Reymond (1931) and Muralt (1966). On Protestantism and science, see, for example, Dillenberger (1960).

2. *Dreyfusards* were partisans of the French Jewish army officer Alfred Dreyfus, convicted of treason and imprisoned on the infamous Devil's Island after a hasty military trial in 1894. He was exonerated in 1906. The affair, one of the most serious political crises of the Third Republic, divided France into a *dreyfusard* camp of socialist-leaning, republican, moderately antimilitaristic intellectuals, and a nationalist, anti-Semitic, and clericalist *antidreyfusard* right wing.

3. As witnessed by the ACSE conferences and the main publications of each movement, social Christians and Christian socialists from France and French-speaking Switzerland were so close that it is not necessary to distinguish them here. I deal with some relevant differences in Chapter 12. For a historical sketch of the movements, see Léonard (1964, 415–422) and especially Baubérot (1985, pt. 2) and Baubérot et al. (1983, pt. 1). The Swiss-French situation is studied by Jules Humbert-Droz (1969) and J.-F. Martin (1976), while Mattmüller (1957–1968) provides a biography of Leonhard Ragaz, the Swiss-German social-Christian leader. Within Catholicism, a social Christian perspective was opened by Leo XIII's encyclical *Rerum novarum* (1891) (on Switzerland, see Ruffieux, 1969).

4. On Flournoy, see Claparède (1921); on Bovet, J.-M. Martin (1986); on Claparède, Trombetta (1976, 1989).

9. The Problem of Religion

1. This information was kindly communicated to me by Ms. N. Gatolliat, of the Secretariat of Neuchâtel's Evangelical Church (Eglise Réformée Evangélique du canton de Neuchâtel).

10. From Catechism to Philosophy

1. Ferdinand Buisson (1841–1932), a major figure in the establishment of the system of public and nonreligious education in France, was remembered in Neuchâtel for his polemical lectures, given at a time when he taught literature at the Academy, against biblical teaching in the schools (Buisson, 1868); he championed "liberal Christianity," which he described as a "lay faith" grounded on a "moral idea" and purged of dogmas, priests, and miracles (Buisson, 1865).

11. *The Mission of the Idea*

1. I have translated the French *conscience* as "conscience" or "consciousness," according to the meaning intended. Sometimes both meanings are simultaneously valid.

2. Monod's letter correcting *The Mission of the Idea* is dated 28 May 1915. No correspondence with Piaget is registered in the cataloged section of the Wilfred Monod Papers at the Bibliothèque de l'Histoire du Protestantisme Français (Paris), and examination of the approximately one hundred boxes of uncataloged archival material revealed no trace of Piaget.

12. The Making of a New Identity

1. I thank Maurice André, of the Leysin communal administration, and Geneviève Heller for useful information and for their help in my (unsuccessful) quest for documentary traces of Piaget's stays in Leysin.

2. Rebecca Piaget sends her good wishes to Jules Humbert-Droz and his wife and mentions her "children in Leysin, the youngest daughter having rejoined her brother." Undated calling card imprinted "Madame Arthur Piaget," Jules Humbert-Droz Papers (henceforth JHDP), no. 003504, Bibliothèque de La Chaux-de-Fonds. Datable December 1916.

3. Rebecca Piaget to Jules Humbert-Droz. Undated calling card imprinted "Madame Arthur Piaget," JHDP, no. 003505. Datable March 1917.

4. The paragraph numbers (§) to which I refer here are absent in the original but were added in my edition of Piaget's text (Vidal, in press [b]).

5. Examination of the manuscript reveals that Piaget inserted "et que la métaphysique est vaine" into the already written phrase (ms. 1917, 4). The existing transcription (1917a, published before the letter was deposited at the Bibliothèque Nationale) has no editorial marks, and one mistake: "c'est la foi" should read "c'est là la foi."

6. Barrère (1955) is a good introduction to Rolland, with numerous excerpts from his works. Valuable documents are gathered in two issues of *Europe:* 10 (1926), 38, and ibid. 32 (1955), 109–110. The key record on Rolland during World War I is his own journal (Rolland, 1952); the essay by the poet Pierre-Jean Jouve (1920) is an indispensable testimony; Starr (1971) is the essential research study. On Rolland and Switzerland, see Baud-Bovy et al. (1966) and Becker (1982). Albertini (1970) includes a useful introduction on Rolland's political commitments and a selection of texts; see also Collart (1963).

7. Rolland's copy of *La Mission de l'Idée* is inscribed "A M. Romain Rolland, hommage d'admiration et de profond respect. [Signed:] J. Piaget." The brochure, now in the R. Rolland Papers at the Bibliothèque Nationale (Paris), is nowhere annotated. Rolland's letter to Piaget has not been found.

8. Information from a letter from Mme. Jenny Humbert-Droz to me (29 August 1990), and from notes of a conversation between her and the historian Marc Perrenoud (15 June 1990), kindly provided by M. Perrenoud.

9. Letter and undated calling card imprinted "Madame Arthur Piaget," JHDP, nos. 003502 and 003505.

10. Neither publications nor archives contain traces of Piaget's participation in the Swiss-French Christian socialist movement other than the ones cited in this chapter. Piaget is not mentioned in the main sources about the movement (Jules Humbert-Droz, 1969; J.-F. Martin, 1976) or in Jenny Humbert-Droz's (1976) biography of her husband. The Swiss National Archives (Archives Fédérales, Bern) possess no relevant documentation on Piaget or his parents. I found no traces of Piaget in the following periodicals: *Voies nouvelles* (La Chaux-de-Fonds; official organ of the Fédération Romande [later, Internationale] des Socialistes-Chrétiens), *La Voix des Jeunes* (La Chaux-de-Fonds; official organ of the Fédération Romande de la Jeunesse Socialiste), *L'espoir du monde* (Paris; official organ of the Union des Socialistes Chrétiens), *Le Phare* (La Chaux-de-Fonds; initially a magazine of "socialist education and documen-

tation" before turning to "communist education and documentation" and becoming the official organ of the Third International in Swiss-French Switzerland), *L'Aube* (Lausanne; "political and literary magazine" of pacifist and internationalist orientation), *Demain* (Geneva; adhered to the principles of Zimmerwald's left), *Les Tablettes* (Geneva; less political, but openly pacifist and internationalist), *Le Carmel* (Geneva; "monthly magazine of literature, philosophy, and art," allegedly "apolitical," unequivocally "Rollandist"), *La revue mensuelle* (Geneva; published for years as *Le carnet de la ménagère. Revue mensuelle,* this magazine of "domestic economy, hygiene, and literary miscellanies" changed its name in 1915 and focused on pacifist propaganda).

13. *Recherche*

1. Piaget (1918a, 46) recommends that Fouillée's philosophy be rendered "entirely positive: in other words, no longer an autonomous philosophy, but a science of life" both biological and psychological. Alfred Fouillée (1838–1912) was a prolific French philosopher. Piaget alludes to his best-known concept, that of *idée-force,* an expression aimed at designating ideas (defined in general as states of consciousness) insofar as they lead to action. Fouillée (1890, 1893) saw his doctrine as fundamental for psychology and metaphysics, and argued that thought-forces were causally efficient factors in evolution (see Ganne de Beaucoudrey, 1936). In October 1914 Piaget read passages from Fouillée to the Friends of Nature (see Chapter 3).

2. *Kreutzer Sonata* (1890), a book that shocked for its boldness, and was forbidden in Russia and in the United States, is a story of a married couple's love, jealousy, and revenge. The phrase Piaget quotes (119) sums up its thesis: "sexual love is only the sign of the non-accomplishment of the law." Tolstoy claimed that the education given to women was aimed at turning them into instruments of pleasure for men, and advocated a "moral marriage" inspired by an ideal of chastity. All passions, and sexual love in particular, were for him an obstacle to the ideal union of human beings. Several French editions would have been available to Piaget; the 1893 edition includes Tolstoy's reply to his critics.

14. The Theory of Equilibrium

1. On this point, Piaget (1952, 241) refers to the "dispute of Durkheim and Tarde," a harsh polemic that lasted about a decade. The influential Sorbonne sociologist Emile Durkheim (1858–1917) viewed society as an irreducible entity, accorded collective phenomena explanatory priority over individuals, and attributed a determinant role to what he called "collective consciousness." For Gabriel Tarde (1843–1904), jurist, criminologist, a founder of social psychology, and from 1900 professor at the Collège de France, "collective consciousness" was an artificial construct; he emphasized that every group is made up of individuals, and saw in "interpsychological" relations the determinant function of social life. Piaget, who was always much closer to Tarde than to Durkheim in his views, discusses the latter at length in *The Moral Judgment of the Child* (1932), largely aimed at refuting the Durkheimian theory of moral authority.

2. A small black notebook found among Reymond's papers (Département des Manuscrits, Bibliothèque Cantonale et Universitaire, Lausanne/Dorigny) includes a

list of his *deuxième* students and their grades. For the literary section (which Piaget attended), a handwritten note states: "Written assignment 11 December [1913]. Subject: The problem of the subconscious." The subject for the scientific section was more general: "Which method in psychology seems to you the best?"

3. "Concentration" corresponds to "condensation," a mechanism Freud described in *The Interpretation of Dreams,* whereby a single idea comes to represent several associative chains. "Displacement," a notion Freud used from the beginning of his theorizing on neurosis and later in connection with the dream-work, denotes the transfer of an idea's interest or intensity to other ideas. Bleuler (1911, 26, 356) defined "condensation" as the contraction of many ideas into one, and "displacement" as the sudden substitution of one idea for another in a chain of thoughts. These definitions highlight the connection the Zurich school established between these mechanisms, the experimental study of word associations for diagnostic purposes, and the theory of the complexes (see the section "Pride, Egoism, and Complexes" earlier in this chapter).

Epilogue

1. Ferrière (1919, 2) claims that before *Recherche* appeared *L'Essor* published an excerpt from "The Crisis," depicting Sebastian's mysticism. I was unable to find it, and wonder whether Ferrière was not thinking about "The Mysteries of Divine Suffering." Two excerpts appeared later under the titles "La foi du peuple" and "Le foyer de l'âme" (*Le Nouvel Essor,* 10 July 1920, 2; ibid., 18 September 1920, 1).

2. In the preface to *Recherche,* Piaget excludes certain events as too recent to discuss, singling out the Russian revolution and Woodrow Wilson's "Christian politics" (which led the American president to formulate the Fourteen Points proposal in January 1918). He also describes himself as cautious regarding such "political and literary movements" as the magazine *Demain* and Gustave Dupin's fiercely anticlerical and antiwar *La guerre infernale* (1917). Finally, Piaget states that, had he modified his text, he would have taken into account Henri Barbusse's *Le Feu* (1916), which offers a realistic depiction of trench-war horrors while advocating pacifism and universal revolution, and his "admirable" *L'Enfer* (1908), the rather graphic story of a lonely individual's moral and sexual torments, as well as *La Religion* (1917), by the modernist Catholic historian of religion Alfred Loisy.

3. Brunschvicg's main publications through the 1920s (all published in Paris) are *La modalité du jugement* (1897), his key statement on judgment as the constitutive act of knowledge; *Introduction à la vie de l'esprit* (1900), which contains an early expression of his religious ideas; *Les étapes de la philosophie mathématique* (1912) and *L'expérience humaine et la causalité physique* (1922), both crucial for understanding Piaget's thinking in the 1920s; and the great synthesis, dedicated to Bergson, *Le progrès de la conscience dans la philosophie occidentale* (1927). In two later books, *De la connaissance de soi* (1931) and *Les âges de l'intelligence* (1934), Brunschvicg cited the results of Piaget's research—which he had himself inspired. Boirel (1964) includes a useful selection of Brunschvicg's writings, as well as a sketch of his life and thought.

"Les récents dragages malacologiques de M. le Prof. Emile Yung dans le lac éman." *Journal de conchyliologie* 60, 205–232.

, "L'albinisme chez la Limnaea stagnalis." *RS* 46, 28. Translated in *EP*, 9.

with Gustave Juvet). "Catalogue des batraciens du canton de Neuchâtel." *BSN* 0, 172–186.

"Malacologie alpestre." *Revue suisse de zoologie* 21, 439–576.

"Premières recherches sur les mollusques profondes du lac de Neuchâtel." *BSN* 0, 148–171.

"Contribution à la faune de la Haute-Savoie: Malacologie de Duingt et des en-irons." *La revue savoisienne* 54, 69–85, 166–180, 234–242.

, "Les mollusques sublittoraux du Léman recueillis par M. le Prof. Yung." *oologischer Anzeiger* 42, 615–624.

"Nouveaux dragages malacologiques de M. le Prof. Yung dans la faune profonde du éman." *Zoologischer Anzeiger* 42, 216–223. Partially translated in *EP*, 10–12.

"La notion de l'espèce suivant l'école mendélienne." Presented 4 December. CAN, no. 617. Edited in Vidal (1992).

"Etude zoogéographique de quelques dépôts coquilliers quaternaires du See-nd et des environs." *Mitteilungen der naturforschenden Gesellschaft in Bern aus em Jahre 1913,* 105–186.

"Notes sur le mimétisme des mollusques marins littoraux de Binic (Bretagne)." *oologischer Anzeiger* 43, 127–133.

"La vie animale dans les profondeurs des océans et de nos lacs." Presented 27 ebruary. PCAN, no. 598.

"Ce que peuvent contenir quelques grammes d'alluvions lacustres." *RS* 47, 4–46.

with Marcel Romy). "Notes malacologiques sur le Jura bernois." *Revue suisse de oologie* 22, 365–406.

, "Malacologie du Vully." *Mémoires de la Société Fribourgeoise des Sciences Naturelles,* Série zoologie 1, no. 3, 69–116.

. "Quelques mollusques de Colombie." In O. Fuhrmann and E. Mayor, *Voyage 'exploration scientifique en Colombie,* Part 2, "Travaux scientifiques." Neuchâtel: ttinger.

, "Notes sur quelques mollusques de la vallée du Doubs." *Mémoire de la Société 'Emulation de Montbéliard* 43, 195–208.

. "Notes sur la biologie des limnées abysales." *Internationale Revue der gesamten Hydrobiologie und Hydrographie,* Biologisches supplement 6. Partially translated a *EP*, 13–18.

. "Un mollusque nouveau pour la faune argovienne." *La feuille des jeunes aturalistes* 44, 148.

"Un nouveau mollusque étranger introduit aux environs de Neuchâtel." *RS* 48, 9–30.

. "Note sur une nouvelle Vivipara subfossile du quaternaire de la plaine 'Annecy." *La revue savoisienne* 55, 59–61.

. "Un mollusque arctique habitant les Alpes suisses." *La feuille des jeunes aturalistes* 44, 5–6.

"Révision de quelques mollusques glaciaires du Musée d'Histoire Naturelle de

Bibliography

In nearly all cases, dates following an author's name correspond to initial publication in the original language.

Abbreviations

AJP Archives Jean Piaget, Geneva
BSN *Bulletin de la Société des Sciences Naturelles de Neuchâtel,* later *Bulletin de la Société Neuchâteloise des Sciences Naturelles*
EP Howard Gruber and Jacques Vonèche, eds., *The Essential Piaget: An Interpretive Reference and Guide* (New York: Basic Books, 1977)
PCAN Papers of the Club des Amis de la Nature, Archives de la Ville, Musée d'Art et d'Histoire, Neuchâtel
PP Paul Pettavel Papers, Bibliothèque de La Chaux-de-Fonds
PV "Procès-verbaux du Club des Amis de la Nature," manuscript notebooks, PCAN
RS *Le rameau de sapin*
RTP *Revue de théologie et de philosophie*

Manuscript Collections

Papers of the Club des Amis de la Nature, Musée d'Art et d'Histoire, Neuchâtel. Includes: "Procès-verbaux du Club des Amis de la Nature," manuscript notebooks containing the records of the Club's meetings, plus "Cahier no. 6. Procès-verbaux des courses, arbres de Noël, déménagements, conférences, 1912–1916," manuscript notebook; several files of correspondence (mainly letters addressed to the club, one by Piaget); manuscripts of presentations by the club's members (ten by Piaget). Materials are chronologically arranged; most manuscripts carry a number. A large manuscript notebook titled "Activité du Club des Amis de la Nature, 1893–1934," based on the "Procès-verbaux," records session number, date, president, location, presentations given, membership issues, and topics of closed-session discussions.

Paul Pettavel Papers, Bibliothèque de La Chaux-de-Fonds. Includes the manuscript of "Les mystères de la douleur divine" and five letters from Piaget to Pettavel (1915–18, 1927). Cataloged.

Arnold Reymond Papers, Département des Manuscrits, Bibliothèque Cantonale et Universitaire, Lausanne/Dorigny. Includes six letters from Piaget to Reymond (1918) and several later pieces (1923–1937). Uncataloged but kept with the correspondence.

Edouard Claparède Papers, Département des Manuscrits, Bibliothèque Publique et Universitaire, Geneva. Includes ten letters from Piaget to Claparède (1916, 1923–1928). Cataloged.

Archives Jean Piaget, Geneva. Approximately 190 letters and postcards addressed to Piaget from 1907 to 1915, for the most part by amateur and professional naturalists, shell collectors, journal editors, or museum directors, mainly from Switzerland and France but also from Italy, Germany, Denmark, Sweden, and the United States. Uncataloged.

Muséum d'Histoire Naturelle, Geneva. Thirteen letters and postcards from Piaget to the museum's director Maurice Bedot (1912–1918). Included in the museum's chronologically arranged administrative correspondence. (Nineteen letters from Bedot to Piaget, dating from 1912 to 1915, are kept at the Archives Jean Piaget.)

Arthur Piaget Papers, Bibliothèque Publique et Universitaire, Neuchâtel. Includes one letter from Wilfred Monod (1915) and one from Fritz de Rougemont (1915), both to Jean Piaget.

Romain Rolland Papers, Département des Manuscrits, Bibliothèque Nationale, Paris. Includes a dedicated copy of *La Mission de l'Idée* and a letter from Piaget to Rolland (1917).

Works by Jean Piaget

Letters

ms. 1912. Letter to Maurice Bedot. Neuchâtel, 10 May. Muséum d'Histoire Naturelle, Geneva. Edited and translated in Vidal (1986b).

ms. 1915a. "Au Club des Amis de la Nature pour son anniversaire." Leysin, 25 September. PCAN, Correspondence, no. 371.

ms. 1915b. To Paul Pettavel. Neuchâtel, 22 December. PP, B$_2$152.

ms. 1916a. To Paul Pettavel. Leysin, 5 February. PP, B$_2$216.

ms. 1916b. To Paul Pettavel. Neuchâtel, 17 May. PP, B$_2$241.

ms. 1916c. To Edouard Claparède. Leysin, Pension Beau Soleil, 17 January. Ms. fr.

4010, f. 68, Département des Manuscrits, Bibliothèque Geneva.

ms. 1917. To Romain Rolland. Les Buts, Leysin, 4 Département des Manuscrits, Bibliothèque Nationale, scribed in Piaget (1917a).

ms. [1917]. To Maurice Bedot. Neuchâtel, 20 March. Mus Geneva.

ms. [1918]. To Paul Pettavel. Neuchâtel, 9 January. PP, B$_2$15

ms. 1918a–f. To Arnold Reymond from Zurich. Reymond Manuscrits, Bibliothèque Cantonale et Universitaire, October; (b) 16 October; (c) 31 October; (d) 1 Novem ten between 1918d and 1918f; (f) 15 December.

ms. 1918g. To Maurice Bedot. Neuchâtel, 27 Septem Naturelle, Geneva.

ms. 1918h. To Maurice Bedot. Zurich, 1 November. Mus Geneva.

ms. 1924. To Arnold Reymond. Geneva, 16 December. Reyr des Manuscrits, Bibliothèque Cantonale et Universitai

ms. 1927. To Paul Pettavel. Monruz, 15 April. PP, A$_{52}$814.

Manuscripts and Published Works

1907. "Un moineau albinos." *RS* 41, 36. Translated in *EP*,

1909. "La *Xerophila obvia* au canton de Vaud." *RS* 43, 13.

1910a. "Un mollusque spécial à notre lac." Presented 9 Ju

1910b. "Deux mollusques trouvés accidentellement à Neu

1910c. "Généralités sur la distribution géographique des M cember. PCAN, no. 539.

1911a. "Les limnées des lacs de Neuchâtel, Bienne, Morat *conchyliologie* 59, 311–332. Partially translated in *EP*,

1911b. "Mollusques recueillis dans la région supérieur Suisse)." *RS* 45, 30–32, 40, 46–47.

1911c. "Les mollusques terrestres et fluviatiles des environ Côtes du Nord–Bretagne)." Presented 23 February. F

1911d. "Quelques observations sur le mimétisme des mo sented 27 April. PCAN, no. 549.

1911e. "Note sur trois variétés nouvelles de mollusqu *chyliologie* 59, 333–340.

1912 (with Marcel Romy). "Les mollusques du Lac de *Société Neuchâteloise de Géographie* 21, 144–161.

1912a. "La vanité de la nomenclature." Presented 26 Sep ited in Vidal (1984).

1912b. "Supplément au catalogue des mollusques du ca 74–89.

Berne." *Mitteilungen der naturforschenden Gesellschaft in Bern aus dem Jahre 1914,* 215–277.

1914j. "L'espèce mendélienne a-t-elle une valeur absolue?" *Zoologischer Anzeiger* 44, 328–331. Also in Vidal (1992). Translated in *EP,* 19–22.

1914k. "Note sur les mollusques de la faune des sommets jurassiens." *La feuille des jeunes naturalistes* 44, 135–138, 152–155.

1914l. "Bergson et Sabatier." *Revue chrétienne* 61, 192–200.

1915a. *La Mission de l'Idée.* Lausanne: La Concorde. Cover dated 1916. Abbreviated translation in *EP,* 26–37. First published as double issue of *Nouvelles de l'Association Chrétienne Suisse d'Etudiants* 6 (2–3), December 1915.

1915b. "Les journées d'Évilard." *Nouvelles de l'Association Chrétienne Suisse d'Etudiants* 5 (7), 198–200.

1916a. "Contribution à la malacologie terrestre et fluviatile de la Bretagne de Saint-Brieuc à Plouha." *BSN* 41, 32–83.

1916b. "Nouvelles recherches sur les mollusques du Val Ferret et des environs immédiats." *Bulletin de la Murithienne* 39, 22–73.

1916c. "Les mystères de la douleur divine." *Supplément de L'Essor. Coin des jeunes,* no. 1, 5 February. Edited in Vidal (in press [a]).

1917a. Letter to Romain Rolland. *Action étudiante* (Geneva) 12 (69) (1966), 7.

1917b. Review of Jeannet (1917). *Nouvelles de l'Association Chrétienne Suisse d'Etudiants* 7 (4), May, 123–124.

1918a. *Recherche.* Lausanne: La Concorde. Chapter-by-chapter summary in *EP,* 43–50.

1918b. "Première neige" and "Je voudrais." *L'Aube* (Lausanne), no. 10, 1 February, 155. Two sonnets. Also in Vidal (in press [b]).

1918c. "La biologie et la guerre." *Feuille centrale de la Société Suisse de Zofingue* 58, 374–380. Translated in *EP,* 38–41.

1918d. Review of Warnery (1917). *Nouvelles de l'Association Chrétienne Suisse d'Etudiants* 8 (4), April, 120–122.

1920a. "Corrélation entre les répartitions des mollusques du Valais et les indices de variations spécifiques." *Revue suisse de zoologie* 28, 125–133.

1920b. "La psychanalyse dans ses rapports avec la psychologie de l'enfant." *Bulletin de la Société Alfred Binet* 20, 18–34, 41–58. Partially translated in *EP,* 55–59.

1921a. *Introduction à la Malacologie Valaisanne.* Sion: Imp. Aymon. Part 1 of Piaget's 1918 doctoral dissertation. Part 2 appeared in *Bulletin de la Murithienne* 42 (1921–1924), 82–112.

1921b. "L'orientation de la philosophie religieuse en Suisse romande." *La semaine littéraire,* 27 August, 409–412.

1921c. *Une forme verbale de la comparaison chez l'enfant.* Geneva: Kundig. Piaget's thesis submitted to the University of Geneva to be allowed to teach as privatdocent. Also in *Archives de psychologie* 18, 141–172.

1923. "La psychologie et les valeurs religieuses." In *Sainte-Croix 1922.* Lausanne: La Concorde.

1924a. "Etude critique, *L'expérience humaine et la causalité physique* de L. Brunschvicg." *Journal de psychologie normale et pathologique* 21, 586–607.

1924b. "Les traits principaux de la logique de l'enfant." *Journal de psychologie normale et pathologique* 21, 48–101.

1925a. "Psychologie et critique de la connaissance." *Archives de psychologie* 19, 193–210.

1925b. "Deux ouvrages récents de psychologie religieuse." *RTP* 13, 142–147.

1925c. "Le réalisme nominal chez l'enfant." *Revue philosophique de la France et de l'étranger* 99, 189–234. Same as chaps. 1–2 of *The Child's Conception of the World.*

1928a. "Immanence et transcendance." In J. Piaget and J. de la Harpe, *Deux types d'attitudes religieuses: Immanence et Transcendance.* Geneva: Association Chrétienne d'Etudiants de la Suisse Romande.

1928b. "Un problème d'hérédité chez la limnée des étangs. Appel aux malacologistes et aux amateurs en conchyliologie." *Bulletin de la Société Zoologique de France* 53, 13–18.

1928c. "Logique génétique et sociologie." *Revue philosophique de la France et de l'étranger* 105, 167–205.

1928d. "La causalité chez l'enfant." *British Journal of Psychology* 18, 276–301.

1929a. "L'adaptation de la *Limnaea stagnalis* aux milieux lacustres de la Suisse romande. Etude biométrique et génétique." *Revue suisse de zoologie* 36, 263–531.

1929b. "Les races lacustres de la *Limnaea stagnalis* L. Recherches sur les rapports de l'adaptation héréditaire avec le milieu." *Bulletin biologique de la France et de la Belgique* 63, 424–455.

1929c. "Encore 'immanence et transcendance.'" *Cahiers Protestants* 13, 325–330. Reply to Reymond (1929).

1930a. *Immanentisme et foi religieuse.* [Geneva:] Groupe Romand des Anciens Membres de l'Association Chrétienne d'Etudiants.

1930b. "Moral Realities in Child Life." *New Era in Home and School* 11, 112–114.

1931. "Introduction psychologique à l'éducation internationale." In *Quatrième cours pour le personnel enseignant. Comment faire connaître la Société des Nations et développer l'esprit de coopération internationale.* Geneva: International Bureau of Education.

1932. *The Moral Judgment of the Child.* Trans. M. Gabain. London: Kegan Paul; Trench: Trubner. Various reprints.

1933. "Social Evolution and the New Education." In T. R. Rawson, ed., *Sixth World Conference of the New Education Fellowship: Full Report.* London: New Education Fellowship.

1936. *The Origins of Intelligence in Children.* Trans. M. Cook. New York: International Universities Press, 1952. Various reprints.

1937. "La philosophie de Gustave Juvet." In *A la mémoire de Gustave Juvet, 1896–1936.* Lausanne: University of Lausanne.

1942. "Psychologie et pédagogie genevoises." *Suisse contemporaine* 2, 427–431.

1944. "L'organisation et l'esprit de la psychologie à Genève." *Revue suisse de psychologie* 3, 97–104.

1945a. Speech. In *Inauguration du buste de M. Arnold Reymond . . . le 16 décembre 1944.* Etudes et documents pour servir à l'histoire de l'Université de Lausanne. Lausanne: F. Rouge.

1945b. "Hommage à C. G. Jung." *Revue suisse de psychologie* 4, 169–171.

Bibliography

In nearly all cases, dates following an author's name correspond to initial publication in the original language.

Abbreviations

AJP   Archives Jean Piaget, Geneva

BSN   *Bulletin de la Société des Sciences Naturelles de Neuchâtel*, later *Bulletin de la Société Neuchâteloise des Sciences Naturelles*

EP   Howard Gruber and Jacques Vonèche, eds., *The Essential Piaget: An Interpretive Reference and Guide* (New York: Basic Books, 1977)

PCAN   Papers of the Club des Amis de la Nature, Archives de la Ville, Musée d'Art et d'Histoire, Neuchâtel

PP   Paul Pettavel Papers, Bibliothèque de La Chaux-de-Fonds

PV   "Procès-verbaux du Club des Amis de la Nature," manuscript notebooks, PCAN

RS   *Le rameau de sapin*

RTP   *Revue de théologie et de philosophie*

Manuscript Collections

Papers of the Club des Amis de la Nature, Musée d'Art et d'Histoire, Neuchâtel. Includes: "Procès-verbaux du Club des Amis de la Nature," manuscript notebooks containing the records of the Club's meetings, plus "Cahier no. 6. Procès-verbaux des courses, arbres de Noël, déménagements, conférences, 1912–1916," manuscript notebook; several files of correspondence (mainly letters addressed to the club, one by Piaget); manuscripts of presentations by the club's members (ten by Piaget). Materials are chronologically arranged; most manuscripts carry a number. A large manuscript notebook titled "Activité du Club des Amis de la Nature, 1893–1934," based on the "Procès-verbaux," records session number, date, president, location, presentations given, membership issues, and topics of closed-session discussions.

Paul Pettavel Papers, Bibliothèque de La Chaux-de-Fonds. Includes the manuscript of "Les mystères de la douleur divine" and five letters from Piaget to Pettavel (1915–18, 1927). Cataloged.

Arnold Reymond Papers, Département des Manuscrits, Bibliothèque Cantonale et Universitaire, Lausanne/Dorigny. Includes six letters from Piaget to Reymond (1918) and several later pieces (1923–1937). Uncataloged but kept with the correspondence.

Edouard Claparède Papers, Département des Manuscrits, Bibliothèque Publique et Universitaire, Geneva. Includes ten letters from Piaget to Claparède (1916, 1923–1928). Cataloged.

Archives Jean Piaget, Geneva. Approximately 190 letters and postcards addressed to Piaget from 1907 to 1915, for the most part by amateur and professional naturalists, shell collectors, journal editors, or museum directors, mainly from Switzerland and France but also from Italy, Germany, Denmark, Sweden, and the United States. Uncataloged.

Muséum d'Histoire Naturelle, Geneva. Thirteen letters and postcards from Piaget to the museum's director Maurice Bedot (1912–1918). Included in the museum's chronologically arranged administrative correspondence. (Nineteen letters from Bedot to Piaget, dating from 1912 to 1915, are kept at the Archives Jean Piaget.)

Arthur Piaget Papers, Bibliothèque Publique et Universitaire, Neuchâtel. Includes one letter from Wilfred Monod (1915) and one from Fritz de Rougemont (1915), both to Jean Piaget.

Romain Rolland Papers, Département des Manuscrits, Bibliothèque Nationale, Paris. Includes a dedicated copy of *La Mission de l'Idée* and a letter from Piaget to Rolland (1917).

Works by Jean Piaget

Letters

ms. 1912. Letter to Maurice Bedot. Neuchâtel, 10 May. Muséum d'Histoire Naturelle, Geneva. Edited and translated in Vidal (1986b).
ms. 1915a. "Au Club des Amis de la Nature pour son anniversaire." Leysin, 25 September. PCAN, Correspondence, no. 371.
ms. 1915b. To Paul Pettavel. Neuchâtel, 22 December. PP, B$_2$152.
ms. 1916a. To Paul Pettavel. Leysin, 5 February. PP, B$_2$216.
ms. 1916b. To Paul Pettavel. Neuchâtel, 17 May. PP, B$_2$241.
ms. 1916c. To Edouard Claparède. Leysin, Pension Beau Soleil, 17 January. Ms. fr.

4010, f. 68, Département des Manuscrits, Bibliothèque Publique et Universitaire, Geneva.

ms. 1917. To Romain Rolland. Les Buits, Leysin, 4 August. Rolland Papers, Département des Manuscrits, Bibliothèque Nationale, Paris. Uncataloged. Transcribed in Piaget (1917a).

ms. [1917]. To Maurice Bedot. Neuchâtel, 20 March. Muséum d'Histoire Naturelle, Geneva.

ms. [1918]. To Paul Pettavel. Neuchâtel, 9 January. PP, $B_2$15.

ms. 1918a–f. To Arnold Reymond from Zurich. Reymond Papers, Département des Manuscrits, Bibliothèque Cantonale et Universitaire, Lausanne/Dorigny: (a) 5 October; (b) 16 October; (c) 31 October; (d) 1 November; (e) undated, but written between 1918d and 1918f; (f) 15 December.

ms. 1918g. To Maurice Bedot. Neuchâtel, 27 September. Muséum d'Histoire Naturelle, Geneva.

ms. 1918h. To Maurice Bedot. Zurich, 1 November. Muséum d'Histoire Naturelle, Geneva.

ms. 1924. To Arnold Reymond. Geneva, 16 December. Reymond Papers, Département des Manuscrits, Bibliothèque Cantonale et Universitaire, Lausanne/Dorigny.

ms. 1927. To Paul Pettavel. Monruz, 15 April. PP, A_{52}814.

Manuscripts and Published Works

1907. "Un moineau albinos." *RS* 41, 36. Translated in *EP*, 6.

1909. "La *Xerophila obvia* au canton de Vaud." *RS* 43, 13. Translated in *EP*, 7.

1910a. "Un mollusque spécial à notre lac." Presented 9 June. PCAN, no. 527.

1910b. "Deux mollusques trouvés accidentellement à Neuchâtel." *RS* 44, 32.

1910c. "Généralités sur la distribution géographique des Mollusques." Presented 8 December. PCAN, no. 539.

1911a. "Les limnées des lacs de Neuchâtel, Bienne, Morat et des environs." *Journal de conchyliologie* 59, 311–332. Partially translated in *EP*, 8.

1911b. "Mollusques recueillis dans la région supérieure du Val-d'Hérens (Valais, Suisse)." *RS* 45, 30–32, 40, 46–47.

1911c. "Les mollusques terrestres et fluviatiles des environs de Binic (Près de St Brieuc, Côtes du Nord–Bretagne)." Presented 23 February. PCAN, no. 546.

1911d. "Quelques observations sur le mimétisme des mollusques neuchâtelois." Presented 27 April. PCAN, no. 549.

1911e. "Note sur trois variétés nouvelles de mollusques suisses." *Journal de conchyliologie* 59, 333–340.

1912 (with Marcel Romy). "Les mollusques du Lac de Saint-Blaise." *Bulletin de la Société Neuchâteloise de Géographie* 21, 144–161.

1912a. "La vanité de la nomenclature." Presented 26 September. PCAN, no. 583. Edited in Vidal (1984).

1912b. "Supplément au catalogue des mollusques du canton de Neuchâtel." *BSN* 39, 74–89.

1912c. "Les récents dragages malacologiques de M. le Prof. Emile Yung dans le lac Léman." *Journal de conchyliologie* 60, 205–232.

1912d. "L'albinisme chez la Limnaea stagnalis." *RS* 46, 28. Translated in *EP*, 9.

1913 (with Gustave Juvet). "Catalogue des batraciens du canton de Neuchâtel." *BSN* 40, 172–186.

1913a. "Malacologie alpestre." *Revue suisse de zoologie* 21, 439–576.

1913b. "Premières recherches sur les mollusques profondes du lac de Neuchâtel." *BSN* 40, 148–171.

1913c. "Contribution à la faune de la Haute-Savoie: Malacologie de Duingt et des environs." *La revue savoisienne* 54, 69–85, 166–180, 234–242.

1913d. "Les mollusques sublittoraux du Léman recueillis par M. le Prof. Yung." *Zoologischer Anzeiger* 42, 615–624.

1913e. "Nouveaux dragages malacologiques de M. le Prof. Yung dans la faune profonde du Léman." *Zoologischer Anzeiger* 42, 216–223. Partially translated in *EP*, 10–12.

1913f. "La notion de l'espèce suivant l'école mendélienne." Presented 4 December. PCAN, no. 617. Edited in Vidal (1992).

1913g. "Etude zoogéographique de quelques dépôts coquilliers quaternaires du Seeland et des environs." *Mitteilungen der naturforschenden Gesellschaft in Bern aus dem Jahre 1913*, 105–186.

1913h. "Notes sur le mimétisme des mollusques marins littoraux de Binic (Bretagne)." *Zoologischer Anzeiger* 43, 127–133.

1913i. "La vie animale dans les profondeurs des océans et de nos lacs." Presented 27 February. PCAN, no. 598.

1913j. "Ce que peuvent contenir quelques grammes d'alluvions lacustres." *RS* 47, 44–46.

1914 (with Marcel Romy). "Notes malacologiques sur le Jura bernois." *Revue suisse de zoologie* 22, 365–406.

1914a. "Malacologie du Vully." *Mémoires de la Société Fribourgeoise des Sciences Naturelles*, Série zoologie 1, no. 3, 69–116.

1914b. "Quelques mollusques de Colombie." In O. Fuhrmann and E. Mayor, *Voyage d'exploration scientifique en Colombie*, Part 2, "Travaux scientifiques." Neuchâtel: Attinger.

1914c. "Notes sur quelques mollusques de la vallée du Doubs." *Mémoire de la Société d'Emulation de Montbéliard* 43, 195–208.

1914d. "Notes sur la biologie des limnées abysales." *Internationale Revue der gesamten Hydrobiologie und Hydrographie*, Biologisches supplement 6. Partially translated in *EP*, 13–18.

1914e. "Un mollusque nouveau pour la faune argovienne." *La feuille des jeunes naturalistes* 44, 148.

1914f. "Un nouveau mollusque étranger introduit aux environs de Neuchâtel." *RS* 48, 29–30.

1914g. "Note sur une nouvelle Vivipara subfossile du quaternaire de la plaine d'Annecy." *La revue savoisienne* 55, 59–61.

1914h. "Un mollusque arctique habitant les Alpes suisses." *La feuille des jeunes naturalistes* 44, 5–6.

1914i. "Révision de quelques mollusques glaciaires du Musée d'Histoire Naturelle de

Berne." *Mitteilungen der naturforschenden Gesellschaft in Bern aus dem Jahre 1914,* 215–277.

1914j. "L'espèce mendélienne a-t-elle une valeur absolue?" *Zoologischer Anzeiger* 44, 328–331. Also in Vidal (1992). Translated in *EP,* 19–22.

1914k. "Note sur les mollusques de la faune des sommets jurassiens." *La feuille des jeunes naturalistes* 44, 135–138, 152–155.

1914l. "Bergson et Sabatier." *Revue chrétienne* 61, 192–200.

1915a. *La Mission de l'Idée.* Lausanne: La Concorde. Cover dated 1916. Abbreviated translation in *EP,* 26–37. First published as double issue of *Nouvelles de l'Association Chrétienne Suisse d'Etudiants* 6 (2–3), December 1915.

1915b. "Les journées d'Évilard." *Nouvelles de l'Association Chrétienne Suisse d'Etudiants* 5 (7), 198–200.

1916a. "Contribution à la malacologie terrestre et fluviatile de la Bretagne de Saint-Brieuc à Plouha." *BSN* 41, 32–83.

1916b. "Nouvelles recherches sur les mollusques du Val Ferret et des environs immédiats." *Bulletin de la Murithienne* 39, 22–73.

1916c. "Les mystères de la douleur divine." *Supplément de L'Essor. Coin des jeunes,* no. 1, 5 February. Edited in Vidal (in press [a]).

1917a. Letter to Romain Rolland. *Action étudiante* (Geneva) 12 (69) (1966), 7.

1917b. Review of Jeannet (1917). *Nouvelles de l'Association Chrétienne Suisse d'Etudiants* 7 (4), May, 123–124.

1918a. *Recherche.* Lausanne: La Concorde. Chapter-by-chapter summary in *EP,* 43–50.

1918b. "Première neige" and "Je voudrais." *L'Aube* (Lausanne), no. 10, 1 February, 155. Two sonnets. Also in Vidal (in press [b]).

1918c. "La biologie et la guerre." *Feuille centrale de la Société Suisse de Zofingue* 58, 374–380. Translated in *EP,* 38–41.

1918d. Review of Warnery (1917). *Nouvelles de l'Association Chrétienne Suisse d'Etudiants* 8 (4), April, 120–122.

1920a. "Corrélation entre les répartitions des mollusques du Valais et les indices de variations spécifiques." *Revue suisse de zoologie* 28, 125–133.

1920b. "La psychanalyse dans ses rapports avec la psychologie de l'enfant." *Bulletin de la Société Alfred Binet* 20, 18–34, 41–58. Partially translated in *EP,* 55–59.

1921a. *Introduction à la Malacologie Valaisanne.* Sion: Imp. Aymon. Part 1 of Piaget's 1918 doctoral dissertation. Part 2 appeared in *Bulletin de la Murithienne* 42 (1921–1924), 82–112.

1921b. "L'orientation de la philosophie religieuse en Suisse romande." *La semaine littéraire,* 27 August, 409–412.

1921c. *Une forme verbale de la comparaison chez l'enfant.* Geneva: Kundig. Piaget's thesis submitted to the University of Geneva to be allowed to teach as privatdocent. Also in *Archives de psychologie* 18, 141–172.

1923. "La psychologie et les valeurs religieuses." In *Sainte-Croix 1922.* Lausanne: La Concorde.

1924a. "Etude critique, *L'expérience humaine et la causalité physique* de L. Brunschvicg." *Journal de psychologie normale et pathologique* 21, 586–607.

1924b. "Les traits principaux de la logique de l'enfant." *Journal de psychologie normale et pathologique* 21, 48–101.

1925a. "Psychologie et critique de la connaissance." *Archives de psychologie* 19, 193–210.

1925b. "Deux ouvrages récents de psychologie religieuse." *RTP* 13, 142–147.

1925c. "Le réalisme nominal chez l'enfant." *Revue philosophique de la France et de l'étranger* 99, 189–234. Same as chaps. 1–2 of *The Child's Conception of the World*.

1928a. "Immanence et transcendance." In J. Piaget and J. de la Harpe, *Deux types d'attitudes religieuses: Immanence et Transcendance*. Geneva: Association Chrétienne d'Etudiants de la Suisse Romande.

1928b. "Un problème d'hérédité chez la limnée des étangs. Appel aux malacologistes et aux amateurs en conchyliologie." *Bulletin de la Société Zoologique de France* 53, 13–18.

1928c. "Logique génétique et sociologie." *Revue philosophique de la France et de l'étranger* 105, 167–205.

1928d. "La causalité chez l'enfant." *British Journal of Psychology* 18, 276–301.

1929a. "L'adaptation de la *Limnaea stagnalis* aux milieux lacustres de la Suisse romande. Etude biométrique et génétique." *Revue suisse de zoologie* 36, 263–531.

1929b. "Les races lacustres de la *Limnaea stagnalis* L. Recherches sur les rapports de l'adaptation héréditaire avec le milieu." *Bulletin biologique de la France et de la Belgique* 63, 424–455.

1929c. "Encore 'immanence et transcendance.'" *Cahiers Protestants* 13, 325–330. Reply to Reymond (1929).

1930a. *Immanentisme et foi religieuse*. [Geneva:] Groupe Romand des Anciens Membres de l'Association Chrétienne d'Etudiants.

1930b. "Moral Realities in Child Life." *New Era in Home and School* 11, 112–114.

1931. "Introduction psychologique à l'éducation internationale." In *Quatrième cours pour le personnel enseignant. Comment faire connaître la Société des Nations et développer l'esprit de coopération internationale*. Geneva: International Bureau of Education.

1932. *The Moral Judgment of the Child*. Trans. M. Gabain. London: Kegan Paul; Trench: Trubner. Various reprints.

1933. "Social Evolution and the New Education." In T. R. Rawson, ed., *Sixth World Conference of the New Education Fellowship: Full Report*. London: New Education Fellowship.

1936. *The Origins of Intelligence in Children*. Trans. M. Cook. New York: International Universities Press, 1952. Various reprints.

1937. "La philosophie de Gustave Juvet." In *A la mémoire de Gustave Juvet, 1896–1936*. Lausanne: University of Lausanne.

1942. "Psychologie et pédagogie genevoises." *Suisse contemporaine* 2, 427–431.

1944. "L'organisation et l'esprit de la psychologie à Genève." *Revue suisse de psychologie* 3, 97–104.

1945a. Speech. In *Inauguration du buste de M. Arnold Reymond . . . le 16 décembre 1944*. Etudes et documents pour servir à l'histoire de l'Université de Lausanne. Lausanne: F. Rouge.

1945b. "Hommage à C. G. Jung." *Revue suisse de psychologie* 4, 169–171.

1946. *The Child's Conception of Time.* Trans. A. J. Pomerans. New York: Ballantine Books, 1971.

1947. *The Psychology of Intelligence.* Trans. M. Piercy and D. E. Berlyne. Totowa, N.J.: Littlefield, Adams, 1972.

1952. "Autobiography." In E. G. Boring, H. Werner, R. M. Yerkes, and H. S. Langfeld, eds., *A History of Psychology in Autobiography.* Vol. 4. Worcester, Mass.: Clark University Press.

1955 (with Bärbel Inhelder). *The Growth of Logical Thinking from Childhood to Adolescence: An Essay on the Construction of Formal Operational Structures.* Trans. A. Parsons and S. Milgram. New York: Basic Books, 1958.

1959a. "Les modèles abstraits sont-ils opposées aux interprétations psycho-physiologiques dans l'explication en psychologie? Esquisse d'autobiographie intellectuelle." *Bulletin de psychologie* 13, 7–13.

1959b. "Lettre." In "Hommage à Arnold Reymond." *Revue de théologie et de philosophie* 9, 44–47.

1961 (with Evert W. Beth). *Epistémologie mathématique et psychologie. Essai sur les relations entre la logique formelle et la pensée réelle.* Paris: Presses Universitaires de France.

1964. *Six Psychological Studies.* Trans. A. Tenzer. New York: Vintage Books, 1968.

1965. *Insights and Illusions of Philosophy.* Trans. W. Mays. New York: New American Library, 1971.

1966 (with Bärbel Inhelder). *The Psychology of the Child.* Trans. H. Weaver. New York: Basic Books, 1969.

1966. "Autobiographie." *Cahiers Vilfredo Pareto (Revue européenne des sciences sociales)* 4, 129–159. Updated version of Piaget (1952).

1967. *Biology and Knowledge: An Essay on the Relations between Organic Regulations and Cognitive Processes.* Trans. B. Walsh. Chicago: University of Chicago Press, 1971.

1970a. *Genetic Epistemology.* Trans. E. Duckworth. New York: Norton.

1970b. *Psychology and Epistemology: Towards a Theory of Knowledge.* Trans. P. A. Wells. Harmondsworth: Penguin, 1972.

1972. *The Child and Reality: Problems of Genetic Psychology.* Trans. A. Rosin. New York: Grossman, 1973.

1973. *Jean Piaget, the Man and His Ideas.* Conversations conducted and edited by Richard I. Evans. New York: Dutton.

1974a. *The Grasp of Consciousness: Action and Concept in the Young Child.* Cambridge, Mass.: Harvard University Press, 1976.

1974b. *Adaptation and Intelligence: Organic Selection and Phenocopy.* Trans. S. Eames. Chicago: University of Chicago Press; Paris: Hermann, 1980.

1975. "L'intelligence selon Alfred Binet." *Bulletin de la Société A. Binet et T. Simon* 75, no. 544, 106–119.

1976a. "Autobiographie." *Cahiers Vilfredo Pareto (Revue européenne des sciences sociales)* 14, 1–43. Updated version of Piaget (1966).

1976b. *Behavior and Evolution.* Trans. D. Nicholson-Smith. New York: Pantheon Books, 1978.

1977. *Conversations with Jean Piaget.* Conducted and edited by Jean-Claude Bringuier. Trans. B. Miller Gulati. Chicago: University of Chicago Press, 1989.

Other Sources

Abauzit Frank. 1922. "Du premier Sainte-Croix au dernier Sainte-Croix. Impressions d'un témoin." *La semaine littéraire,* 4 November, 548–550.

A. J. 1916. Review of P. Jeannet, *La première semaine de Jacques Leber. Nouvelles de l'Association Chrétienne Suisse d'Etudiants* 6 (6), 203–204.

Albertini, Jean, ed. 1970. *Romain Rolland. Textes politiques, sociaux et philosophiques choisis.* Paris: Editions Sociales.

——— 1971. *Romain Rolland. L'esprit libre. Au-dessus de la mêlée, Les précurseurs.* Geneva: Edito-Service (Cercle du Bibliophile).

Album des internés de guerre en Suisse. Les alliés. 1917. Geneva: Atar.

Allen, Garland. 1978. *Life Science in the Twentieth Century.* Cambridge: Cambridge University Press.

Amiel, Henri-Frédéric. 1978. *Journal intime* (entry for 12 November 1852). Ed. B. Gagnebin and P. Monnier. Vol. 2. Lausanne: L'Age d'Homme.

Amiet, Albert, Jules Vincent, and Maurice Vuilleumier. 1922. *Vers la vie! Entretiens d'un pasteur avec ses catéchumènes.* Lausanne: La Concorde.

Anonymous. 1912. "Les limnées du Léman." *Gazette de Lausanne,* 13 November, [p. 3], cols. 3–4. Summary of Blanc's presentation of Roszkowski (1912).

——— 1915. Report of the Neuchâtel group. *Nouvelles de l'Association Chrétienne Suisse d'Etudiants* 5 (8), June, 234–235.

——— 1916a. Answer of the Swiss Christian Students' Association to the question "What have been the effects of the War on your Movement?" *Student World* (New York) 9, 165.

——— 1916b. "Sommation." *L'Essor,* 18 March, 1.

——— 1916c. "La Voix des Jeunes." *La Voix des Jeunes* 1, 2d ser., July, [p. 1].

——— 1923. Report on the 1922 Sainte-Croix meeting, *Cahiers de "Jeunesse"* 7 (April–May), 185–186.

Attinger, Victor, Marcel Godet, and Henri Türler, eds. 1921–1934. *Dictionnaire historique et biographique de la Suisse.* Neuchâtel: Attinger.

Autorités, professeurs, étudiants. 1916–1919. Brochure published annually by the University of Neuchâtel.

Baldwin, James Mark, ed. 1901. *Dictionary of Philosophy and Psychology.* 3 vols. New York: Macmillan.

Balestra, Dominic J. 1980. "The Mind of Jean Piaget: Its Philosophical Roots." *Thought* 55, 412–427.

Barrère, Jean-Bertrand. 1955. *Romain Rolland par lui-même.* Paris: Seuil.

Barrès, Maurice. 1912. *The Sacred Hill.* Trans. M. Cowley. New York: Macaulay, 1929.

Barth, Karl. 1922. "La parole de Dieu, tâche de la théologie." In *Parole de Dieu et parole humaine.* Trans. P. Maury and A. Lavanchy. Paris: Je Sers; Geneva: Labor.

——— 1947. *Protestant Theology in the Nineteenth Century: Its Background and History.* Valley Forge: Judson Press, 1973.

Bateson, William. 1894. *Materials for the Study of Variation.* New York: Macmillan.

Battro, Antonio M. 1966. *Piaget: Dictionary of Terms.* Trans. E. Rütschi-Hermann and S. F. Campbell. New York: Pergamon Press, 1973.

——— 1969. *El pensamiento de Jean Piaget. Psicología y epistemología.* Buenos Aires: Emecé.

Baubérot, Jean. 1985. *Le retour des huguenots.* Paris: Cerf; Geneva: Labor et Fides.

Baubérot, Jean, et al. 1983. *Itinéraires socialistes chrétiens.* Geneva: Labor et Fides.

Baud-Bovy, Samuel, Alfred Berchtold, Daniel Anet, and Sven Stelling-Michaud. 1966. *Romain Rolland en Suisse.* Geneva: Musée d'Art et d'Histoire.

Becker, Jean-Jacques. 1982. "Romain Rolland, la Suisse et la France pendant la Première Guerre Mondiale." In R. Poidevin and L.-E. Roulet, eds., *Aspects des rapports entre la France et la Suisse de 1843 à 1939.* Neuchâtel: La Baconnière.

Bedot, Maurice. ms. 1913. Letter to J. Piaget. Geneva, 20 September. AJP.

Béguin, Albert, and Pierre Thévenaz, eds. 1943. *Henri Bergson. Essais et témoignages.* Neuchâtel: La Baconnière.

Béguin, Jacques. ms. 1910. "Critique officielle du travail de Jean Piaget." PCAN, with manuscript of Piaget (1910a).

Benda, Julien. 1913. *Une philosophie pathétique. Cahiers de la Quinzaine* 2, 15th ser.

Berchtold, Alfred. 1963. *La Suisse romande au cap du XXe siècle. Portrait littéraire et moral.* Lausanne: Payot.

Bergson, Henri. 1889. *Essai sur les données immédiates de la conscience.* In Bergson (1963).

——— 1896. *Matière et mémoire. Essai sur la relation du corps à l'esprit.* In Bergson (1963).

——— 1907. *Creative Evolution.* Trans. A. Mitchell. New York: Henry Holt, 1911.

——— 1934. *La pensée et le mouvant.* In Bergson (1963).

——— 1963. *Oeuvres,* ed. A. Robinet. Paris: Presses Universitaires de France.

——— 1972. *Mélanges,* ed. A. Robinet. Paris: Presses Universitaires de France.

Berguer, Georges. 1914. "Revue et bibliographie générales de psychologie religieuse." *Archives de psychologie* 14, 1–91.

Berman, Antoine. 1983. "Bildung et Bildungsroman." *Le temps de la réflexion* 4, 141–159.

Bersot, Henri. 1932. *La femme nerveuse.* Neuchâtel: Delachaux et Niestlé.

Binet, Alfred. 1908. "Une enquête sur l'évolution de l'enseignement de la philosophie." *L'année psychologique* 14, 152–231.

Binet, Alfred, and Théodore Simon. 1910. "La folie systématisée." *L'année psychologique* 16, 215–265.

Blaisdell, Muriel L. 1992. *Darwinism and Its Data: The Adaptive Coloration of Animals.* Harvard Dissertations in the History of Science. New York: Garland.

Blanc, Henri. 1913. "Limnées de la faune profonde du Léman." *Archives des sciences physiques et naturelles* (Geneva) 35, 187–188. Blanc's presentation of Roszkowski (1912).

Bleuler, Eugen. 1911. *Dementia Praecox or the Group of Schizophrenias.* Trans. J. Zinkin. New York: International Universities Press, 1952.

Boden, Margaret. 1980. *Jean Piaget.* Harmondsworth: Penguin.

Boirel, René. 1964. *Brunschvicg. Sa vie, son oeuvre, avec un exposé de sa philosophie.* Paris: Presses Universitaires de France.

Borel, V[irgile]. 1873. *Nervosisme ou neurasthénie. La maladie du siècle et les divers moyens de la combattre.* 2d ed. Lausanne: Payot, 1894.

Boring, Edwin G., Heinz Werner, Robert M. Yerkes, and Herbert S. Langfeld, eds. 1952. *A History of Psychology in Autobiography.* Vol. 4. Worcester, Mass.: Clark University Press.

Bourguignat, Jules-René. 1880–81. *Matériaux pour servir à l'histoire des mollusques acéphales du système européen.* Poissy: Imp. S. Lejay.

Boutroux, Emile. 1874. *De la contingence des lois de la nature.* Paris: Alcan, 1895.

———— 1895. *De l'idée de loi naturelle dans la science et dans la philosophie contempo-raine.* Paris: Alcan, 1913.

———— 1908. *Science et religion dans la philosophie contemporaine.* Paris: Flammarion, 1917.

Bovet, Pierre. 1911. *Quelqu'un: John Mott.* Saint-Blaise: Foyer Solidariste.

———— 1920. "Théodore Flournoy." *La semaine littéraire,* 13 November, 532–535.

———— 1925. *Le sentiment religieux et la psychologie de l'enfant.* Neuchâtel: Delachaux et Niestlé.

———— 1943. "La fondation et les quatre premières années (1893–97) des Amis de la Nature." Lecture given at the fiftieth anniversary of the Club of the Friends of Na-ture, 12 June. Duplicated for private distribution; bound with Ducommun (1943).

Bowler, Peter. 1983. *The Eclipse of Darwinism: Anti-Darwinian Evolution Theories in the Decades around 1900.* Baltimore: Johns Hopkins University Press.

———— 1984. *Evolution: The History of an Idea.* Los Angeles: University of California Press.

Brenner, Heinrich. 1929. *Samuel Cornut.* Ph.D. diss., University of Zurich. Gais: J. Kern.

Buican, Denis. 1984. *Histoire de la génétique et de l'évolutionnisme en France.* Paris: Presses Universitaires de France.

Buisson, Ferdinand. 1865. *Le Christianisme libéral.* Paris: Cherbuliez.

———— 1868. *Une réforme urgente dans l'instruction primaire.* Neuchâtel.

———— 1882. "Club Jurassien." In Buisson, ed., *Dictionnaire de pédagogie et d'instruction primaire.* 2 vols. Paris: Hachette. Part 1, vol. 1.

Burian, Richard M., Jean Gayon, and Doris Zallen. 1988. "The Singular Fate of Genet-ics in the History of French Biology, 1900–1940." *Journal of the History of Biology* 21, 357–402.

Burnand, René. 1936. *Une ville sur la montagne.* Neuchâtel: Attinger.

Buscarlet, Daniel. 1920. "Notre inspiration. La Fédération Universelle des Associations Chrétiennes d'Etudiants." In *L'Association Chrétienne d'Etudiants. Aux étudiants des universités.* Lausanne: La Concorde.

Cardot, H. 1912. "Polymorphisme de l'Unio tumidus Phil. dans la Meuse aux environs de Mézières (Ardennes)." *Journal de conchyliologie* 60, 197–205.

Carl, J[ean]. 1932. "Henri Blanc." *Compte-rendu des séances de la Société de Physique et d'Histoire Naturelle de Genève* 49, 6–7.

Carlson, Elof Axel. 1966. *The Gene: A Critical History.* Philadelphia: W. B. Saunders.

Cary Agassiz, Elizabeth. 1885. *Louis Agassiz: His Life and Correspondence.* 2 vols. Boston: Houghton Mifflin.

Chapman, Michael. 1988. *Constructive Evolution: Origins and Development of Piaget's Thought.* New York: Cambridge University Press.

Chopard, Wilfred. 1918. "Recherche." Review of Piaget (1918a). *La revue romande,* October, 7–10.

Cifali, Mireille. 1983. "Théodore Flournoy, la découverte de l'inconscient." *Le Bloc-notes de la psychanalyse* 3, 111–131.

———— 1984. "Le fameux couteaux de Lichtenberg." *Le Bloc-notes de la psychanalyse* 4, 171–188.

Le cinquantenaire de l'Académie. Speeches delivered on 26 October 1916. Neuchâtel: Attinger, 1917.

Claparède, Edouard. 1921. "Théodore Flournoy. Sa vie et son oeuvre. 1854–1920." *Archives de psychologie* 18, 1–125.

———— 1930. "Autobiography." In Murchison (1930).

Clerc, Charly. 1916. "Le renouvellement des pensées." In *Sainte-Croix 1915.* Lausanne: La Concorde.

———— 1923. "Affirmation et recherche." *Journal de Genève,* 29 September, 1.

———— 1950. *L'âme d'un pays.* Neuchâtel: Delachaux et Niestlé.

Le Club Jurassien, 1865–66 à 1891. Histoire, activité, statistique. Neuchâtel: Comité Central, Club Jurassien, 1891.

Collart, Yves. 1963. "Romain Rolland et le mouvement socialiste contre la guerre." In *Mélanges d'histoire économique et sociale en hommage au professeur Antony Babel.* Vol. 1 of 2 vols. Geneva.

Compayré, Gabriel. 1909. *L'adolescence. Etudes de psychologie et de pédagogie.* Paris: Alcan.

Conry, Yvette. 1974. *L'introduction du darwinisme en France au XIXe siècle.* Paris: Vrin.

Cornut, Samuel. 1903. *Le testament de ma jeunesse.* Lausanne: Payot.

———— 1910. *Essais et Confessions.* Lausanne: Payot.

Coulon, Cécile de. 1913. "Ce qui nous manque." *Nouvelles de l'Association Chrétienne Suisse d'Etudiants* 4 (1), 1–9.

Courvoisier, Jean. 1963. *Panorama de l'histoire neuchâteloise.* Neuchâtel: La Baconnière.

Coutagne, G. 1895. *Recherches sur le polymorphisme des mollusques de France.* Lyons: Imp. A. Rey.

Cresson, André. 1913. *L'espèce et son serviteur (sexualité, moralité).* Paris: Alcan.

Crook, D. P. 1989. "Peter Chalmers Mitchell and Antiwar Evolutionism in Britain during the Great War." *Journal of the History of Biology* 22, 325–356.

Cuendet, William. 1916. "Tendances actuelles." In *Sainte-Croix 1916.* Lausanne: La Concorde.

Dardel, Otto de. 1916. Review of Piaget (1915b). *La Suisse libérale,* 9 February.

Dartigue, Henry. 1916. "De l'état d'esprit de la jeunesse intellectuelle avant la Guerre." *Revue chrétienne* 63, 278–293, 464–474, 570–588.

Darwin, Charles. 1859. *On the Origin of Species.* Facsimile of 1st ed. Cambridge, Mass.: Harvard University Press, 1964.

Dautzenberg, P. 1912. Obituary of P. Godet. *Journal de conchyliologie* 60, 358–360.

Delachaux, Théodore, and Jean-G. Baer. 1945. "Otto Fuhrmann. 1871–1945." *BSN* 69, 147–167.

Delage, Yves. 1903. *L'hérédité et les grands problèmes de la biologie générale.* Paris: C. Reinwald.

Delage, Yves, and Marie Goldsmith. 1909. *Les théories de l'évolution.* Paris: Flammarion.

Demos, John, and Virginia Demos. 1972. "Adolescence in Historical Perspective." In D. Rogers, ed., *Issues in Adolescent Psychology.* New York: Appleton-Century-Crofts.

Dietrich, Suzanne de. n.d. *Cinquante ans d'histoire. La Fédération Universelle des Associations Chrétiennes d'Etudiants (1895–45).* Paris: Ed. du Semeur.

Digeon, Claude. 1959. *La crise allemande de la pensée française, 1870–1914.* Paris: Presses Universitaires de France.

Dillenberger, John. 1960. *Protestant Thought and Natural Science.* Westport, Conn.: Greenwood Press.

Dollfus, Gustave F. 1911. "Recherches critiques sur quelques genres et espèces d'*Hydrobia* vivants ou fossiles." *Journal de conchyliologie* 13, 179–240.

Dubois, Georges. 1976. *Naturalistes neuchâtelois du XXe siècle.* Neuchâtel: La Baconnière.

Du Bois, Pierre. 1980. "Le mal suisse pendant la première guerre mondiale. Fragments d'un discours sur les relations entre Alémaniques, Romands et Tessinois au début du vingtième siècle." *Cahiers Vilfredo Pareto (Revue européenne des sciences sociales)* 18, 43–66.

——— 1983. "Mythe et réalité du fossé pendant la Première Guerre mondiale." In P. Du Bois, ed., *Union et division des suisses. Les relations entre alémaniques, romands et tessinois aux XIXe et XXe siècles.* Lausanne: L'Aire.

Ducommun, Paul. 1943. "Historique du Club des Amis de la Nature." Lecture given at the fiftieth anniversary of the club, 12 June. Duplicated for private distribution; bound with Bovet (1943).

Ducret, Jean-Jacques. 1984. *Jean Piaget, savant et philosophe. Les années de formation, 1907–1924. Etude sur la formation des connaissances et du sujet de la connaissance.* 2 vols. Geneva: Droz.

Dunn, L. C. 1965. *A Short History of Genetics.* New York: McGraw-Hill.

Du Pasquier, Armand. 1923. "Une figure neuchâteloise: Arthur Piaget." In *Nouvelles étrennes neuchâteloises.*

Du Pasquier, Marc. 1920. "Quelques souvenirs de jeunesse." *Cahiers de "Jeunesse"* 4, 120–133. On Pierre Jeannet.

Duplain, J. ms. 1913. Letter to J. Piaget, 27 November. AJP.

Eakin, Paul John. 1985. *Fictions in Autobiography: Studies in the Art of Self-Invention.* Princeton: Princeton University Press.

Ecklin, Robert. 1914. Report of the Neuchâtel high school group. *Nouvelles de l'Association Chrétienne Suisse d'Etudiants* 4 (5), 177–178.

Elkind, David. 1986a. Review of Vander Goot (1985). *Contemporary Psychology* 31, 153–154.

——— 1986b. Reply to Vander Goot (1986). *Contemporary Psychology* 31, 1010.

Encrevé, André. 1985. *Les protestants en France de 1800 à nos jours. Histoire d'une réintégration.* Paris: Stock.

Faessler, François. 1969. "De 1848 à nos jours." In *Neuchâtel et la Suisse.* Neuchâtel: Conseil d'Etat.

Farber, Paul Lawrence. 1982. "The Transformation of Natural History in the Nineteenth Century." *Journal of the History of Biology* 15, 145–152.

Favre, Jules. 1927. "Les mollusques post-glaciaires et actuels du bassin de Genève." *Mémoires de la Société de Physique et d'Histoire Naturelle de Genève* 40:171–434.

Favre, Louis. 1883. "Histoire abrégée de la Société Neuchâteloise des Sciences Naturelles depuis sa fondation." *BSN* 13, 3–33.

Favre, Louis, A[uguste] Bachelin, and Dr. [Louis] Guillaume. 1874. "A nos lecteurs." *RS* 8, 1.

Feliksiak, Stanisław. 1987. "Roszkowski, Wacław Andrzej Remigiusz." In S. Feliksiak, ed., *Słownik biológow polskich.* Warsaw: Polska Akademia Nauk.

Ferrière, Adolphe. 1919. "Recherche." Review of Piaget (1918a). *L'Essor,* 28 June, 2–3.

Fischer-Homberger, Esther. 1970. *Hypochondrie. Melancholie bis Neurose: Krankheiten und Zustandsbilder.* Bern: Huber.

Flournoy, Théodore. ca. 1884. "Fragments sur Kant. (Introduction à la philosophie pratique. Philosophie religieuse.)" *RTP* 9, n.s. (1921), 293–319.

———— 1890. *Métaphysique et psychologie.* 2d ed. Geneva: Kündig; Paris: Fischbacher, 1919.

———— 1900. *From India to the Planet Mars: A Study of a Case of Somnambulism with Glossolalia.* Trans. D. B. Vermilye. New York: Harper.

———— 1903. *Les principes de la psychologie religieuse.* Geneva: Kündig. Also in *Archives de psychologie* 2 (1902), 33–57.

———— 1905. *Le génie religieux.* Lausanne: La Concorde. Also in *Sainte-Croix 1904.* Lausanne: La Concorde, 11–57.

———— 1911a. *La philosophie de William James.* Saint-Blaise: Foyer Solidariste.

———— 1911b. "Aux étudiants suisses. Quelques mots à l'occasion de la prochaine visite de John Mott." *Nouvelles de l'Association Chrétienne Suisse d'Etudiants* 1 (3), 29–32.

———— 1913a. "Au seuil de la vie universitaire." *Cahiers de "Jeunesse"* 9 (1926), 472–480. Notes for a lecture given at a meeting of high school groups of the Swiss Christian Students' Association, 18 May 1913.

———— 1913b. Review of A. Keller, "Ruhige Erwägungen im Kampf um die Psychoanalyse," *Kirchenblatt für die reformierte Schweiz,* 3 and 10 February 1912. *Archives de psychologie* 13, 202–203.

———— 1915. "Une mystique moderne (Documents pour la psychologie religieuse)." *Archives de psychologie* 15, 1–224.

———— 1916. "Religion et psychoanalyse." *Le Bloc-notes de la psychanalyse* 4 (1984), 191–199. Notes for a lecture given at Sainte-Croix, 1916.

Forel, François-Alphonse. 1873. "Faune profonde du lac Léman." *Actes de la Société Helvétique des Sciences Naturelles,* 136–152.

———— 1885. "La faune profonde des lacs suisses." *Nouveaux mémoires de la Société Helvétique des Sciences Naturelles* 29, no. 2.

Fouillée, Alfred. 1890. *L'évolutionnisme des idées-force.* Paris: Alcan.

———— 1893. *La psychologie des idées-force.* 2 vols. Paris: Alcan.

Froidevaux, Anita. 1990. *Bibliographie neuchâteloise.* Hauterive: Attinger.

Frommel, Gaston. 1900. "Protestantisme en Suisse romande." In Seippel (1899–1901), vol. 2.

———— 1915. *La vérité humaine. Un cours d'apologétique.* 3 vols. Neuchâtel: Attinger.

G. 1915. Review of Jeannet (1914). *Nouvelles de l'Association Chrétienne Suisse d'Etudiants* 5 (7), 202–203.

Gagnebin, Laurent. 1987. *Christianisme spirituel et christianisme social. La prédication de Wilfred Monod (1894–1940).* Geneva: Labor et Fides.

Gagnebin, Samuel. 1919. "Recherche." Review of Piaget (1918a). *RTP* 7, n.s., 131–135.

Galland, Emmanuel. 1916. "Les 'Volontaires du Christ.'" *Nouvelles de l'Association Chrétienne Suisse d'Etudiants* 6 (7), 214–222.

Ganne de Beaucoudrey, Elisabeth. 1936. *La psychologie et la métaphysique des idées-forces chez Alfred Fouillée.* Paris: Vrin.

Gerber, Rémy, et al. 1981. *Autour de Ferrière et de l'éducation nouvelle. Cahiers de la Section des Sciences de l'Education,* no. 25. University of Geneva.

Gilbert, Muriel. 1988. "Utilisation de métaphores dans les écrits poétiques du jeune Piaget: Une étude de cas." Personal communication.

Godet, Ernest. 1911. "Prof. Dr Paul Godet, 1836–1911." *Actes de la Société Helvétique des Sciences Naturelles,* 58–66.

Godet, Paul. 1872. "Les anodontes du canton de Neuchâtel." *BSN* 9, 141–151.

———— 1874. "Les collections d'histoire naturelle." *RS* 8, 45–47.

———— 1875. "Les collections d'histoire naturelle." *RS* 9, 5–6. Continues previous article.

———— 1879. "Charles-Henri Godet, botaniste neuchâtelois." *BSN* 12, 166–175.

———— ms. 1894. Letter, "A Messieurs les Membres du Club des Amis de la Nature," 26 October. PCAN, Correspondence, no. 5.

———— 1904. "Palées et bondelles." *RS* 38, 25–27.

———— ms. 1907. Letter to J. Piaget, 5 October. AJP.

———— 1907a. "Catalogue des Mollusques de Neuchâtel et des régions limitrophes des Cantons de Berne, Vaud et Fribourg." *BSN* 34, 97–158.

———— 1907b. "Le Prof. Louis Agassiz et le Musée d'Histoire Naturelle de Neuchâtel." *BSN* 34, 288–294.

———— ms. 1909. Letter to J. Piaget, 19 March. AJP.

Godet, Philippe. 1890. *Histoire littéraire de la Suisse française.* Neuchâtel: Delachaux et Niestlé.

———— 1900. "La littérature dans la Suisse française." In Seippel (1899–1901), vol. 2.

———— 1901. *Neuchâtel pittoresque. La ville et le vignoble.* Sécheron-Genève: S. A. des Arts Graphiques.

———— 1902. "La journée de Peseux." *Musée neuchâtelois* 39, 267–272. Reports on the debate between A. Piaget and E. Perrenoud at a meeting of the Neuchâtel Historical Society.

Gounelle, Elie. 1919. "Nos visées spirituelles et sociales." *Le Christianisme social,* 7–15.

La Grande Encyclopédie. Paris: C. Lamirault, 1886–1902.

Grin, Edmond. 1930. *Les origines et l'évolution de la pensée de Charles Secrétan.* Cahiers de la Faculté de Théologie de l'Université de Lausanne, IV. Lausanne.

Grogin, Robert C. 1988. *The Bergsonian Controversy in France.* Calgary: University of Calgary Press.

Gruber, Howard. 1974. *Darwin on Man: A Psychological Study of Scientific Creativity.* New York: E. P. Dutton.

———— 1980a. "Cognitive Psychology, Scientific Creativity, and the Case Study Method." In M. D. Grmek et al., eds., *On Scientific Discovery.* Boston: Reidel.

———— 1980b. "The Evolving Systems Approach to Creativity." In S. and C. Modgil, eds., *Toward a Theory of Psychological Development.* Windsor: NFER.

Gruber, Howard, and Jacques Vonèche, eds. 1977. *The Essential Piaget: An Interpretive Reference and Guide.* New York: Basic Books.

Guillaume, Dr. [Louis]. 1881. *Coup d'oeil sur la vie sociale dans le canton de Neuchâtel. Liste des institutions et des sociétés libres de bienfaisance, d'utilité publique, d'éducation, d'instruction et de récréation.* Neuchâtel, Bureau du Comité de la Société Neuchâteloise d'Utilité Publique.

Guillaume, Dr. [Louis], et al. 1864. *Trois jours de vacances. Voyage des écoles industrielles dans le Jura neuchâtelois, les 3, 4 et 5 juillet 1864.* Neuchâtel: Delachaux et Sandoz.

Gunter, Pete Addison Yancey. 1986. *Henri Bergson: A Bibliography.* 2d ed. Bowling Green, Ohio Philosophy Documentation Center, Bowling Green University.

Gusdorf, Georges. 1956. "Conditions and Limits of Autobiography." In Olney (1980b).

Gymnase cantonal de Neuchâtel, 1873–1973. Neuchâtel, 1974.

Hall, G. Stanley. 1904. *Adolescence: Its Psychology and Its Relations to Physiology, Anthropology, Sociology, Sex, Crime, Religion, and Education.* 2 vols. New York: Appleton.

———— 1917. *Jesus, the Christ, in the Light of Psychology.* 2 vols. Garden City, N.Y.: Doubleday, Page.

Hankins, Thomas L. 1979. "In Defence of Biography: The Use of Biography in the History of Science." *History of Science* 17, 1–16.

Heller, Geneviève. 1979. *"Propre en ordre." Habitation et vie domestique 1850–1930: L'exemple vaudois.* Lausanne: Ed. d'En-Bas.

———— 1990. "Leysin et son passé médical." *Gesnerus* 47, 329–344.

Hirsch, Marianne. 1979. "The Novel of Formation as Genre: Between Great Expectations and Lost Illusions." *Genre* 12, 293–311.

Histoire de l'instruction publique dans le canton de Neuchâtel. 1914. Neuchâtel: Attinger.

Histoire de l'Université de Neuchâtel. 1 vol. to date. Hauterive: Attinger, 1988–.

Histoire du pays de Neuchâtel. 2 vols. to date. Hauterive: Attinger, 1989–.

Holmes, Frederic L. 1981. "The Fine Structure of Scientific Creativity." *History of Science* 19, 60–70.

———— 1986. "Patterns of Scientific Creativity." *Bulletin of the History of Medicine* 60, 19–35.

Hommage à Jean Piaget. 1982. Geneva: University of Geneva. Includes speeches delivered at a tribute to Piaget's memory on 3 November 1981, and newspaper articles published upon Piaget's death.

Hubendick, Bengt. 1951. "Recent Lymnaeidae. Their Variation, Morphology, Taxonomy, Nomenclature, and Distribution." *Kungliga Svenska Vetenskapsakademiens Handlingar* 3, 1–223.

Humbert-Droz, Jenny. 1976. *Une pensée, une conscience, un combat. La carrière politique de Jules Humbert-Droz retracée par sa femme.* Neuchâtel: La Baconnière.

Humbert-Droz, Jules. 1916. *Guerre à la guerre. A bas l'armée.* La Chaux-de-Fonds: Edition des Jeunesses Socialistes Romandes.

—— 1969. *Mon évolution du tolstoïsme au communisme, 1891–1921.* Neuchâtel: La Baconnière.

L'instruction religieuse de la jeunesse dans les Eglises réformées de la Suisse romande. Basel: Gasser, 1908.

Jaccottet, G[eorges], Marcel de Fourmestraux, D[aniel] Baud-Bovy, and [John] Locking. 1918. *Au soleil et sur les monts. L'étape libératrice. Scènes de la vie des soldats alliés internés en Suisse.* Geneva: Sadag.

James, Henry, ed. 1920. *The Letters of William James.* 2 vols. Boston: Atlantic Monthly.

James, William. 1902. *The Varieties of Religious Experience: A Study in Human Nature.* New York: New American Library, n.d.

—— 1907. *Pragmatism: A New Name for Some Old Ways of Thinking.* New York: Longmans, Green.

Jaurès, Jean. 1895. "La 'nuée dormante' de la guerre." In M. Bonnafous, ed., *Oeuvres de Jean Jaurès. Pour la paix,* vol. 1: *Les alliances européennes (1887–1903).* Paris: Rieder, 1931.

Jeannet, Pierre. 1914. *Les deux maisons.* Saint-Amans-Soult (Tarn): privately published.

—— 1915. "Sainte-Croix 1915." *L'Essor,* 16 October, 2–3.

—— 1917. *Le Christ. (Très insuffisante esquisse).* Lausanne: La Concorde.

Jones, Leonard Chester. 1929. *Arnold Guyot et Princeton.* Neuchâtel: Secrétariat de l'Université.

—— 1931. "The Neuchâtel Group and Science in the United States." *Amerikanische-Schweitzer Zeitung* (New York), no. 4–10 (18 November–30 December).

[Joseph, Jules]. 1896. *Les Ecoles du Dimanche de la Suisse romande.* Lausanne: Comité des Ecoles du Dimanche du Canton de Vaud.

—— 1915. "Aux catéchumènes et à leurs parents." *Journal religieux des Eglises indépendantes de la Suisse romande* 58, 183.

Jost, François. 1969. "La tradition du Bildungsroman." *Comparative Literature* 21, 97–115.

Jouhaud, Michel. 1992. "Bergson et la création de soi par soi." *Etudes philosophiques,* no. 2, 196–215.

Journet, Charles. 1925. *L'esprit du protestantisme en Suisse.* Paris: Nouvelle Librairie Nationale.

Jouve, Pierre-Jean. 1920. *Romain Rolland vivant, 1914–1919.* Paris: P. Ollendorf.

Jung, Carl Gustav. 1907. *The Psychology of Dementia Praecox.* In Jung, *Collected Works,* vol. 3: *The Psychogenesis of Mental Disease.* Trans. R. F. C. Hull. Princeton: Princeton University Press, 1960/1989.

—— 1910. "The Association Method." In Jung, *Collected Works,* vol. 2: *Experi-*

mental Researches. Trans. L. Stein. Princeton: Princeton University Press, 1973/ 1990.

———— 1911. "On the Doctrine of Complexes." In Jung, *Collected Works,* vol. 2 (see Jung, 1910).

———— 1963. *Memories, Dreams, Reflections.* Ed. A. Jaffé, trans. R. and C. Winston. New York: Random House/Vintage Books.

Junod, Emmanuel. 1923. "Les étapes de la Société d'Histoire." In *Nouvelles étrennes neuchâteloises.*

Juvet, Gustave. ms. 1913. "Le transformisme." Presented 13 February. PCAN, no. 596.

———— ms. 1914. "Le finalisme." Presented 26 February. PCAN, no. 623.

———— ms. 1915a. "La tendance néo-darwinienne en Biologie." Presented 29 April. PCAN, unnumbered.

———— ms. 1915b. "Langage et précision." Presented 9 December. PCAN, no. 666.

Käppeli, Anne-Marie. 1990. *Sublime croisade. Ethique et politique du féminisme protestant, 1875–1928.* Geneva: Zoé.

Kaye, Kenneth. 1980. "Piaget's Forgotten Novel." *Psychology Today,* November, 102.

Kesselring, Thomas. 1988. *Jean Piaget.* Munich: C. H. Beck.

Kimler, William C. 1983. "Mimicry: Views of Naturalists and Ecologists before the Modern Synthesis." In M. Grene, ed., *Dimensions of Darwinism: Themes and Counterthemes in Twentieth-Century Evolutionary Theory.* Cambridge: Cambridge University Press; Paris: Maison des Sciences de l'Homme.

Kolakowski, Leszek. 1985. *Bergson.* New York: Oxford University Press.

Kurtz, Hans Rudolf. 1970. *Dokumente der Grenzbesetzung 1914–1918.* Frauenfeld and Stuttgart: Verlag Huber.

Lademacher, Horst, ed. 1967. *Die Zimmerwalder Bewegung. Protokolle und Korrespondenz.* 2 vols. Paris and The Hague: Mouton.

La Vergata, Antonello. 1985. "Guerre, biologie et évolution." In P. Viallaneix and J. Ehrard, eds., *La bataille, l'armée et la gloire.* Clermont-Ferrand: Association des Publications de Clermont II.

———— In press. "Biology and War, 1870–1918." *Nuncius. Annali di storia della scienza* 10.

Le Dantec, Félix. 1896. *Théorie nouvelle de la vie.* Paris: Alcan.

———— 1899a. "Les néo-darwiniens et l'hérédité des caractères acquis." *Revue philosophique* 47, 1–41.

———— 1899b. *Lamarckiens et Darwiniens.* Paris: Alcan.

———— 1906. *La lutte universelle.* Paris: Flammarion.

———— 1907. *De l'homme à la science. Philosophie du XXe siècle.* Paris: Flammarion.

———— 1908. *Science et conscience. Philosophie du XXe siècle.* Paris: Flammarion.

———— 1912a. *Contre la métaphysique. Questions de méthode.* Paris: Alcan.

———— 1912b. *L'égoïsme, base de toute société. Etude des déformations résultant de la vie en commun.* Paris: Flammarion.

———— 1912c. *La science de la vie.* Paris: Flammarion.

Lejeune, Philippe. 1971. *L'autobiographie en France.* Paris: Colin.

Léonard, Emile G. 1964. *Histoire générale du protestantisme.* Vol. 3. Paris: Presses Universitaires de France.

Le Roy, Edouard. 1899–1900. "Science et philosophie." *Revue de métaphysique et de morale* 7, 375–425, 503–562, 706–731; 8, 37–72.

———— 1907. *Dogme et critique.* Paris: Bloud.

Liniger, Jean. 1980. *En toute subjectivité. Cent ans de conquêtes démocratiques locales et régionales, 1880–1980.* Neuchâtel: Messeiller.

López Piñero, José M. 1983. *Historical Origins of the Concept of Neurosis.* Trans. D. Berrios. Cambridge: Cambridge University Press.

Lovejoy, Arthur. 1936. *The Great Chain of Being.* Cambridge, Mass.: Harvard University Press. Various reprints.

Lurie, Edward. 1960. *Louis Agassiz: A Life in Science.* Chicago: University of Chicago Press.

———— 1974. *Nature and the American Mind: Louis Agassiz and the Culture of Science.* New York: Science History Publications.

Lutz, Tom. 1991. *American Nervousness, 1903: An Anecdotal History.* Ithaca: Cornell University Press.

Marcacci, Marco. 1986. "Statistiques retrospectives, 1825–1985." In *Dies Academicus 1986.* Geneva: University of Geneva.

Margot, W[illy]. 1913. "Qu'est-ce que l'Association?" *Nouvelles de l'Association Chrétienne Suisse d'Etudiants* 4 (3), 86–90.

Maritain, Jacques. 1913. *La philosophie bergsonienne. Etudes critiques.* Paris: P. Téqui, 1948.

Martin, Jean-François. 1976. "Les socialistes chrétiens de Suisse romande, 1910–1976." Mémoire de licence en théologie, University of Lausanne.

Martin, Jean-Michel. 1986. *Pierre Bovet, l'homme du seuil. Sa position par rapport à la pédagogie, à la psychanalyse et à la psychologie religieuse.* Cousset: Del Val.

Marx, Karl, and Friedrich Engels. 1848. *Manifesto of the Communist Party.* Excerpts in Marx and Engels, *On Religion.* New York: Schocken Books, 1971.

Mattmüller, Markus. 1957–1968. *Leonhard Ragaz une die religiöse Sozialismus. Eine Biographie.* 2 vols. Zollikon: Evangelischer Verlag.

Mauriac, François. 1926. *Le jeune homme.* Paris: Hachette.

Maury, Léon. 1892. *Le réveil religieux dans l'Eglise réformée à Genève et en France (1810–1850). Etude historique et dogmatique.* 2 vols. Paris: Fischbacher.

Mayr, Ernst. 1976. *Evolution and the Diversity of Life: Selected Essays.* Cambridge, Mass.: Harvard University Press.

McLaughlin, Judith A., ed. 1988. *Bibliography of the Works of Jean Piaget in the Social Sciences.* Lanham, Md.: University Press of America.

Mémoire Juvet: A la mémoire de Gustave Juvet, 1896–1936. Lausanne: University of Lausanne, 1937.

Mermod, Gaston. 1930. *Gastéropodes. Catalogue des invertébrés de la Suisse,* vol. 18. Geneva: Muséum d'Histoire Naturelle.

Meystre, P[ierre] E[rnest]. 1980. "Quelques souvenirs de Jean Piaget." *Feuille d'avis de Neuchâtel,* 19 September. Also in *Hommage à Jean Piaget,* 32.

Miéville, Henri-L. 1956. "Société romande de philosophie. Rapport du président." *RTP* 6, 3d ser., 280–284.

Monastier, Hélène. 1916. "Nouvelles des groupes socialistes-chrétiens suisses." *L'espoir du monde* 9 (5) (May), 44–47.

———— 1918. "Réponse des socialistes chrétiens." *L'Essor,* 19 January, 1–2.

Monod, Wilfred. 1908. *"Que ton règne vienne!" Essai de catéchisme évangélique*. 2d ed. Paris: Fischbacher.

———— 1914a. *Comment on devient chrétien social ou même socialiste chrétien*. Lausanne: La Concorde.

———— 1914b. *Aux croyants et aux athées*. 3d ed. Paris: Fischbacher.

———— ms. 1915. Letter to J. Piaget. Paris, 28 May. Arthur Piaget Papers, ms. 2103 2^n, Bibliothèque Publique et Universitaire, Neuchâtel.

———— 1915a. *Le manifeste des quatre-vingt-treize (Un cas psychologique)*. Paris: Fischbacher.

———— 1915b. *Vers l'Evangile, sous la nuée de guerre. Courtes méditations pour commencer chaque semaine*. 2 vols. Paris: Fischbacher.

———— 1919. "Après la victoire." In J.-E. Roberty, W. Monod, and J. Viénot, *Victoire et délivrance*. Paris: Fischbacher.

———— 1929. *La nuée de témoins*. 2 vols. Paris: Fischbacher.

———— 1938. *Après la journée, 1867–1937 (Souvenirs et visions)*. Paris: B. Grasset.

Monvert, Charles. 1898. *Histoire de la fondation de l'Eglise évangélique neuchâteloise indépendante de l'état*. Neuchâtel: Attinger.

Mossé-Bastide, Rose Marie. 1959. *Bergson et Plotin*. Paris: Presses Universitaires de France.

Muralt, André de. 1966. *Philosophes en Suisse française*. Neuchâtel: La Baconnière.

Murchison, Carl, ed. 1930. *A History of Psychology in Autobiography*. Vol. 1. Worcester, Mass.: Clark University Press.

Murisier, P. 1930. "Professeur Dr Henri Blanc, 1859–1930." *Actes de la Société Helvétique des Sciences Naturelles*, 487–492.

Nakhimovsky, Alexander D., and Alice Stone, eds. 1985. *The Semiotics of Russian Cultural History: Essays by Iurii M. Lotman, Lidiia Ia. Ginsburg, and Boris A. Uspenskii*. Ithaca: Cornell University Press.

Neeser, Maurice. 1917. *La théologie des Eglises et de l'Evangile à la lumière des événements actuels*. Lausanne: La Concorde.

Neubauer, John. 1992. *The Fin-de-Siècle Culture of Adolescence*. Cambridge, Mass.: Harvard University Press.

[Nicod, Gustave]. 1915. Review of Jeannet (1914). *Jeunesse* 62, 29.

———— 1916. Review of Piaget (1915a). *Jeunesse* 63, 36.

North, Marcel. 1960. *Neuchâtel, petite ville rangée*. Neuchâtel: Ides et Calendes.

Notre Association. Par quelques-uns des nôtres. Lausanne: La Concorde, 1913.

Nouvelle histoire de la Suisse et des suisses. 3 vols. 2d ed., 1 vol., 1986. Lausanne: Payot, 1982–83.

Nouvelles étrennes neuchâteloises. Neuchâtel: Imp. J. Guinchard, 1923.

O'Brien, Justin. 1937. *The Novel of Adolescence in France: The Study of a Literary Theme*. New York: Columbia University Press.

Olney, James. 1972. *Metaphors of Self: The Meaning of Autobiography*. Princeton: Princeton University Press.

———— 1980a. "Autobiography and the Cultural Moment: A Thematic, Historical, and Bibliographical Introduction." In Olney (1980b).

————, ed. 1980b. *Autobiography: Essays Theoretical and Critical*. Princeton: Princeton University Press.

Oppenheim, Janet. 1991. *"Shattered Nerves": Doctors, Patients, and Depression in Victorian England*. New York: Oxford University Press.

Pascal, Roy. 1960. *Design and Truth in Autobiography*. Cambridge, Mass.: Harvard University Press.

Paul, Harry. 1972. *The Sorcerer's Apprentice: The French Scientist's Image of German Science, 1840–1919*. Gainesville: University of Florida Press.

Le pays de Neuchâtel. 8 vols. Neuchâtel, 1948.

Perrenoud, J.-L. 1936. *Paul Pettavel. Pasteur, unioniste, journaliste*. Genèva: Labor.

Perrenoud, Marc. 1988. "De la 'Fédération jurasienne' à la 'commune socialiste.' Origines et débuts du parti socialiste neuchâtelois (1885–1912)." In C. Cantini et al., *Les origines du socialisme en Suisse romande*. Lausanne: Association pour l'Etude du Mouvement Ouvrier.

Perriraz, Louis. 1961. *Histoire de la théologie réformée française (de Calvin à la fin du XIXe siècle)*. Vol. 4: *Histoire de la théologie protestante au XIXe siècle*. Neuchâtel: Messeiller.

Perrochet, Edouard. 1914. *Etude sur la Chronique des Chanoines de Neuchâtel*. Neuchâtel: Attinger. Against A. Piaget (1896).

Perrot, Charles. 1979. *Jésus et l'histoire*. Paris: Desclée.

Pettavel, Paul. ms. 1915. Letter to J. Piaget, 31 December. AJP.

———— 1916a. Review of Piaget (1915b). *L'Essor*, 29 January, 3.

———— 1916b. "Aux jeunes." *Supplément de L'Essor. Coin des jeunes*, no. 1, 5 February.

———— 1916c. "Contre-sommation (réponse aux jeunes)." *L'Essor*, 25 March, 1.

———— 1916d. "Vous exagérez! Aux jeunes." *L'Essor*, 1 April, 1.

———— 1918a. "Il vaudrait mieux s'entendre (A nos amis socialistes-chrétiens)." *L'Essor*, 5 January, 2–3.

———— 1918b. "Réplique du rédacteur de *L'Essor*." *L'Essor*, 9 January, 1. Reply to Monastier (1918).

P. F. 1923. Report on the meeting. In *Sainte-Croix 1922*. Lausanne: La Concorde.

Pfister, Oskar. 1920. "Jean Piaget: La psychanalyse et la pédagogie." *Imago* 6, 294–295. Review of Piaget (1920b). French translation by J. Moll, *Le Bloc-notes de la psychanalyse* 1 (1980), 89–92.

Piaget, Arthur. 1896. *La Chronique des Chanoines de Neuchâtel*. Neuchâtel: Imp. Wolfrath.

———— 1917. "Histoire d'une promesse." In *Cinquantenaire*.

———— 1935. *Pages d'histoire neuchâteloise*. Neuchâtel: Société d'Histoire et d'Archéologie.

Piaget, Rebecca. 1914a. "Une visite aux réfugiés de Thonon et Evian." *Feuille d'avis de Neuchâtel*, 27 October, 3–4.

———— 1914b. "A propos de quelques soeurs de la Croix-Rouge allemande." *Feuille d'avis de Neuchâtel*, 12 December, 6.

Picot, Albert. 1920. "Théodore Flournoy, médecin de l'âme." *La semaine littéraire*, 11 December, 582–584.

Pictet, Arnold. 1918. "Professeur Dr. Emile Yung (1854–1918)." *Actes de la Société Helvétique des Sciences Naturelles*, 143–158.

———— 1925. *Emile Yung (1854–1918). L'influence de son oeuvre sur la science de son époque*. Geneva: Imp. Centrale.

———— 1928. "Dr. Maurice Bedot. 1859–1927." *Actes de la Société Helvétique des Sciences Naturelles*, 3–13.

Pilkington, A. E. 1976. *Bergson and His Influence: A Reassessment*. Cambridge: Cambridge University Press.

Poujol, P. 1965. "Bio-bibliographie du Christianisme Social. IV. Le pasteur Wilfred Monod." *Christianisme social* 73, 199–209.

Programme des cours du gymnase cantonale de Neuchâtel. Annual brochure. Neuchâtel: Attinger.

Quartier-la-Tente, Edouard. 1898. *Le district de Neuchâtel*, vol. 2 of Quartier-la-Tente, ed., *Le canton de Neuchâtel. Revue historique et monographique des communes du canton, de l'origine à nos jours*. Neuchâtel: Attinger.

Rambert, Eugène. 1875. *Alexandre Vinet. Histoire de sa vie et de ses ouvrages*. Lausanne: G. Bridel.

Reardon, Bernard M. G. 1966. *Religious Thought in the Nineteenth Century, Illustrated from Writers of the Period*. Cambridge: Cambridge University Press.

———— 1968. *Liberal Protestantism*. London: Adam and Charles Black.

Revilliod, Pierre. 1928. "Maurice Bedot. 1859–1927." *Revue suisse de zoologie* 35, 1–16.

Rey, Abel. 1908. *La philosophie moderne*. Paris: Flammarion.

———— 1909. "Vers le positivisme absolu." *Revue philosophique* 67, 461–479.

Reymond, Arnold. 1900. *Essai sur le subjectivisme et le problème de la connaissance religieuse*. Thèse de licence, Faculté de Théologie de l'Eglise Libre du Canton de Vaud. Lausanne: G. Bridel.

———— 1903. "La notion de mystère dans les sciences et dans la religion chrétienne." In *Sainte-Croix 1903*. Lausanne: La Concorde.

———— 1905. "Sciences et philosophie religieuse." *RTP* 38, 5–17.

———— 1908. *Logique et mathématiques. Essai historique et critique sur le nombre infini*. Ph.D. diss., University of Geneva. Saint-Blaise: Foyer Solidariste.

———— 1910. "Science et religion." *Feuille centrale de Zofingue* 50, 551–567.

———— 1913a. *La philosophie de M. Bergson et le problème de la raison*. Lausanne: La Concorde. Inaugural lesson at the University of Neuchâtel, 18 April. Also in *RTP* 1, n.s., 329–343.

———— 1913b. "La notion de miracle et son importance." *RTP* 1, n.s., 112–124.

———— 1913c. *Vérité scientifique et vérité religieuse*. Lausanne: La Concorde. Also in *Sainte-Croix 1913*. Lausanne: La Concorde, 18–38.

———— ms. 1914. Letter to J. Piaget. Vauseyon (Neuchâtel), 14 July. AJP.

———— 1914. "Lois scientifiques et réalités spirituelles." *RTP* 2, n.s., 178–190.

———— 1918a. *Le protestantisme et ses caractères objectifs*. Lausanne: La Concorde. Also in *Sainte-Croix 1917*. Lausanne: La Concorde, 31–60.

———— 1918b. "A propos d'une 'recherche.'" Review of Piaget (1918a). *La semaine littéraire*, 23 November, 550–551.

———— 1919. "La question des confessions de foi." *RTP* 7, n.s., 140–141.

———— 1921. "Flournoy, logicien et philosophe." *RTP* 9, n.s., 246–270.

———— 1929. "Transcendance et Immanence." *Cahiers Protestants* 13, 161–170. Critique of Piaget (1928a); followed by Piaget's reply (1929c) and a short response by Reymond, 331–333.

———— 1931. "La pensée philosophique en Suisse romande de 1900 à nos jours." *RTP* 19, n.s., 364–377. With a "Post-Scriptum" on Reymond by Piaget, 377–379.

———— 1937. Memorial statement about Gustave Juvet. *RTP* 25, n.s., 42–44.

———— 1945. Speech. In *Inauguration du buste de M. Arnold Reymond . . . le 16 décembre 1944*. Lausanne: F. Rouge.

———— 1950. "L'épistémologie génétique selon Jean Piaget." *Studia Philosophica* 10, 153–163.

Reymond, Arnold, and René Guisan. 1902. "A propos des confessions de foi." *RTP* 35, 37–49.

———— 1904. *La confession de foi de l'Eglise libre du canton de Vaud.* Moudon: Imp. de l'Eveil.

Reymond, Bernard. 1990. *A la redécouverte d'Alexandre Vinet.* Lausanne: L'Age d'Homme.

Reymond, Maurice. 1913. "Convalescence. Rapport du groupe gymnasien de Neuchâtel." *Nouvelles de l'Association Chrétienne Suisse d'Etudiants* 4 (2), 51–52.

Ritter, William. 1891. *Aegyptiacque.* Paris: A. Savine.

Rolland, Romain. 1903–1912. *Jean-Christophe.* 10 vols. Paris: P. Ollendorf.

———— 1913. *Vie de Tolstoï.* Paris: Hachette.

———— 1914. "Au-dessus de la mêlée." In Albertini (1971).

———— 1917. "Tolstoy: L'esprit libre." *Les Tablettes,* no. 9, 3–4 (special issue on Tolstoy). Also in Albertini (1971).

———— 1952. *Journal des années de guerre, 1914–1919.* Paris: Albin Michel.

Romanes, George John. 1897. *Darwin, and after Darwin,* vol. 3. Chicago: Open Court.

Rossel, Virgile. 1903. *Histoire littéraire de la Suisse romande des origines à nos jours.* Neuchâtel: F. Zahn.

Rossetti, Etienne. ms. 1913. "Scientistes et pragmatistes." Presented 6 November. PCAN, no. 613.

———— ms. 1914. "L'évolution et la théorie des mutations." Presented 26 March. PCAN, no. 629.

Roszkowski, Wacław. 1912. "Notes sur les Limnées de la faune profonde du lac Léman." *Zoologischer Anzeiger* 40, 375–381.

———— ms. 1912. Letter to J. Piaget, 12 December. AJP.

———— ms. 1913a. Letter to J. Piaget, Lausanne, 17 May. AJP.

———— ms. 1913b. Letter to J. Piaget, Lausanne, 23 May. AJP.

———— 1913. "A propos des Limnées de la faune profonde du lac Léman." *Zoologischer Anzeiger* 43, 88–90.

———— 1914. "Contribution à l'étude des Limnées du lac Léman." *Revue suisse de zoologie* 22, 457–539.

———— 1915. "Les coquilles de Limnaea ovata Drap." *Comptes-rendus de la Société des Sciences de Varsovie* 8, 386–388. French summary of a Polish text.

———— 1922. "Contributions à l'étude de la famille des *Lymnaeidae.*" *Disciplinarum Biologicarum Archivum Societatis Scientiarum Varsaviensis* 1. French summary of a Polish text.

Rougemont, Denis de. 1948. *Suite neuchâteloise.* Neuchâtel: Ides et Calendes.

Rougemont, Fritz [Frédéric] de. ms. 1915. Letter to J. Piaget, Lausanne, 16 October.

Arthur Piaget Papers, ms. 2103 2^r, Bibliothèque Publique et Universitaire, Neuchâtel.

——— 1921. "De Saint-Croix 1895 à Neuchâtel 1920." In *Conférence d'étudiants 1920*. Lausanne: La Concorde.

——— n.d. "L'appel des universités." In *Les ministères chrétiens. Union des étudiants volontaires pour les ministères chrétiens*. Lausanne: La Concorde.

Rt. 1941. "Ch[arles]-Daniel Junod. 1865–1941." *Le messager de l'Eglise neuchâteloise indépendante de l'état*, 2 December.

Ruchti, Jacob [et al.]. 1928–1930. *Geschichte der Schweiz während des Weltkrieges 1914–1919*. 2 vols. Bern: P. Haupt.

Ruffieux, Roland. 1969. *Le mouvement chrétien-social en Suisse romande, 1891–1949*. Fribourg: Ed. Universitaires.

——— 1974. *La Suisse de l'entre-deux-guerres*. Lausanne: Payot.

Sabatier, Auguste. 1880. "Jésus-Christ." In F. Lichtenberger, ed., *Dictionnaire des sciences religieuses*. Vol. 7. Paris: Sandoz and Fischbacher.

——— 1897. *Esquisse d'une philosophie de la religion d'après la psychologie et l'histoire*. Paris: Fischbacher. Abridged trans. by T. A. Seed: *Outlines of a Philosophy of Religion Based on Psychology and History*. London: Hodder and Stoughton, n.d.

——— 1899. *The Apostle Paul: A Sketch of the Development of His Doctrine*. Trans. A. M. Hellier. London: Hodder and Stoughton.

——— 1904. *Religions of Authority and the Religion of the Spirit*. Trans. L. S. Houghton. New York: McClure, Phillips.

Schepeler, Eva M. 1993. "Jean Piaget's Experiences on the Couch: Some Clues to a Mystery." *International Journal of Psycho-Analysis* 74, 255–273.

Schmidt, Lucie. 1913. "Un témoignage." *Nouvelles de l'Association Chrétienne Suisse d'Etudiants* 4 (3), 90–95.

——— 1915. Report of the Neuchâtel group. *Nouvelles de l'Association Chrétienne Suisse d'Etudiants* 5 (5), 133–135.

Schmitt, Ariane. 1980. *L'Essor, 1905–1980. Un journal de précurseurs*. La-Chaux-de-Fonds: L'Essor.

Schnegg, Alfred. 1953. "Arthur Piaget, 1865–1952." *Revue suisse d'histoire* 3, 119–123.

Schweitzer, Albert. 1913. *The Quest of the Historical Jesus*. Trans. W. Montgomery. New York: Macmillan, 1968.

Schweizerische Hochschulstatistik, 1890–1935. Bern: Eidgenösisches Statistisches Amt, 1935.

Seiler, D.-L., and René Knüssel, eds. 1989. *Vous avez dit Suisse romande?* Lausanne: Editions 24 Heures.

Seippel, Paul, ed. 1899–1901. *La Suisse au XIXe siècle*. 3 vols. Lausanne: Payot.

——— 1912. *Adèle Kamm*. Lausanne: Payot.

Sérieux, P[aul], and J. Capgras. 1909. *Les folies raisonnantes. Le délire d'interprétation*. Paris: Alcan.

Sheets-Pyenson, Susan. 1990. "New Directions for Scientific Biography: The Case of Sir William Dawson." *History of Science* 28, 399–410.

Shore, Miles F. 1981. "Biography in the 1980s: A Psychoanalytic Perspective." *Journal of Interdisciplinary History* 12, 89–113.

Shortland, Michael. 1988. "Exemplary Lives: A Study of Scientific Autobiographies." *Science and Public Policy* 15, 170–179.

Söderqvist, Thomas. Forthcoming. "Should Science Biography Be an Edifying Genre? Towards an Existential Approach to Science Biography." In R. Yeo and M. Shortland, eds., *Telling Lives in Science: Studies of Scientific Biography*. New York: Cambridge University Press.

Sokal, Michael M. 1990. "Life Span Developmental Psychology and the History of Science." In *Beyond History of Science: Essays in Honor of Robert E. Schofield*. Bethlehem, Pa.: Lehigh University Press.

Spearman, Charles. 1930. "Autobiography." In Murchison (1930).

Starobinski, Jean. 1966. "The Idea of Nostalgia." *Diogenes,* no. 54, 81–103.

——— 1970a. "The Style of Autobiography." In Olney (1980b).

——— 1970b. "L'écart romanesque." In *Jean-Jacques Rousseau. La transparence et l'obstacle.* Paris: Gallimard, coll. Tel, 1971.

Starr, William Thomas. 1956. *Romain Rolland and a World at War.* Reprint, New York: AMS Press, 1971.

Statuts de l'Association Chrétienne Suisse d'Etudiants et reglément de la branche romande. Lausanne: La Concorde, 1911.

Steiner, Andreas. 1964. *"Das nervöse Zeitalter." Der Begriff der Nervosität bei Laien und Ärtzen in Deutschland und Österreich um 1900.* Zurich: Juris.

Sublet, Paul. 1911. *Idéal spirituel et préoccupations économiques.* Saint-Blaise: Foyer Solidariste. Lecture given at Sainte-Croix, 1910.

——— 1914. *La situation sociale en Suisse.* Lausanne: La Concorde.

Suleiman, Susan. 1979. "La structure d'apprentissage. *Bildungsroman* et roman à thèse." *Poétique* 10, 24–42.

Sulloway, Frank J. 1979. "Geographic Isolation in Darwin's Thinking: The Vicissitudes of a Crucial Idea." *Studies in the History of Biology* 3, 23–65.

Toepffer, Rodolphe. 1858. *Nouveaux voyages en zigzag.* Paris: Garnier.

Traz, Robert de. 1934. *Les "heures de silence."* Paris: Bernard Grasset.

Tribolet, Maurice de. 1899. *Le mouvement scientifique à Neuchâtel au XIXe siècle.* Neuchâtel: Attinger.

——— 1905. *L'Académie d'hier et l'Académie d'aujourd'hui. Coup d'oeil sur le développement de l'enseignement supérieur à Neuchâtel.* Neuchâtel: Attinger.

Trombetta, Carlo. 1976. *Edouard Claparède. La famiglia. L'infanzia. Gli studi. Bibliografia.* Rome: Bulzoni.

——— 1989. *Edouard Claparède psicologo.* Rome: Armando.

Trouessart, E[douard-Louis]. 1898. "Mimétisme." In *La Grande Encyclopédie,* vol. 23.

Valéry, Paul. 1930–31. *Cahiers.* 2 vols. Paris: Gallimard, 1973.

——— 1960. *Oeuvres.* 2 vols. Paris: Gallimard.

Vallette, Pierre. 1929. *La cité douloureuse. (Croquis de Leysin).* Geneva: Jullien.

Vandenberg, Brian. 1991. "Piaget and the Death of God." *Theory and Philosophy of Psychology* 11, 35–42.

Vander Goot, Mary. 1985. *Piaget as a Visionary Thinker.* Bristol, Ind.: Wyndham Hall Press.

——— 1986. Reply to Elkind (1986a). *Contemporary Psychology* 31, 1010.

Verzeichnis der Vorlesungen an der Universität Zürich in Wintersemester 1918/1919. Zurich: Aschmann & Scheller, 1918. Includes lists of courses, professors, and students.

Vidal, Fernando. 1984. "*La vanité de la nomenclature*. Un manuscrit inédit de Jean Piaget." *History and Philosophy of the Life Sciences* 6, 75–106.

———— 1986a. "Jean Piaget et la psychanalyse: Premières rencontres." *Le Bloc-notes de la psychanalyse* 6, 171–189.

———— 1986b. "'I would eagerly leave Neuchâtel . . .' A 1912 letter by Jean Piaget." *Journal of the History of the Behavioral Sciences* 22, 23–26.

———— 1988. "Piaget adolescent, 1907–1915." Ph.D. diss., University of Geneva.

———— 1992. "Jean Piaget's Early Critique of Mendelism: 'La notion de l'espèce suivant l'école mendélienne' (A 1913 Manuscript)." *History and Philosophy of the Life Sciences* 14, 113–135.

———— In press (a). "Piaget poète. Avec deux sonnets oubliés de 1918." *Archives de psychologie*.

———— In press (b). "'Les mystères de la douleur divine.' Une prière du jeune Jean Piaget pour l'année 1916." *RTP*.

Virieux-Reymond, Antoinette, Robert Blanché, Gabriel Widmer, and Fernand Brunner. 1956. *Arnold Reymond*. Turin: Ed. de "Filosofia."

Visages du pays de Neuchâtel. Cahiers de l'Institut Neuchâtelois, vol. 16. Neuchâtel, 1973.

Vonèche, Jacques. 1992. "La première théorie de l'équilibre de Jean Piaget (1918)." *Cahiers de la Fondation Jean Piaget* 12, 11–29.

Vries, Hugo de. 1906. *Species and Varieties: Their Origin by Mutation*. 2d ed. Chicago: Open Court.

Vuilleumier, Marc. 1977. "La grève générale de 1918 en Suisse." In Marc Vuilleumier et al., *La grève générale de 1918 en Suisse*. Geneva: Gronauer.

Vuilleumier, Maurice. 1913. "L'instruction religieuse des catéchumènes en face des exigences actuelles." *RTP* 1, n.s., 125–143.

Wagner, Moritz. 1882. *De la formation des espèces par la ségrégation*. Paris: O. Doin.

Warnery, Renée. 1917. *Via Crucis*. Lausanne: La Concorde.

Wavre, Rolin. 1937. "Gustave Juvet, le mathématicien et l'ami." In *Mémoire Juvet* (1937).

Weber, Max. 1905. "Critical Studies in the Logic of the Cultural Sciences." In E. A. Shils and H. A. Finch, eds., *Max Weber on the Methodology of the Social Sciences*. Glencoe, Ill.: Free Press, 1949.

Weck, René de. 1912. *La vie littéraire dans la Suisse française*. Paris: Fontemoing.

Weintraub, Karl J. 1978. *The Value of the Individual: Self and Circumstance in Autobiography*. Chicago: University of Chicago Press.

Welch, Claude. 1972. *Protestant Thought in the Nineteenth Century: 1799–1870*. New Haven: Yale University Press.

———— 1985. *Protestant Thought in the Nineteenth Century: 1870–1914*. New Haven: Yale University Press.

Williams, L. Pearce. 1991. "The Life of Science and Scientific Lives." *Physis* 28, 199–213.

Wohl, Robert. 1979. *The Generation of 1914*. Cambridge, Mass.: Harvard University Press.

Wyler, Roger. 1917. "A propos de la vie religieuse de nos Associations." *Nouvelles de l'Association Chrétienne Suisse d'Etudiants* 7 (3), 67–70.

Young, Robert M. 1988. "Biography: The Basic Discipline for Human Science." *Free Associations* 11, 108–130.

Yung, Emile. 1904. "Discours prononcé par le Prof. Emile Yung, président d'honneur, au banquet de la Société zoologique de France." *Bulletin de la Société Zoologique de France* 29, 40–46.

——— 1917. "Les variations de la coquille d'Helix pomatia." *Archives des sciences physiques et naturelles* (Geneva) 44, 74–75.

Zeldin, Theodore. 1977. *France 1848–1945*. 2 vols. Vol. 2: *Intellect, Taste and Anxiety*. Oxford: Clarendon Press.

Zobrist, T. ms. 1913a. Letter to J. Piaget. Porrentruy, 14 July. AJP.

——— ms. 1913b. Letter to J. Piaget. Porrentruy, 1 September. AJP.

Index

Absolute: theory of, 55, 56, 126, 128, 129, 143, 190; humanity, 135, 136, 169–170, 203; moral, 144, 146; ideal, 187; value, 187, 188, 190, 192, 201, 202, 204, 210

Abyssal (deep-water) fauna, 39, 40, 41. *See also Limnaea*: deep-water

Acclimatization, 37–38

Acquired characteristics, 216–217, 226

ACSE. *See* Swiss Christian Students' Association

Action, concept of, 171–172, 173

Adaptation, 1, 2, 25, 56, 63, 88; evolution and, 37–40, 67; biometric approach to, 38; environment and, 39–40, 42, 226; direct, 40, 69, 70; mimicry and, 64; active and passive, 65, 70, 88, 131, 147, 172, 224; and intelligence, 227

Adaptation and Intelligence (Piaget), 227

Aesthetics, 200, 201, 202

Agassiz, Louis, 17, 18, 25

"Albino Sparrow" (Piaget), 8

Altruism, 200, 212–213, 217

Amiel, Henri-Frédéric, 104

Analysis, 55, 61. *See also* Intuition

Anatomy, 74, 81

Anti-intellectualism, 54, 127, 207–208

Aristotle, 89, 201

Arms race, 147, 232

Assimilation, 197, 198, 215, 216, 217, 223, 227

Atheism, 191

Autism and autistic thinking, 200, 201, 206, 209–210, 211, 212

Autobiographical pact, 6–7

Autobiography (Piaget's), 5–9; religion in, 52, 113–114, 119; psychology in, 91

Autonomy, 202, 210, 211. *See also* Individuality

Barrès, Maurice, 111, 112, 188

Barth, Karl, 95

Bates, Henry Walter, 62

Beauty, concept of, 201, 205, 212

Bedot, Maurice, 34, 35–36, 37

Behavior and Evolution (Piaget), 227

Belgium, 148

Benda, Julian, 55

Bergson, Henri, 46–47, 61, 223; influence on Piaget, 2, 7, 8, 32, 33, 49–52, 54, 57, 58, 62, 65–67, 69–71, 78, 83–86, 90–92, 113, 114, 120, 127, 198, 224; life and work, 54–56; on duration, 59, 68, 69, 70, 128, 214, 226; on science and metaphysics, 59–60, 72–73; on evolution, 84–85, 144, 145; on Lamarckism, 88; on genera, 88–89, 90; on religion, 92, 110, 120, 173; influence on generation of 1914, 110; Piaget's break with, 123–124; Piaget, Sabatier, and, 127–131; on *élan vital*, 128–129; on God, 130–131

"Bergson and Sabatier" (Piaget), 123, 124, 127–128, 130, 145, 150, 172

Bersot, Henri, 14, 15

Bildungsroman, 165, 166, 173, 184–185, 190

Binet, Alfred, 225

Biography, 3–5

Biology, 47, 87, 195, 197; Piaget's study of and work in, 1–2, 23, 37, 40–41, 57, 71, 89–91, 131, 196, 199, 226; adaptation and, 39, 40–

Biology *(cont.)*
  43; of species, 41, 78–79, 80; metaphysics
  and, 44; evolutionary, 48, 62; explanation of
  knowledge through, 52, 57; mechanistic, 66,
  129; equilibrium of, 200, 215
Biology and Knowledge (Piaget), 227
"Biology and Philosophy" (Piaget), 50
"Biology and War" (Piaget), 215, 217, 218
Blanc, Henri, 73, 74
Bleuler, Eugen, 206, 207, 209, 211, 212, 225
Bouglé, Célestin, 99
Bourget, Paul, 188
Bourguignat, Jules-René, 31
Boutroux, Emile, 102, 222–223
Bovet, Félix, 98
Bovet, Pierre, 16, 20–22, 101, 102, 105,
  107, 123, 222, 225, 228; as Piaget's mentor,
  96, 115; as director of Rousseau Institute,
  153
Breeding experiments, 67, 68, 81, 83
Breuer, Joseph, 211
Bringuier, Jean-Claude, 5, 183
Brunschvicg, Léon, 222, 229, 231
Buisson, Ferdinand, 127, 239n1

Capitalism, 98, 99, 100, 149
Catholicism, 54, 121, 185, 187, 188
Cendrars, Blaise, 11
Chance, concept of, 48
Chapman, Michael, 202
Characteristics: external, 24; fixed specific, 25,
  32–33; stability of, 28; hereditary, 31, 38, 48,
  72, 76; specific, 32; variability of, 32, 76, 80,
  82; acquired, 48, 69, 70; conchological, 72,
  75, 82
Child development, 1, 4, 7, 8, 224
Child psychology, 225, 228
Child's Conception of Physical Causality, The
  (Piaget), 230
Chopard, Wilfred, 221
Christ: in liberal Protestantism, 93–95; and
  Jesus, 143–144; as thinker's model, 193–
  194. *See also* Jesus
Christianity: social(ist), 98–100, 103, 112, 133,
  153, 154, 155, 156, 176, 177, 178; rebirth of,
  132, 140–142, 148, 159, 161, 202; Piaget on,
  134, 151
Christian Socialist Federation, 98, 176, 177
Chromosomes, 83, 145, 238n3
Church(es), 115–116, 139; Piaget's condemna-
  tion of, 140, 142, 149–150; ideal, 202
Claparède, Edouard, 101, 102, 153, 164
Classification of species, 20, 21, 24, 26, 43, 59;
  of mollusks, 2, 35, 72–81; by form, 29–30,

31, 40; by Piaget, 37, 90. *See also* Taxonomy
Clerc, Charly, 103–104, 105, 152
Collection of specimens, 20, 23, 24
Collège Latin, 16, 44
Communist Manifesto, The (Marx and Engels),
  100
Compayré, Gabriel, 106
Complexes, 210–213
Comte, Auguste, 55–56, 94, 192
Conscience: moral, 94–95, 98, 103, 104, 128,
  129, 142–143, 146; individual, 97–98, 120
Conscientious objectors, 153, 154, 180
Consciousness, 145; stream of, 55, 199; grasp
  of, 172–173, 181, 184, 231
Conservatism, 140, 144, 149, 200
Constructivism. *See* Epistemology
Continuity, 2, 7, 69; morphological, 30–32, 58,
  67; variability and, 30–32; continuous series
  of species, 31, 58; graduated notion of, 76,
  77–78; and discontinuity, 127
Continuous series method, 31–32
Conventionalism, 188
Conversion: spiritual, 95, 107, 116, 118, 119,
  140, 143, 190; Plotinian, 137, 170; of Piaget,
  141, 183
Cope, Edward Drinker, 227
Cornut, Samuel, 51–54, 99, 104, 184, 185
Creative Evolution (Bergson), 2, 49, 50, 54, 55,
  56, 88, 198, 226; life/matter theory in, 59,
  60; adaptation in, 65; influence on Piaget,
  57, 71, 72, 123, 127; on genera, 86–87; on
  immutability, 129; on consciousness, 145
Crisis, 112; inner/moral, 103–104, 107–108,
  222; religious, 116, 120, 162, 184; world,
  148, 152; in *Recherche*, 182, 190–194; conversion and, 183–184

Dardel, Otto de, 152–153, 157
Darwin, Charles/Darwinism, 3, 215, 217; the-
  ory of evolution, 25, 30–31, 62; species con-
  cept, 30, 32, 58, 68, 80; Lamarckism and,
  47, 48, 50; theory of natural selection, 48,
  62–68, 70, 80, 147, 172; neo-Darwinism, 50;
  mechanisms, 64–65, 70; Piaget's rejection
  of, 65, 144, 147; anti-Darwinism, 144
Deep-Water Fauna of Swiss Lakes, The (Forel),
  41
Delage, Yves, 48
De la Harpe, Jean, 96
Democracy, 171, 177
De Montherlant, Henry, 11
De Pourtalès, Guy, 11
De Rougemont, Denis, 12
De Traz, Robert, 165

De Vries, Hugo, 81
Diary (Piaget's), 185, 190
Discontinuity, 79–80, 82, 127
Disequilibrium, 210, 213
Distribution of species, 27, 38, 40
Dogma, 101, 118, 139, 141; Christian/religious, 93, 94, 102, 103, 120, 121, 127, 131, 134, 138–140; symbols as, 113–114; evolution of, 127, 128, 130; transformation of, 146
Doubt, 138, 189, 190–191, 208
Dream analysis, 203, 224
Duration: concept of, 55, 57, 60, 61, 69, 137; Bergsonian, 59, 68, 69, 70, 128, 214, 224, 226; Piaget and, 61–62, 69, 91; intuition of, 90, 128; as psychological process, 130, 172
Durkheim, Emile, 4, 241–242n1

Education: Piaget's, 16–17, 25; in *Recherche,* 202. *See also* Religious instruction
Ego, 208, 210–213, 231
Egocentrism, 229, 230–231
Egoism, 201
Elan vital, 49, 52, 54, 55, 57, 70, 145, 187; in creative evolution, 65, 66, 127; heredity and, 87; the idea and, 139
Environment, 217, 218, 226; influence on variability, 37, 38; adaptation and, 39–40, 42, 66, 75
Epistemology, 1, 7, 56, 91; Piaget's interest in, 2, 3, 4, 8, 60, 173, 216; constructivist, 173
Equilibration, 215
Equilibration of Cognitive Structures, The (Piaget), 226
Equilibrium/disequilibrium: concept of, 7, 89, 91, 149; in *Recherche,* 91, 182–184, 188, 191, 192, 193, 195, 211, 218; between parts and wholes, 179, 183, 195–197, 198–200, 212, 214; Piaget's theory of, 181, 194, 196, 197, 202, 203, 212, 216, 219, 222, 223, 225–226; ideal, 196, 200, 202, 212; psychology and, 196–197, 200, 230
Essential Piaget, The (Gruber and Vonèche), 8
Ethics, 118, 146, 147
Evangelicalism, 92–96, 105, 116, 153
Evans, Richard L., 5
Evil, 141, 144, 147, 162, 168–171, 212
Evolution, 7, 43, 48, 136, 171, 215; Piaget's theory of, 2, 39, 144, 146–147, 157, 227; variation in, 24, 30–31; Darwinian, 25, 30–31, 62; taxonomy and, 31, 32, 56, 58–59; adaptation and, 37–40; teleological theory of, 47, 49, 50; creative, 49, 50, 54, 57, 65, 66, 67, 70, 90–91, 123, 127, 131, 137, 145, 172,

224, 227; mechanistic theory of, 49, 50, 56; nominalism and, 57–62; gradual, 58, 79–80; Bergson's theory of, 84–85, 144, 145; probability of, 84, 85; biological, 127, 227; religious, 128, 130; symbolic, 143; as moral concept, 147; equilibrium and, 199

Faith, 93, 94, 96, 106, 120, 139, 229; science and, 102, 103, 110, 121, 122, 125, 182, 188, 189, 192, 202, 220–221, 222; metaphysics and, 138, 160–161, 200, 210; personal, 184, 201, 217–218; Piaget's, 188, 201–202. *See also* Religion
Fatherland, 143, 148, 151, 180. *See also* Nationalism
Federalism, 179, 202
Ferrière, Adolphe, 153, 222
Flournoy, Théodore, 101–102, 105, 107, 118, 125, 185, 206–208, 228, 229
Forel, François-Alphonse, 20, 41, 75–76, 77
Fouillée, Alfred, 50, 188, 241n1
France, 12, 53, 56, 62, 66, 83, 94; in World War I, 98–99
Freud, Sigmund, 206, 207, 211
Friends of Nature, 18, 19–20, 21, 24, 34, 45, 107; Piaget's participation in, 44, 62, 73, 152; philosophical debates, 46, 48, 50
Frommel, Gaston, 97, 98, 101
Fuhrmann, Otto, 20, 34–35, 36–37, 41

Gagnebin, Samuel, 220–221
Genera, science of, 86–89, 127, 197–198. *See also* Laws of science and nature
General strike of 1918, 13, 175
Genetics, 62, 66, 81, 83, 226
Genotype, 2, 37, 81, 226
Germany, 12, 53, 98–99, 155, 220
Gide, André, 11
Godet, Charles-Henri, 24
Godet, Paul, 16, 18, 20, 21, 73; Piaget and, 19, 23, 24, 25–27, 30, 32, 33, 35, 70; as Christian, 24–25; as taxonomist, 25, 27, 31, 32, 82
Godet, Philippe, 16, 21, 103, 115
God: for Sabatier, 47; proofs of existence, 113, 114, 118; for Bergson, 130–131; in *Mission of the Idea,* 142–144; in "Mysteries of Divine Suffering," 168–172; as thought, 173, 229; in *Recherche,* 193, 201–202
Good, concept of, 140, 141, 144, 146, 201, 215; evolution and, 147; in *Recherche,* 191, 200
Gospel(s), 154, 156, 160, 204
Gounelle, Elie, 99
Gruber, Howard, 3, 8, 132, 133, 217

Guillaume, Louis, 18, 19

Habits of species, 40–41, 42, 64
Hall, G. Stanley, 106–107
Hankins, Thomas, 3
Heredity, 24, 70, 84, 216; of characteristics, 31, 38, 80, 82–83
History, 134, 143, 229, 233
History of Psychology in Autobiography, A (Piaget), 5–6
Holmes, F. L., 3
"Hours of Silence," The (Traz), 165–166
Hubendick, Bengt, 79
Humanity, 156, 205, 208; absolute, 135, 136, 206; religion and, 140, 168–170, 171; and the Idea, 144; history of, 146; effect of war on, 173
Humbert-Droz, Jules, 176, 177

Idea, concept of, 156–158. *See also Mission of the Idea, The* (Piaget)
Ideal, 192, 197, 209, 214, 215, 221; vs. reality, 195, 210
Identity, personal, 161, 166–167, 194, 202, 215, 217
Illness, Piaget's, 162, 163–164, 165, 167, 179, 192. *See also* Mountain health resort at Leysin
Imitation, 215, 216, 217
Immanentism/immanence, 92, 93, 94, 96, 227, 228–229, 231, 232; Piaget's belief in, 162, 173
Individuality, 104, 180–181, 190, 202, 227; evolution and, 89; in theology, 93, 96, 97, 100; society and, 200–201, 203–204, 206, 210–211; equilibrium and, 203–204; loss of, 205
Insights and Illusions of Philosophy (Piaget), 5, 6, 57, 183
Instinct, 64, 65, 66, 146
Intellect and intelligence, 55, 57, 60, 61, 66, 125, 126, 127, 146, 152, 227; in *Recherche*, 187, 189
Introduction to Genetic Epistemology (Piaget), 8
Introspection, 94, 116, 183. *See also* Self
Intuition, 55, 57, 59–62, 128, 137, 221; religious, 93, 94; of the idea, 142–143; of duration, 199, 226
Isolation of species, 66–70; geographic, 67, 68, 70, 78, 79, 84, 90; of abyssal *Limnaea*, 76, 77, effect on migration, 83

James, William, 46–47, 55, 86, 101, 102, 199, 207
Janet, Pierre, 225

Jean Barois (Martin du Gard), 185
Jean-Christophe (Rolland), 106, 174, 184, 220
Jeannet, Pierre, 24, 180, 184, 185
Jesus, 141, 143–144, 153, 157, 159–160; mission of youth to follow, 107, 110, 132, 133, 134. *See also* Christ
Judgment and Reasoning in the Child (Piaget), 230
Jung, Carl Gustav, 206, 207, 212, 225
Junod, Charles-Daniel, 116, 118
Jura Club, 18–19, 24
Juvet, Gustave, 40, 83, 96; friendship with Piaget, 45, 47, 124; philosophical debates with Piaget, 46, 47, 48–50

Kant, Immanuel, 56, 93, 94, 97, 102, 118, 228, 229
Kinetogenesis, 227
Knowledge, 121, 129; biological theory of, 52, 57, 114; theory of life and, 60, 89; scientific vs. religious, 125, 188; of self, 173; reform of, 186; qualitative vs. quantitative, 200
Kropotkin, Peter, 147

Lake Annecy, France, 51–52
Lake Geneva, Switzerland, 35, 41, 72–81
Lake Neuchâtel, Switzerland, 25–26, 35, 41, 73, 78
Lamarckism/neo-Lamarckism, 35, 38, 62, 65; vs. Darwinism, 47, 48, 50, 68, 70; Piaget and, 63, 87–88; on acquired characteristics, 216–217
Language and Thought of the Child, The (Piaget), 230
Laws of science and nature, 86–87, 197, 223. *See also* Genera
Learned societies in Neuchâtel, 16, 17–21, 45
Le Dantec, Félix, 47, 48, 49, 65, 197, 198, 215, 216
LeGrand Roy, Eugène, 21
Lejeune, Philippe, 6
Lenin, V. I., 149
Le Roy, Edouard, 102
L'Essor journal, 153–154, 167, 177–178, 222
Leysin, Switzerland. *See* Mountain health resort at Leysin
Liberalism, 92–96, 121, 155, 184
Libido, 22, 214, 216
Life, 52, 129, 140, 215, 223; understanding of, through duration, 55, 61; /matter theory of evolution, 59–60; theory of knowledge and, 60; project, Piaget's, 132, 134–135, 145, 158, 161, 177, 202–203; the idea and, 139, 146; true life concept, 140–141, 144; struggle for,

146–148, 171, 215–216, 217; science of, 197; logic of, 214, 218

Limnaea, 25; variability, 26, 30; classification, 27, 41–42, 72–81, 84; number of species, 29; biology, 35, 41; adaptation, 37, 226, 227; deep-water, 39, 40, 41–42, 68, 72, 74–81, 84, 90; shallow-water, 39–40, 41–42, 74–81, 84

Limnology, 20, 35, 67, 78

Linnaean binominal system, 24, 28

Lipps, Gotthold-Friedrich, 224, 225

Logic, 8, 57, 188, 195, 201, 209, 214, 218, 228–231

Logico-mathematical structures, 8, 85, 86

Loosli, Carl-Albert, 20

Love, xii, 192–193, 216, 217; in *Recherche*, 191, 192, 208–209

Magic Mountain, The (Mann), 165

Malacology, 23, 26, 36, 38–39

Mann, Thomas, 165

Maritain, Jacques, 131

Martin du Gard, Roger, 185

Materialism, 105

Materialist reductionism, 49

Mathematics, 47–48, 57, 60, 125, 127, 196, 197, 223

Matter, 55, 56, 61, 65; inert, 57, 66, 70, 88; /life theory of evolution, 59–60

Matter and Memory (Bergson), 56, 88

Mauriac, François, 106

Mendel's laws/Mendelism, 48, 80; Piaget's criticism of, 81–85, 86, 90, 145

Metaphor, 137, 138, 147

Metaphysics, 172; biological, 44; intuition and, 55, 60; dualism of, 126–127; Piaget's, 132, 133–139, 147, 159, 160–161, 167, 168, 190, 201, 206, 208; faith and, 138, 160–161, 200, 210

Migration, 38, 67, 68, 75–79, 83

Mimicry, 2, 29, 62–66, 88; Piaget's discussion of, 63–65, 66, 70, 147, 172

Mission of the Idea, The (Piaget), 3, 7, 100, 111, 132–133, 168, 169, 179, 180, 200, 203, 231; metaphysics in, 133–139, 147, 160–161; religion in, 139–144; morality in, 144–150, 227; reform in, 149; local context of, 150–157; themes, 150–151; reviews and critical reception of, 152, 153, 154, 155, 157, 174; idea and life images in, 158–159; Gospels and, 160; truth concept, 172. *See also* God

Mollusk(s), 24, 33; taxonomy, 2, 23, 27–32, 226; morphology, 26, 72; variation, 27, 28–

29, 30–32; mimicry in, 62, 64. *See also* *Limnaea*

Monastier, Hélène, 178

Monod, Wilfred, 100, 118–119, 132, 171; critique of Piaget, 155–157

Moral enterprise of Piaget, 3, 4, 7

Morality and moral conduct, 97, 102, 191–192, 231; conscience, 94–95, 98, 103; in literature, 103–104; religious, 118, 201; Piaget on, 135, 144–150, 161, 200–201; absolute, 144; science and, 161, 168, 201, 213–214, 223, 227; equilibrium and, 200, 212; individual, 212, 232; biological, 213; judgment, 232–233

Moral Judgment of the Child, The (Piaget), 231, 232

Morphology, 26, 28–30, 33, 39–40, 72, 74, 79, 226–227

Morsier, Auguste de, 153

Mott, John, 104

Mountain health resort at Leysin, 162–167, 168, 169, 178, 179, 185, 190, 191, 192, 193. *See also* Illness, Piaget's

Musée neuchâtelois journal, 18

Museum of Fine Arts, Neuchâtel, 16

Museum of Natural History, Neuchâtel, 20, 23, 32, 34

Music, 137, 142

Mutation. *See* Species: mutation of

"Mysteries of Divine Suffering, The" (Piaget), 167–173, 179, 180, 181. *See also* God

Mystical experiences, 141, 142, 167, 170

Mysticism, 94, 102, 111, 112, 117, 180, 201; metaphysics and, 142; Piaget's interpretation of, 187, 190, 206, 208–210. *See also* Sensuality

Nationalism, 147, 149, 174, 175, 179, 232

Natural history, 19, 20, 24; Piaget's study of, 2, 23, 33, 34, 51, 227

Natural sciences, 17, 19, 34, 51

Natural Sciences Society of Neuchâtel, 17–18, 34, 35

Natural selection, 48, 62–68, 70, 80, 147, 172

Naturphilosophie, 93, 135

Neeser, Maurice, 100

"Neo-Darwinian Trend in Biology, The" (Juvet), 50

Nervousness *(nervosisme)*, 14–15

Nervous Woman, The (Bersot), 14, 15

Neuchâtel, Switzerland (canton), 10–14; churches in, 115–116

Neuchâtel, Switzerland (city), 8, 10, 11, 16–17

Nomenclature, 26, 28, 29–30; vanity of, 51, 57, 58, 59, 69

Nominalism, 57–62, 86, 87, 90, 195; evolutionary, 66, 70, 76, 89

"Note on the Biology of Deep-Water *Limnaea*" (Piaget), 42–43

"Notion of the Species according to the Mendelian School, The" (Piaget), 83

Observation of nature, 17, 19, 20

"On the History of the Psychoanalytic Movement" (Freud), 206

Organization, 196, 199, 200, 201

Origins of Intelligence in Children (Piaget), 227

"Outline of a Neo-Pragmatism" (Piaget), 86

Outlines of a Philosophy of Religion Based on Psychology and History (Sabatier), 94, 113, 116–117, 118, 120, 127, 128

Pacifism, 53, 154, 176, 178

Pantheism, 54, 55

Parallelism, 199, 229, 230

Pascal, Blaise, 136, 193

Passion, 175, 187, 189, 191, 192, 205–206, 213; as disequilibrium, 201; ideal and, 203; in *Recherche*, 208, 209; concept of good and, 214

Patriotism, 148, 151, 200, 202. *See also* Nationalism

Péguy, Charles, 121, 188

Personality, 202, 203, 204, 210–211, 212

Pettavel, Paul, 153, 154, 157, 167, 176, 222; socialist youth and, 177–178. *See also* L'*Essor*

Pfister, Oskar, 206, 207, 225

Phenotype, 2, 37, 226

Piaget, Arthur, 13–14, 21, 53, 115, 157

Piaget, Rebecca (née Jackson), 13, 14–16, 114, 176–177

Pietism, 93, 98

Plato, 136, 137

Plotinus, 136, 137

Poet, Piaget as, 139

Poincaré, Henri, 102

Pragmatism, 46, 102, 188

Pride, 201, 210–213

Progress, 129, 135, 146, 158, 171, 172, 222, 229; moral, 147, 148

Protestantism, 105–106, 121, 139, 202, 231; evangelical, 92–93; liberal, 92–93, 94, 95, 102, 125, 207, 228, 233; Swiss-French, 92, 96, 98, 110–111, 112, 114, 118, 120, 149, 185, 228; individualism and, 97, 100; World War I and, 98–99; in *Recherche*, 187–188

Psychoanalysis, 14, 203, 206, 213–214, 224, 225; Piaget's psychoanalytic discourse, 205–208

Psychobiography, 4–5

Psychology, 14, 60; biography and, 4–5; Piaget's theory of, 8, 88, 90, 91, 130, 199; in Bergson's philosophy, 55, 56; religion and, 92, 94, 100–103, 188, 201, 210, 227, 228; genetic, 106; equilibrium theory and, 196–197, 200, 230; as key science, 223–224; child, 225, 228; empirical, 229; development and, 230

Quality (vs. quantity), 198, 200, 210

Ragaz, Leonhard, 100

Rameau de sapin, Le (magazine), 18, 24, 26, 44

Realism, 90, 195, 196, 199

"Realism and Nominalism in the Life-Sciences" (Piaget), 86

Reason, 125–126, 204, 205

Recherche (Piaget), 2, 3, 51, 56, 61, 104, 149, 157, 161, 171, 211; science of genera in, 89; theory of equilibrium/disequilibrium in, 91, 182–183, 184, 187, 188, 189; religion in, 106, 120–122, 140; metaphysics in, 136, 139, 172; illness and self-discovery as theme, 166–167; socialism in, 178, 179; crisis theme in, 182, 190–194, 208; literary construction of, 182–183, 188–189; preparation theme in, 182, 186–190, 191, 208; reconstruction theme in, 182–183, 195–196, 200, 209; socialism in, 182; in Piaget's autobiography, 183; Swiss-French *Bildungsroman* and, 183–185; as autobiographical novel, 184; critical reviews of, 219–222; motivation for, 185–186; structure of the self and, 216; psychology in, 223. *See also* God

Religion: psychology of, 92, 94, 100–103, 188, 201, 207, 227, 228; conflict of science with, 102, 103, 110, 112, 113–114, 115, 120, 185; Swiss-French, 119, 228; evolution and, 130; of Piaget, 139–144, 200, 201; as moral consciousness, 145; theology as separate from, 156; metaphysics and, 159

Religious instruction, 51, 52, 113–120, 123; catechism, 116, 118–119, 125

Research program, Piaget's, 196–203

Revelation, 121, 184, 190, 191

Revival, 95, 112, 116, 152

Revue de metaphysique et de morale, 219–220

Revue suisse de zoologie, 36

Rey, Abel, 46, 47

Reymond, Arnold, 16, 125–126; Piaget and,

86, 96, 123, 124, 126, 130, 195, 219, 228–229, 231–232; critique of Bergson, 125–127; review of *Recherche*, 185, 186, 220, 221
Ritter, William, 11
Rolland, Romain, 97, 106, 168, 176, 188–189, 220; on Christianity, 153–154; youth movement and, 174–175, 215; Piaget and, 203–205, 210
Romanes, George John, 67
Romy, Marcel, 46, 49
Rossetti, Etienne, 46–47, 48, 49
Roszkowski, Wacław, 84; debate with Piaget on definition of species, 72–81, 85, 89, 123, 145, 226, 238n4
Rousseau, Jean-Jacques, 11, 104
Rousseau Institute, 10, 21, 94, 97, 101, 153, 225; Piaget at, 227–228

Sabatier, Auguste, 51, 93–94, 113, 116–118, 123; Piaget, Bergson, and, 127–131
Sacrifice, 191, 192
Salvation, 95, 96, 140, 143, 158, 170, 171; social, 192, 193, 202; universal, 217
Schizophrenia, 206, 209, 212
Schleiermacher, Friedrich, 93, 95, 128
Science, 61, 171, 180–181; mechanistic, 89–90, 138, 197, 199; religion and, 102, 103, 110, 121, 122, 125, 160–161, 182, 185, 188, 189, 192, 200, 201, 202, 210, 220–221, 222; socialism and, 149, 175; morality and, 161, 201, 213–214, 223, 227; of genera, 182, 183, 188, 197; in *Recherche*, 188; Piaget and, 196, 221; value and, 229
Science and Hypothesis (Poincaré), 102
Scientism, 46, 47, 50, 55
Secrétan, Charles, 97–98
Self, 3, 6, 184, 215; -analysis (Piaget's), xii, 190, 203–204; -discovery, 166–167, 191; creation, 168–171, 181, 186; -criticism, 180–181, 209; -examination, 183, 186, 190, 191; -awareness, 193–194; collective makeup of, 205–206; -understanding, 209; perception, 211; logic of, 214; faith and, 217–218
Sensuality, 208, 209, 213
Separation of church and state, 96, 97, 115, 154
Sexuality, 192–193, 208, 214
Sheets-Pyenson, Susan, 3
Simon, Théodore, 225
Socialism, 97; Christian, 98–100, 103, 112, 133, 153, 154, 155, 156, 173, 177, 178; and science, 149, 175; of Piaget, 153, 176, 179–180, 182, 189; wartime, 175–180; radical, 176, 179, 180; liberal, 179; cooperative, 202; individualism and, 221

Socialization, 2, 4, 34, 36, 232
Sociology, 200–201, 223
Söderqvist, Thomas, 3
Solidarism, 99
Solidarity, 146, 147, 149, 205, 211
Spearman's rank order correlation coefficient, 226
Speciation, 39, 67, 68, 70, 76, 78–79, 88
Species, 37, 41; problem, definition of, 24, 26, 32–33, 57, 68–69, 72–81, 85, 89; origins of, 25, 28, 38; formation of (new, nascent), 28, 32, 48, 56, 58, 65, 66, 67, 68, 72, 75, 88; morphology of, 28–29; delimitation of, 29, 61; mutation of, 29–30, 62–63, 72, 80–81, 82, 84; type, 30, 32; nominalistic concept of, 30–31, 57–62; method of continuous series, 31, 58; isolation of, 66–70; hereditary, 68; Piaget/Roszkowski debate over, 72–81. *See also* Taxonomy
Spencer, Herbert, 55–56
Starobinski, Jean, 5, 104
Stream of consciousness, 55, 199
Subconscious, 208, 210
Sublet, Paul, 99
Sublimation, 213–214, 216
Suffering: religious dimension of, 166; divine, 167–173; metaphysical, 167–168, 172; physical, 167; human, 168–169, 170
Swiss Christian Students' Association (ACSE), 22, 101, 104–107, 229, 231; religion and, 92, 125; Piaget's participation in, 96, 109, 120, 145, 148, 150–152; socialism in, 99, 100; member profiles, 107–108; World War I and, 108–110; anti-intellectualism, 110–111; Sainte-Croix meetings, 111–112, 141, 154; science/religion conflict in, 118
Swiss-French tradition, 96, 125, 185; theology, 97–98; social philosophy, 98–100; psychology and religion, 100–103; literature, 103–104, 125; *Bildungsroman*, 183–185
Swiss Natural Sciences Society, 27, 34
Swiss Zoological Society, 34, 35
Symbolism, 94, 121, 127, 129, 187; dogma and, 113–114; vs. revelation, 190; of dreams, 200; autism and, 201
Systematics, 28, 32, 38, 81. *See also* Taxonomy

Taxonomy, 20, 57; malacological, 2, 23, 27–32, 36, 56, 70, 74, 81; evolution and, 31, 32, 56; categories of, 56, 58; link with evolution, 58–59; nominalism and, 66
Theology, 92, 103, 156, 167; Swiss-French tradition and, 97–98. *See also* Religion
Tendency, 64, 65; to evolve, 66, 78, 147; to

Tendency *(cont.)*
vary, 69–70; life as, 158; toward equilibrium, 198, 200
Testament of My Youth, The (Cornut), 184, 185
Time, 55, 59, 62, 68, 69, 70, 226; psychological, 128, 129
Time and Free Will: An Essay on the Immediate Data of Consciousness (Bergson), 56
To Believers and Atheists (Monod), 155, 171
Toepffer, Rodolphe, 20
Tolstoy, Leo, 175, 192, 193, 204, 205, 208, 241n2
Transcendence, 92, 96, 101, 125, 168, 194, 228, 230, 232
Trouessart, Edouard-Louis, 63
Truth, 188, 191–192, 201

Unconscious, 191, 206, 208, 211–212
Union of Christian Socialists, 98, 176
Universal Federation of Christian Students' Associations, 104–105. *See also* Swiss Christian Students' Association
University of Neuchâtel, 10, 17, 219
University of Zurich, 224

Valéry, Paul, xi, 56
Values, 191–192, 200, 214–215; absolute, 187, 188, 190, 192, 201, 202, 204
"Vanity of Nomenclature, The" (Piaget), 51, 57, 58, 59, 66, 123
Variation and variability: evolutionary, 24, 25, 26, 39–40, 48; of mollusks, 27, 28–29, 30, 37, 38; continuity and, 30–32, 58; proliferation of species and, 31; environment and, 37, 38; mimicry and, 63; fluctuation in, 83, 84
Varieties of Religious Experience, The (James) 101
Varieties of species, 25, 28, 30–31, 38; as nascent species, 67, 75

Vinet, Alexandre, 97, 98, 104, 128, 166
Vitalism, 53, 54, 57. *See also Elan vital*
Voies nouvelles, 176, 177–178
Vonèche, Jacques, 8, 84, 132, 133, 217, 223

Wagner, Moritz, 68, 69
Wallace, Alfred Russel, 62
War, 144, 189, 217, 220; Piaget on, 147–148, 173–175, 179. *See also* World War I
Warnery, Renée, 180
Wavre, Rolin, 47, 124
Weber, Max, 3
Weismann, August, 48, 73, 216
Will, 63, 64, 65, 66, 201
Williams, P. Pearce, 4
Women: rights of, 148, 149, 153; nervousness *(nervosisme)* in, 14–15
World War I, 12, 140, 147, 149, 186; effect on Piaget, 91, 92, 141, 148, 167; socialism and, 98–99; youth movement and, 108–109, 152
Wreschner, Arthur, 224

Young, Robert L., 4
Young Men's Christian Association (YMCA), 105, 108, 153–154
Youth, 110–111, 116–117, 152; missionary spirit of, 104, 106, 107, 108–110, 112, 157–161, 173–175; groups/movement, 107, 178; mission to follow Jesus, 107, 110, 132, 133, 134; socialism and, 175–180; progressive, 215. *See also* Swiss Christian Students' Association
Yung, Emile, 34, 35, 36–37, 41

Zeno of Elea, 60–61
Zofingue society, 215
Zurich, 13, 207–208, 211; Piaget in, 2, 222, 224–225, 226